MEDICINE
OF THE
PROPHET

MW00851483

Ibn Qayyim al-Jawziyya

MEDICINE OF THE PROPHET

Translated by Penelope Johnstone

THE ISLAMIC TEXTS SOCIETY

Available from:
www.IslamicBookstore.com
Baltimore. Maryland. USA

English language translation © Penelope Johnstone 1998

This edition published 1998 by The Islamic Texts Society
22a Brooklands Avenue, Cambridge CB2 2DQ, UK

Reprinted 2001 / 2004

ISBN 0 946621 19 5 cloth
ISBN 0 946621 22 5 paper

British Library Cataloguing in Publication Data

A catalogue record for this book is available from
The British Library.

No part of this book may be reproduced
in any form without prior permission of
the publishers. All rights reserved.

Printed and bound in Malaysia
by CS Multi Print Sdn. Bhd.

Cover illustration:

From manuscript Ee.5.7 by permission
of the Syndics of Cambridge University Library

NOTE: The material appearing in this book is for
information purposes only and is not intended as a
replacement for medical advice.

Contents

PART TWO · SIMPLE DRUGS AND FOODS

Hamza

Bā'

Tā'

Thā'

Qāf

Kāf

Lām

Mīm

Nūn

Hā'

Wāw

Yā'

Foreword

In the Name of Allāh, the Compassionate, the Merciful

ISLAM, as a guide for all facets of human life, has had to concern itself with the general principles of medicine. There are several verses of the Qur'ān in which medical questions of a very general order are discussed, and there are also many Sayings of the Prophet ﷺ (*ḥadīth*) dealing with health, sickness, hygiene and other problems pertaining to the field of medicine. Diseases such as leprosy, pleurisy and ophthalmia are mentioned—remedies such as cupping, cautery and the use of honey and other home remedies are proposed. This body of *ḥadīth* on medical questions was systematized by later Muslim writers and became known as *al-Ṭibb al-Nabawī* or *Medicine of the Prophet*.

The Qur'ān and *sunna* are the basic sources of knowledge in Islam and the importance of *sunna* is emphasized in the Qur'ān. The section of *sunna* which contains the very words of the Prophet ﷺ is known as *ḥadīth*. Following the *ḥadīth* in general and the art of therapeutics specifically is, like other branches of conduct among the Muslims, based on the customs of the Arab Muslims modified by what the Prophet ﷺ himself said and did.

Of course *al-Ṭibb al-Nabawī* is a specialised field and can only be dealt with in depth by someone with specialised knowledge of Islamic theology and philosophy as well as having a mastery of the medical profession. Certainly what follows here is the English translation of such an author's book. His full name was Shams al-Dīn Abū ʿAbd-Allāh Muḥammad ibn Abī Bakr Ibn Qayyim al-Jawziyya al-Ḥanbalī, and he was a Muslim theologian as well as a practising physician, a fact which no doubt coloured his version of the *Medicine of the Prophet*. His *al-Ṭibb al-Nabawī* is not mentioned in the *Kashf al-Ẓānūn* (Lexicon composed by Ḥajjī Khalīfa in 1658 AH) which seems surprising at first. However, an answer to this problem has been supplied by the editor of a printed edition off *al-Ṭibb al-Nabawī* published in Aleppo (in 1927, as mentioned by Cyril Elgood). The editor suggests that Ḥajjī Khalīfa remained ignorant of the existence of this collection because it lay hidden within another work of the same author and escaped his notice.

Ibn Qayyim al-Jawziyya also wrote a large book which he entitled *Zād al-Maʿād fī Hadī Khayr al-ʿIbād*, or *The Victuals of Pilgrimage and the Guide to the Good of Mankind*. This was published in Cairo in 1906 and within it is a large section on the Medicine of the Prophet ﷺ which has now been extracted and published separately, with no acknowledgement (until the 1927 edition) of the fact that it forms part of a larger work. Ibn Qayyim was probably born in Damascus in January 1292. In 1310 he joined Ibn Taimiyya and became his ardent disciple, sharing his labours and to some extent his sufferings. They were put in prison together in Cairo. Ibn Qayyim died in September 1350. Some fifty treatises are ascribed to him, most of which are devoted to the defence of Ḥanbalī theology in the spirit of his master Ibn Taimiyya.

Cyril Elgood has mentioned that it was Ḥajjī Khalīfa, the great bibliographer of his age who arranged the titles of Arabic, Persian and Turkish books in *Kashf al-Ẓānūn* wherein, among the sub-divisions of works on medicine, is to be found a speciality which he entitled '*ʿIlm al-Ṭibb al-Nabawī*' or 'The Science of the Medicine of the Prophet'. In the days when Ḥajjī Khalīfa wrote his encyclopaedia (*Kashf al-Ẓānūn*), he was able to record some six works, all bearing the title *al-Ṭibb al-Nabawī* all purporting to give the *ipissima verba* and views of the Prophet ﷺ on various aspects of medicine. The oldest version among those is that of Abū Nuʿaym Aḥmad of Isfahan, others being authored by Abū'l-ʿAbbās Jaʿfar Mustaghfirī, Jalāl al-Dīn al-Suyūṭī, Abū'l-Ḥasan ʿAlī al-Razā, Ḥabīb Nīshāpūrī, and ʿAbd al-Malik bin Ḥabīb. ʿAbd al-Muʿṭī Amīn Qalʿajī, editor to Muwaffaqu'l-Din ʿAbd al-Laṭīf al-Baghdādī's *al-Ṭibb min al-Kitāb wa'l-Sunna* has given the names of four authors (the fifth being unknown to him) who have written manuscripts under the same title. In addition to Ibn Qayyim, he mentioned Ḍiyā' al-Dīn al-Maqdissī, Muḥammad ibn Musāʿid al-Anṣārī and Muḥammad al-Ṣiftī al-Zīnī. In the postscript to one of his review articles (n.d.) on Medicine of the Prophet ﷺ, Cyril Elgood has reported two more versions, *viz*, *Al-Sirr al-Muṣṭafā fī Ṭibb al-Nabī* by Nūr al-Dīn Abū'l-Ḥasan ibn Jazzār (numbered 3035 in the catalogue of the Bibliothéque Nationale, Paris) and *Risāla fī Ṭibb al-Nabī* by Abū'l-Qāsim Nīshāpūrī (also mentioned by *Hajjī Khalīfa*).

The subject matter of the English text of *al-Ṭibb al-Nabawī* of Ibn Qayyim al-Jawziyya varies from the treatment of individual diseases as recommended by the Prophet ﷺ to medico-legal matters, such as malpractice, the hallmarks of a competent physician, and so forth. Matters such as enchantment and parapsychology are discussed very little in the book, although the treatment for the evil eye is dealt with at length. It is apparent from the study of the following text that the Prophet ﷺ had a knowledge so wide that his remarks upon many common diseases were remembered, and this fact has been well illustrated by Ibn Qayyim.

The text indicates in the broadest sense all that regards preventive medicine and general treatment procedures, and in view of this Ibn Qayyim divided the book in two parts, the first dealing with medicine and the second with simple foods and drugs. The overall work makes us aware of the firm religious belief of the author who has discussed everything with reference to *ḥadīth* including the common ailments like fevers, diarrhoea, epilepsy, sciatica, headache, etc; as well as contagious diseases like plague and leprosy, and has mentioned the incantations for bites, scorpion sting, itching, ulcers, and so on. In general, the preservation of health as regards the use of foods and drinks and common traditional treatment techniques, like cupping and cautery, etc. are discussed under Prophetic traditions (*ḥadīth*).

The second part of the text deals with *materia medica* including common mineral, inorganic, organic, animal and vegetable remedies used and recommended by the Prophet ﷺ like *ithmid* (collyrium), *tamr* (dates), *ḥinnā'* (henna), *shūnīz* (black cumin, *Nigella sativa*), *ḥulba* (fenugreek), *rayḥān* (basil), *dhahab* (gold), *siwāk* (toothbrush tree twig), *qusṭ* (costus), *misk* (musk), *mā'* (water) etc. These simple drugs and foods are discussed accordingly under Arabic alphabetial arrangement.

I have gone through the translated manuscript of *Medicine of the Prophet* and observed the hard work done by Dr. Penelope Johnstone. The Islamic Texts Society has done a good service in commissioning the translation and making it available to English readers, especially English-speaking Muslims who have had little or no access to the original sources. We hope that the Muslim readers of this work will judge it in the light of their experience which will include familiarity with the Qur'ān and Prophetic traditions as well as their faith in Islam.

I hope that this book will be favourably reviewed and will find wide acceptance, for I myself have found this masterly translation a significant and welcome addition to the treasury of translated Islamic medico-religious literature and to the historical and cultural heritage of Islam.

May Allāh bless and reward the author, the translator, the editor, the publisher and, of course, the readers of this monumental publication.

Hakim Mohammed Saʿīd
Hamdard Foundation
Pakistan

Preface

THE body of works known in the Islamic world as 'Prophetic medicine' or the 'medicine of the Prophet', of which the present work is one of the best examples, is not simply a type of 'folk medicine' with religious connotations. Rather, it is a compilation and systematization of an aspect of the legacy of the Prophet ﷺ in the domain of diet, health and illness complementing the legal, intellectual and spiritual dimensions of the legacy he left to the Islamic community through his *sunna* or wonts and traditions. A revelation implies the penetration of a divine message into a whole cosmic sector embracing the humanity for which the revelation is destined. In the case of Islam the revelation itself is the Qur'ān while the recipient, the Prophet ﷺ, represents the perfect human receptacle who has received that revelation in a perfect mode and disseminated it into the world about him. As a consequence, something of the soul, 'person' and actions of the Prophet ﷺ have remained within the Islamic community over the ages, and complement the Qur'ān in providing guidelines for human life and bestowing meaning upon existence and the existents which the Muslim encounters in the journey of life. The Prophet ﷺ has sanctified certain actions and objects through his own acts and *dicta* and by virtue of being a prophet has bestowed upon such acts and objects a permanent value, significance and power within the Islamic universe.

It is in the light of the prophetic function in Islam that the 'medicine of the Prophet' must be understood, not through an external historicism based upon the assumption of the irrelevance of revelation and its effect upon the world which receives it. A particular instruction of the Prophet ﷺ concerning a dietary practice or the use of a particular substance in times of illness must be understood in the light of who the Prophet ﷺ is for Muslims and what efficacy his teachings have had and continue to have precisely by virtue of their being *his* teachings. No amount of 'scientific' detraction from such kind of medical instruction can diminish its significance or for that matter efficacy for those who live in the world of faith (*al-īmān*) and who see the Prophet ﷺ as the Perfect Man through whom God revealed His final revelation to the world. The 'medicine of the Prophet' is in a sense part and parcel of the Prophetic *sunna* with all that this participation implies.

Early in Islamic history, the sayings and actions of the Prophet ﷺ

concerning medicine were assembled into collections which came to be known as *al-ṭibb al-nabawī*. This medicine remained distinct while interacting with the medicine which was then being learned from Greek, Persian and Indian sources, the latter process resulting in that synthesis in the hands of such masters as al-Ṭabarī, al-Rāzī and Ibn Sīnā which is known as Islamic medicine. In the translator's preface, the history of Islamic medicine in its relation to the 'medicine of the Prophet' has been discussed and we therefore do not need to delve into it here. Suffice it to say that the great Muslim physicians who developed the so-called 'scientific medicine' were themselves men of faith and operated within a religious universe. Most of them were aware of the 'medicine of the Prophet' and some wrote about it. In most cases in fact there was a complementarity between the two schools rather than confrontation. If there was an occasional opposition, it usually came from certain jurists opposed to the pre-Islamic (*awā'il*) sciences but even such cases are overshadowed by the much more frequent instances of accord wherein 'scientific medicine' associated with al-Rāzī, Ibn Sīnā and the like was cited as support for the 'medicine of the Prophet' while 'the medicine of the Prophet', especially as it dealt with diet, was integrated into the teachings of Islamic 'scientific medicine'.

Because of the strong faith of Muslims in the tenets of Islam and their love of the Prophet ﷺ, the tenets of the 'medicine of the Prophet', especially its dietary injunctions, became integrated into daily life as one can observe to this day. Many of the sayings of the Prophet ﷺ concerning the care of the body such as the necessity to leave the table before feeling full or to eat in a calm atmosphere without agitation became repeated in numerous forms through not only the original *ḥadīth*, but also proverbs, poems and the like in numerous languages throughout the Islamic world. The 'medicine of the Prophet' became an integral part of the life of the Islamic community, not only complementing the 'scientific' medical tradition, but in a sense providing the framework and affecting the very human element for that medical tradition.

Needless to say, traditional Islamic medicine functioned in a world in which unity reigned, and spirit, soul, and body had not become totally separated with the former two being cast aside as irrelevant, as is the case of much of modern medicine. This medicine saw an integral relationship between the spirit and the soul on the one hand, and the soul and the body on the other as seen in the classical works of Ibn Sīnā. Herein is to be found another dimension of the significance of the 'medicine of the Prophet' in which the concerns of the spirit and the soul are naturally even more central than those of the body whose health is nevertheless of great importance according to Islamic teachings, bodily health being itself closely linked to the health of the soul as the health of the soul depends upon the degree to which it is able to conform itself to the world of the Spirit.

The interrelation between the domains of the spirit, the soul and the body is to be seen directly in works devoted to the 'medicine of the Prophet' themselves.

In the present book by Ibn Qayyim sickness with which medicine is concerned is itself divided into the sickness of the heart and sickness of the body. The sickness of the heart, which being the centre of the human microcosm is also the 'locus' of the spirit and the soul, is without doubt concerned with the reality of God and the afterlife, and temptation to commit evil. The cure of such an illness is given by God to the prophets only, and physicians are helpless before this most dangerous of all sicknesses. As for the sickness of the body, either it can be in accordance with the creation of animals in which case again the treatment of a physician is not necessary, or it is an illness which requires thought and reflection. Only in the latter case, according to Ibn Qayyim, is the service of a physician necessary. All human medicine is therefore made subservient to the tenets of religion which cure the ailments of the soul and to the world of nature itself which reflects directly the wisdom of the Creator who is also the Supreme Curer, one of His Names being *al-Shāfī*.

This perspective which emphasizes the limitations of the power and domain of efficacy of any human medicine and which begins the work of Ibn Qayyim is far from being limited to either authors of works on the 'medicine of the Prophet' or jurists. This view in fact dominates over the whole of the traditional Islamic world, where no human medicine, no matter how efficacious, is absolutized. It is with this principle in mind that the supreme Persian poet Ḥāfiẓ says,

> It is better to hide my pain from pretentious physicians
> Perhaps I will be cured from the 'Treasury of the Invisible'.

The 'Treasury of the Invisible' (*khazāna-yi ghayb*) is of course in reference to the Divine Order where the archetypes of all manifestation are to be found. It also refers to the vertical cause in contrast to the 'horizontal causes' with which the ordinary physician is concerned.

One of the important functions of the 'medicine of the Prophet' has, therefore, been to prevent any human medicine from being able to make claims to absoluteness as has happened in so much of modern medicine with the accompanying reduction of the human microcosm to merely the body which itself is then simply reduced to a complex machine as if life were incidental to the living body. Moreover, the 'medicine of the Prophet' has kept alive before the Islamic community the principles of religion as they pertain to medicine and health besides providing teachings concerning hygiene, diet and the cure of individual ailments on the basis of Prophetic teachings as the text of Ibn Qayyim testifies.

The work of Ibn Qayyim being translated here is not of course simply a repetition of earlier works on the 'medicine of the Prophet'. The well-known authority on Islamic medicine, Hakim Mohammed Saʿid, has dealt with the genre of works on the 'medicine of the Prophet' from the beginning of Islamic history to Ibn Qayyim in his foreword and there is no need to deal with the relation between the present work and earlier texts on this subject here. Despite many differences, however, this work shares with earlier writings on the 'medicine of the Prophet' in situating 'scientific' medicine within the layer framework of what constitutes the well-being of man taken in his totality and in relating the well-being of the body to that of the soul. It also shares with earlier texts of this kind its concern to disseminate knowledge almost as instructions for the care of the body and treatment of numerous illnesses according to practices and sayings which go back to the Prophet ﷺ himself.

Some have spoken of this kind of medicine and especially the astronomy used for specific religious purposes such as finding the direction of the *qiblah* as a folk science in the service of religion. It is interesting to study in fact the possible parallelism between the mathematical astronomy of Muslims in relation to the more popular 'folk astronomy' used often in orienting mosques and determining times of prayers on the one hand and the 'scientific' tradition of Islamic medicine in relation to the 'medicine of the Prophet' on the other hand. Although in both cases one may speak of science in the service of religion, there are major differences in the two cases. In the case of astronomy a wider chasm is to be seen between the astronomy of the mathematical astronomers and the so-called folk astronomy than in the case of medicine. In the former case those who practiced the simple methods of determining the direction of the *qiblah* and the times of prayers were almost totally ignorant of or impervious to the mathematical astronomy which was available to them although there are some exceptions. In the case of medicine, in contrast, there was much greater interaction between the two medical traditions, the 'scientific' and the Prophetic, and the fruit of the efforts and studies of the Avicennan tradition was more available to the public at large than the mathematical astronomy of let us say his contemporary al-Bīrūnī. Despite these differences, however, the relation between the 'medicine of the Prophet' and the 'folk astronomy' used in conjunction with Islamic religious rites in the history of Islamic science is of some interest. It should be studied further in order to understand better the whole question of the use of science in the service of religion in the case of Islam. One should, however, always keep in mind that the 'medicine of the Prophet' despite its very wide usage throughout the Islamic world must not be simply identified with 'a folk medicine' as this term is usually understood.

Ibn Qayyim al-Jawziyya was a close disciple of Ibn Taymiyya and is identified especially in modern times with anti-Sufi tendencies of Islamic thought, although it is now known that Ibn Taymiyya was himself a member of the Qādiriyya Order while opposing many of the theses of the school of Ibn ʿArabī. In any case neither Ibn Qayyim nor his master can be associated with that inner perspective in Islam which seeks to 'see' God as not only the Transcendent but also the Immanent, as not only Truth but also Presence and most of his works, like those of Ibn Taymiyya, deal with jurisprudence and the study of the Qur'ān and *ḥadīth* from the juridical point of view rather than dealing with the inner dimension of Islam with its emphasis upon the sacred character of all existence seen as theophany rather than veil. Yet, Ibn Qayyim was also a practicing physician and his interest in medicine is clearly reflected in the present work which deals in a sense with the sanctification of certain aspects of everyday life. Prophetic medicine brought the *sunna* of the Prophet ﷺ into the daily life of Muslims, contributing on the deepest level to making more manifest for the faithful the vestiges (*āyāt*) of God in all things. The person who followed the directives contained in works on Prophetic medicine identified his actions with the *sunna* of the Prophet ﷺ and derived not only medical but also religious benefit from such medical practices. In fact the two, the medical and the religious, were never separated in his mind and the latter often helped the former when medical treatments involved control and discipline. In the mind of many a patient the following of medical advice based on Prophetic medicine was made easier because it was related in that person's mind to the example and wont of the Prophet ﷺ rather than being based on ordinary human opinion and being of only physical importance. How many a devout Muslim leaves the table still partly hungry because it is an injunction of the Prophet ﷺ and how many do so because some physician has told them that it is better for the digestive system to do so!

Sharīʿite injunctions sanctify the life of the Muslim by having him perform this or that act according to the Divine Law which is none other than the concrete Will of God. Although not directly the Will of God or part of the *sharīʿa*, Prophetic medicine has shared something of this character by relating particular treatments, diets, substances, etc. to the *sunna* of the Prophet ﷺ which is itself the second source of the *sharīʿa* after the Qur'ān. In this sense the practice of Prophetic medicine in traditional Islamic society has been seen as almost an extension of the *sharīʿa* and has been intertwined with the everyday life of the practitioners of the *sharīʿa* as seen in the field of diet or the use of the bath which in its traditional form has had an important role to play both from the sharīʿite point of view and medically.

In any case the study of the 'medicine of the Prophet' and the texts devoted to it such as the one translated here are of great importance for the comprehension of an important dimension of the life of traditional Islamic society. Such a study will reveal an important aspect of a theory and practice of medicine which complemented the medical theories and practices of a Rāzī or an Ibn Sīnā and which became united in an organic whole with the latter in many instances. On the deepest level, however, the study of the 'medicine of the Prophet' makes manifest yet another aspect of the reality of the Prophet of Islam ﷺ as this reality has affected the life of generations of Muslims through his *sunna* which, being all pervasive, could not neglect such an important area of human life as that of health and medicine. By means of this medicine of a Prophetic origin, Muslims were reminded, because of the association of this medicine with the

Prophet ﷺ, of God's Presence everywhere and the ubiquitousness of His Will which reigns supreme over all things, for the Prophet ﷺ, the beloved of God, lived and spoke in such a way that all that is associated with him bears the perfume of the remembrance of God in which he always lived and in whose embrace he departed from this world of impermanence.

Seyyed Hossein Nasr

Translator's Introduction

MEDICINE OF THE PROPHET

Medicine of the Prophet by Ibn Qayyim al-Jawziyya (691–751 AH/1292–1350 AD) is about spiritual and physical health. It deals with the preservation and restoration of health of soul and body, chiefly by religious means and the recommendation of the Prophet Muḥammad. Despite its medical content, it is not a medical textbook in the present-day sense, but shows the combination of medicine and religion available to the general public at the time. In *Medicine of the Prophet* we see the point of view of a theologian of orthodox belief and practice, one more concerned with piety than medical theory.

Ibn Qayyim aims to give 'Guidance', stemming from the Prophet—therefore ultimately divine guidance—whereby the Muslim could conduct his affairs especially in matters of health and illness. Ibn Qayyim looks first at Qur'ānic verses and *ḥadīth*, which he holds more important than scientific considerations which must come under the judgement of religion.

In his concern for practical guidance, he considers what is permissible and why; what is in accordance with Islamic law; the Qur'ān's ruling, if such exists; the Prophet's teaching or practice on the subject; any special concessions, and their reasons; whether medicine itself is in accordance with the Divine decree; the possibility and the availability of cures; and the status of medicine. On this last point, he concludes that medicine is not only permitted but is recommended, or even obligatory.

There is little reference to the material which is found in writings of earlier physicians, such as al-Rāzī, al-Ṭabarī, Ibn Sīnā; and Ibn Qayyim cannot be judged by the same criteria. He gives the religious aspects, reflecting orthodox teaching and also actual practice. Ibn Qayyim's book is of great interest in its own right, at the side of more scientific works, inasmuch as it gives a wide range of customs and attitudes current at the time, and the practices of ordinary people.

WHY MEDICINE OF THE PROPHET

How does this differ from what is commonly known as 'Islamic Medicine' or 'Arabic Medicine'? In general terms, the more usual sort of book on medicine would be concerned primarily with health and disease of the body, starting from philosophical principles and physiological data. Elements, humours, their interactions, together with information and instruction for the physician, scholar and student, formed the study of medicine, which was closely allied to metaphysical philosophy. The two main divisions were between Theory and Practice; the aims of medicine were 'the preservation of health and its restoration when disturbed'. Medical teachings were inherited mainly from the Greeks. At the same time, in India, Egypt, China and elsewhere, Islam came into contact with the medical teachings of those civilisations and incorporated much from their traditions.

Ibn Qayyim is aware of all this, but considers it secondary to his main theme. This becomes apparent at the outset of his work, where reference to the Qur'ānic description of 'those in whose hearts is sickness' is intended to show a different division of illness and medicine: that of the body and the heart.

His pronouncements are not subject to changes in medical theory or practice, slight though they would be at the period when he was writing, but have a timeless quality about them. If divine teachings are for all time then any apparent divergences must be reconciled through adapting practice to religious teaching. So 'scientific' medicine is cited in support of teachings derived from religious sources, while at times Ibn Qayyim is at pains to point out how the physicians have strayed from the true path.

One example of such harmonisation is seen in Ibn Qayyim's discussion of the plague in chapter five and in particular its spread and control. The starting-point is the *ḥadīth* on this subject: the instruction not to flee from a place where the plague is, nor to go deliberately to a city where it has broken out. This seems well in accord with the need to avoid contagion or infection. Yet he constructs another argument to show the excellence of this advice: any violent movement would disturb the humours, weaken the constitution and thus render the person more susceptible to illness. Here, a physical aspect is cited to reinforce the *ḥadīth*, which itself cannot be questioned but only explained and expanded.

Within a total way of life such as Islam, medicine must be compatible with religious teaching if it is to be accepted. In theory, since there is no division between the religious and the secular, all learning either follows or contradicts Islamic principles. Teachings must fit into the received framework.

Given that the guidance of the Prophet is stressed more than his knowledge of therapeutics, the author's reasoning and his method of procedure can be better understood. No remedy must be used if it seems to contradict Islamic law. Qur'ān and *ḥadīth* together give guidance which must always be preferred to secular medicine; this latter can be resorted to, and indeed is recommended, once it is seen to accord with Islamic teachings.

The book of *Medicine of the Prophet* is divided into two main parts:

1. General and particular medicine,
2. *Materia medica.*

In the first division come such matters as fevers, jaundice, eye diseases in general, plague, the evil eye, incantations and the preservation of health. The book begins, as do so many medical works, by stating the purpose and divisions of medicine. But our author differs by at once making the distinction between bodily and spiritual health and sickness. Thus the heart, *qalb*, used in the metaphorical sense, is at once distinguished from the body, *badn*.

In the second, we find an alphabetical list of all medicinal substances mentioned by the Qur'ān or in any way recommended by the Prophet. The term 'medicinal' includes many kinds of foodstuffs; water, and Zamzam water, with its religious significance; religious practices, especially prayer and fasting; in short, all that can be seen as beneficial to the health of 'heart and body'.

MEDICINE AT THE TIME OF THE PROPHET

Apart from the Greeks, Ibn Qayyim quotes from such writers as al-Rāzī, Ibn Sīnā, al-Ghāfiqī the herbalist, al-Zahrāwī the physician-surgeon, Thābīt b. Qurra, Ibn Juljul the herbalist and Ibn Riḍwān; but their contributions are minor and confirmatory.

Even so, the medical theories of such persons are assumed and accepted. These theories are philosophical-medical, derived from the Greeks, and although not explained in detail they clearly form the background to the *Medicine of the Prophet* whenever a precept needs to be elaborated or justified.

Illnesses of any kind are, in general, due to a disturbance of the humours (*akhlāṭ*) which compose the human body. These humours, blood, bile, black bile and phlegm, are combined in certain proportions: in equality, forming the mean (*iʿtidāl*), or when one predominates, a temperament (*mizāj*, literally 'mixture') characterised by one or other of the humours. Excess of any one leads to an imbalance, which needs correction. A medicine will be chosen in accordance with its capacity to rectify this, generally by evacuating the excess of humour.

Behind the humours are the qualities, hot, cold, moist, dry. From a mixture of either of the first two with either of the second two, four variations are possible: hot and moist, hot and dry, cold and moist, cold and dry. These variations correspond, respectively, with the elements air, fire, water, earth. A medicine will be characterised by a combination of qualities; each one can be at a 'degree' of one to four. A medicine to combat a cold disease should predominate in warmth; for a mainly moist disease, there should be a dry quality, and so on. Thus any description of a drug had to include the degree of its chief quality or qualities.

Some mediaeval textbooks of medicine illustrate this method of prescribing in Tables, where, on a grid, the disease with its characteristic qualities can be matched up with the appropriate drug to combat it. Beyond this, certain drugs were considered specific for certain illnesses. Precisely how this came about probably owed at least as much to centuries of experience as it did to the humoral theory. The credentials of a medicine were not such as would be expected today, although in a great many cases common sense, theory and experience would coincide. To take a simple example from the Chapter on Fevers, the relief afforded by cold water—drunk or applied externally—does not rely upon the connection made between fever and hell, though the *ḥadīth* is taken as the starting-point.

MATERIA MEDICA

As is usual in Arabic medicine as well as many other traditional medicinal systems, *materia medica* include both simple drugs and foods, some items being capable of inclusion under either category, especially since treatment by diet could move gradually to treatment by simples. The majority are of plant origin, with some animal and some mineral items. In accordance with the spirit of the book, material is selected for its appearance in Qur'ān and *ḥadīth*, and relevant quotations are given. Foods such as fish and meat, water of various kinds and origins, are described in some detail.

Apart from foods and medicines, there are items which are chosen for their effect upon the soul and so the whole person. Fasting and prayer have obvious effects upon the body, but even more they are seen as purifying and strengthening the spirit, which in turn strengthens the body. In fact it is hardly valid to separate the two; the human being is one. 'Guidance' is to keep the soul and body in health and harmony.

Identification of plants is notoriously difficult, especially inasmuch as classification has developed since some of the earlier books dealing with Arabic *materia medica* appeared (eg. Issa, Siggel). Often 'drugs' from the further east are more straightforward, while plants with local variations of species and name, collected in the wild then prepared and sold in the city, are more difficult to identify with precision.

Where possible, identifications have been taken from Miki, *Index*, with reference to Ghaleb, *Dictionnaire*, and to Levey, *Formulary* and *Pharmacology*. It is unlikely that, in a book devoted to the religious aspects of medicine, Ibn Qayyim would have been over interested in sub-species of plants; he concentrated on what was available and familiar, and we shall therefore do the same. Readers wishing for more specific detail are referred to the books mentioned above, and to Arabic writers such as Ibn al-Bayṭār, Abū Ḥanīfa, al-Ghāfiqī (see bibliography).

DISEASES

As we see at the outset, Ibn Qayyim divides medicine into two parts: for hearts (*qulūb*) and bodies (*abdān*). The spiritual aspect he considers more important.

However, the very nature of the subject he is discussing means that he deals with specific bodily ailments, despite the concentration upon preservation of health. 'Guidance' is for all the Muslims, so this includes advice and instructions concerning everyday matters of health and hygiene.

In general, the ailments and diseases he discusses are the same as are common today, especially in the Middle East. Identification and description were less sophisticated, although Arab physicians were well-known for their careful clinical descriptions. As Ibn Qayyim's interest lies in the guidance needed, he does not generally go into great detail. One cannot always identify a disease in such cases with precision, partly because of the greater detail and advanced classification of today.

English terms have been obtained largely from the dictionaries of Sharaf and Hitti. From these it is apparent that many concepts and details were simply unknown in Ibn Qayyim's day. In the translation we have taken what seems the closest and most feasible English term, as well as the one most likely to convey the meaning to the average English reader. Ibn Qayyim was writing for educated persons, not specialists, and on the whole he uses terms both current and general.

The difficulties of finding equivalents are apparent, eg. in:

(a) skin diseases: Ibn Qayyim refers to *baraṣ, bahaq, judhām* and *dā' al-fīl.* Concerning the first two in particular, European scholars have been in dispute, as indeed were earlier Arabic writers. Taking the majority consensus, we have translated as follows: *baraṣ* = vitiligo, *bahaq* = leukoderma, *judhām* = leprosy, *dā' al-fīl* = elephantiasis, keeping consistently to these terms so that the original Arabic can be retrieved by those who are interested.

(b) Pleurisy: there are three names, with their descriptions, for pain affecting the pleural region. *Dhāt al-janb,* generally translated 'pleurisy', can, as Ibn Qayyim points out, refer simply to pain in the rib cage (*bahw*). *Shawṣa* has been translated as 'pleurisy', though it can also be rendered 'pleuralgia' (Hitti). *Birsām,* used less frequently, is another term for pleurisy.

(c) Headaches: Ibn Qayyim explains *ṣudāᶜ* as pain in the head, and *shaqīqa* as pain in 'one of the two sides' of the head, ie. hemicrania, migraine. In another place he refers to the use of two words which really mean 'helmet', *bayḍa* and *khūdha,* which are by analogy used to describe pain which involves the entire head area.

MANUSCRIPTS AND EDITIONS

Of the editions of *al-Ṭibb al-Nabawī* which are available, the present translation has relied chiefly upon that of ᶜAbd al-Muᶜṭi Amīn Qalᶜajī, Dār al-Turāth, Cairo 1398/1978.

Others include that printed at al-Maṭbaᶜ al-ᶜIlmiyya, Aleppo 1346/1927.

The editor of the Cairo edition tells us that he himself relied upon the following manuscripts from Dār al-Kutub al-Miṣriyya, Cairo:

1. Ṭibb 1627, written 1163 AH (his main source)
2. Ṭibb Taymur 439, written 1191 AH
3. al-Zahiyya 552, written 1070 AH
4. Ṭibb Ṭalʿat 503, written 1084 AH

Other manuscripts are indicated by Ullmann, *Medizin* 187: Chester Beatty 3292, 11; by Brockelmann, GAL II 106 n. 19: Paris 3045, Uppsala 348. Supp. II 127 n. 20, he signals the Aleppo edition.

PHYSICIANS

For a concise account of the development of Arabic medicine, from the time of the translations from Greek into Arabic—mainly in the eighth and ninth centuries AD—to the thirteenth and fourteenth centuries, the reader is referred to works which give such an outline (see Bibliography).

Ibn Qayyim in his *Medicine of the Prophet* is aware of this heritage of medical learning and practice, but in some ways he distances himself from it; the 'popular' or 'prophetic' takes precedence over the 'scientific'; however, during the course of his work he refers to a number of physicians. The brief notes which follow are therefore centred around those mentioned in his book, indicating their place in the history of medicine.

Hippocrates of Cos, the 'Father of Medicine', lived from around 460 to 360 BC. His works were translated early in the ʿAbbāsid period, or even earlier, and were widely available for study and commentary. His *Aphorisms* (*Fuṣūl*) were particularly popular. Ibn Qayyim quotes from several of his works, including *Acute Diseases*, in Chapter 28, and *Prognostics* in Chapter 35c. (Ullman, *Medizin*, 25–35, 50f, 61f; Levey, *Pharmacology*, 19). Hippocrates' works are available in English translation by W.H.S. Jones, Loeb editions; and several in Arabic and English in the series *Arab Technical and Scientific Texts*, Cambridge.

Galen, c. 129–199 AD, was one of the most prolific of writers on medicine; his works include commentaries on Hippocrates, and lengthy treatises on every aspect of medicine including pharmacology and surgery. The majority of his works were translated into Arabic, and together constituted virtually a complete library of medical texts, some of which the Arabic medical student was obliged to learn by heart. (Ullman, *Medizin*, 35–68; Levey, *Pharmacology*, 20–21). A number of Galen's works also appear in the Cambridge series. Ibn Qayyim quotes him several times, e.g. on fevers, Chapter 3, on figs (*tīn*), cress (*ḥurf*) in Part II.

Translations from these works were already being made into Syriac, before the spread of Islam, in Jundishapur in South-west Persia. As the importance of the Arabic language increased, the Syriac versions were translated into Arabic, and in time the practice was to translate direct into Arabic from Greek. With the rise of the ʿAbbāsid dynasty, who founded their new capital of Baghdad, this city became the centre for the study and translation of the Greek works of philosophy, science and medicine. In 820 AD the caliph al-Ma'mūn founded the *Bayt al-ḥikma* (house of wisdom) for this specific purpose, the chief translator being Ḥunayn b. Isḥāq, a Nestorian Christian.

During the early years of the ʿAbbāsid dynasty (from 750 AD) members of the family of Bukhtīshūʿ were summoned to Baghdad from Jundishapur to act as personal physician to the caliph, a task which they carried out for several generations. Jibrīl b. Bukhtīshūʿ, son of Bukhtīshūʿ b. Jīrjīs, grandson of Jirjis b. Jibrīl b. Bukhtīshūʿ, to whom Ibn Qayyim refers in the final section, was physician to Hārūn al-Rashīd (765–809), later to al-Ma'mūn (813–33). It is possibly he who is quoted elsewhere as 'physician to al-Ma'mūn'. He died in 827. (Ullman, *Medizin*, 111).

Yūḥannā b. Māsawayh, c. 777–857, from Jundishapur, spent most of his working-life in Baghdad as director of the hospital and personal physician to the caliphs, including al-Ma'mūn. He translated from Greek and wrote his own works on various medical subjects. Among his students was Ḥunayn b. Isḥāq. He is quoted once by Ibn Qayyim on the citron (*utrujj*). (Ullman, *Medizin*, 112–15).

Yaʿqūb b. Isḥāq al-Kindī, d. circa 873, a philosopher with a wide range of interests, wrote several works on medicine, of which not many survive. His *Formulary* of compound medicines has been translated by M. Levey; quoted on Indigofera (*katam*).

Thābit b. Qurra, 834–901, a Sabian ('star-worshipper') from Ḥarrān, a mathematician, wrote on medicine, but not a great deal of his writing is extant. The 'Treasury' (*al-dhakhīra*), according to Ullman (*Medizin*, 123, 136) is incorrectly attributed to him. Quoted on food and drink, in Chapter 32c.

ʿAli b. al-ʿAbbās al-Majūsī, d. 944, came from a Persian Mazdean family, hence the name Majūsī, and worked for the Būyid ʿAḍud al-Daūla (949–82). For the ruler he composed *Kāmil al-ṣināʿa al-ṭibbiyya* (Perfection of the art of medicine), also known as *al-kitāb al–malakī* (the royal book). This is a huge work arranged into many chapters, dealing with diseases classified according to the parts of the body and with medicaments. Ibn Qayyim quotes from him once, as 'author of *al-Kāmil*', in Chapter 28. (Ullman, *Medizin*, 140–46, Levey, *Pharmacology*, 106).

Abū ʿAbd Allāh Muḥammad b. Aḥmad b. Saʿīd al-Tamīmī came from Jerusalem. In 970 he went to Egypt to work as physician for the vizier Yaʿqūb b. Killis, and died there in 980. He wrote a 'guide' on foods and medicines, as well as a book concerning plague, *māddāt al-baqā' bi-iṣlāḥ fasād al-hawā'*, to which Ibn Qayyim refers in Chapter 5 (cf. n. 4).

Isḥāq b. Sulayman al-Isrā'īlī, c. 855–950, was both physician and philosopher. He first worked as an oculist in Cairo, but emigrated to Kairouan in Tunisia, where he studied medicine under Isḥāq b. ʿImrān and later became court physician to Ziyādat Allāh III, the last of the Aghlabid dynasty. He is best known for his *Kitāb al-ḥummayāt*, 'Book of fevers', of which the third discourse, on hectic fever (consumption) has been edited and translated by J.D. Latham and H. Isaacs (*Arabic Technical and Scientific Texts*,volume 8, Cambridge 1981). He is quoted on camel's milk, in Chapter 6.

Sharaf al-Dīn ʿAlī b. ʿĪsā al-Kaḥḥāl (the oculist), who died after 1010, practised as an oculist and physician in Baghdad. He wrote one of the most famous of all Arabic works on the eye, its disease and treatment, *Kitāb tadhkirat al-kaḥḥālīn*, 'oculists' notebook', from which Ibn Qayyim quotes in Chapter 19. (Ullman, *Medizin*, 208–9).

Abū Sahl ʿĪsā b. Yaḥyā al-Masīḥī al-Jurjānī, d. 1010, a student of Ibn Sīnā, wrote on medicine in general. He worked in Khurasan and later in Khwarizm. Ibn Qayyim cites him once, concerning the use of clay for ulcers, in Chapter 31d. (Ullman, *Medizin*, 151).

Abū'l-Ḥasan ʿAlī b. Riḍwān, d. 1068, despite a childhood spent in poverty, studied and then worked first as an astrologer and later as physician, becoming personal physician to the Fāṭimid Caliph al-Mustanṣir of Egypt (1035–94). He carried on a controversy with Ibn Buṭlān (edited and translated by J. Schacht and M. Meyerhof, Egyptian University Faculty of Arts Publication no. 13, Cairo 1937). He wrote many works on medicine, including commentaries on Hippocrates and Galen; *Kitāb al-nāfiʿ fī kayfiyyat taʿlīm ṣināʿat al-ṭibb* (the useful book on the method of teaching the art of medicine); *Kitāb dafʿ maḍarr al-abdān bi-arḍ Miṣr*, which has been translated and annotated by M. Dols, *Medieval Medicine*. (Ullman, *Medizin*, 158–59). Ibn Qayyim quotes him on Salvadora persica (*kabāth*).

Perhaps the best-known of all Arabic philosopher-physicians were al-Rāzī (Rhazes) and Ibn Sīnā (Avicenna). They combined a thorough knowledge of both disciplines with a careful attention to detail, skill in practice and a power of observation and description. Their works greatly influenced later medical writers, became the subject of numerous commentaries, were later translated into Latin, and continued to influence medical work until the eighteenth or even nineteenth century.

Abū Bakr Muḥammad b. Zakariyā al-Rāzī, circa 865–923, a native of Rayy in Khurasan, studied philosophy, literature, alchemy as well as medicine. He moved to Baghdad where he became personal physician to the Caliph al-Muqtadir. His chief works include *al-Manṣūrī*, written for an earlier patron the Sāmānid Abū Ṣāliḥ al-Manṣūr b. Isḥāq, ruler of Kirman and Khurasan, and a posthumous compilation of his notes on every branch of medicine, *al-Ḥāwī fī l-ṭibb* (the 'Comprehensive'), later translated into Latin as *Continens*. Al-Rāzī is especially noted for his clinical observations, a collection of which was edited and translated by M. Meyerhof (*Isis*, 1935). Ibn Qayyim quotes from *al-Ḥāwī* on fevers, in Chapter 3, and in several other places. (Ullman, *Medizin*, 128–36).

Abū ʿAlī b. Sīnā, 980–1037, born near Bukhara, worked as both physician and statesman for several rulers, and during his travels wrote an astonishing amount on every aspect of medicine. His chief work is *al-Qānūn fī l-ṭibb*, a comprehensive encyclopaedia, later translated into Latin as *Canon Medicinae*. Ibn Sīnā is famous as a philosopher, but when quoting from his medical work Ibn Qayyim mostly refers to him as 'author of the *Qānūn*'; he refers to him on numerous occasions, eg. on cupping in Chapter 8. (Ullman, *Medizin*, 152–56, 333–37).

PHYSICIANS IN MUSLIM SPAIN

In the western end of the Islamic empire, the Umayyads of Andalus (Islamic Spain) established themselves after the downfall of the Umayyads of Damascus in 750, and made their capital at Cordoba. When ʿAbd al-Raḥmān III in 929 declared himself caliph, he sought equal footing with the ʿAbbāsid Caliphs in Baghdad. Science, arts and medicine flourished under the Umayyads of Cordoba. Andalus was especially noted for its botanists, three of whom are quoted by Ibn Qayyim: Ibn Juljul, Ibn Samajūn, al-Ghāfiqī.

Sulaymān b. al-Ḥasan ibn Juljul, d. after 994, worked at the court of ʿAbd al-Raḥmān III, and assisted in the translation of Dioscorides' herbal into Arabic. He wrote a Commentary on Dioscorides, and a Supplement on 'Drugs which Dioscorides did not mention'. In 987 AD he completed a history of medicine and of physicians, *Ṭabaqāt al-aṭibbā' wa-l-ḥukamā'*, which has been edited by Fu'ad Sayyid, Cairo 1955. (Ullman, Medizin, 229, 268). Ibn Qayyim quotes him once, on Salvadora persica (*kabāth*).

His contemporary Ibn Samajūn compiled a large herbal, *al-Kitāb al-jāmiʿ li-aqwāl al-qudamā' wa'l-mutaḥaddithīn min al-aṭibbā' wa'l-mutafalsifīn fi'l-adwiya al-mufrada*, the 'comprehensive book of sayings of ancient and modern physicians and philosophers concerning simple drugs', quoting previous authorities on plants and medicines. Not all of this has survived, but a sample is given in P. Kahle, 'Ibn Samagun und sein Drogenbuch: ein Kapitel aus den Anfangen der arabischen Medizin', *Documenta Islamica Inedita*, Berlin 1952, 25–44. Ibn Qayyim quotes him on aloes wood (*ʿūd*). (Ullman, *Medizin*, 267).

A century or more later, Abū Jaʿfar Aḥmad b. Muḥammad al–Ghāfiqī, d. 1135 AD, originally from Ghāfiq near Cordoba, compiled an even larger herbal and drug book, *Kitāb al-adwiya al-mufrada*, 'Book of simple drugs'. Much of this has been lost, but parts, in the recension made by Bar Hebreaus in the thirteenth century, were edited and translated by M. Meyerhof and G.P. Sobhy. (*The Abridged Version of 'The Book of Simple Drugs' of Aḥmad ibn Muḥammad al-Ghāfiqī, Egyptian University,* The Faculty of Medicine, publication No. 4, Cairo 1932). This work cites Greek and Arabic authors, and gives synonyms in the various languages. It was used extensively by Ibn al-Bayṭār of Malaga, d. 1248 AD, whose work *al-Jāmiʿ li-mufradāt al-adwiya wa'l-*

aghdhiya is probably the best-known of all Arabic herbals; it exists in numerous manuscripts, and an edition was printed in Cairo (Bulāq) in 1291 AH. Ibn Qayyim quotes al-Ghāfiqī on citron (*utrujj*), truffles (*kam'a*), and indigofera (*katam*). (Ullman, *Medizin*, 276; 280 f).

Also in Andalus, Ibn Zuhr (Avenzoar), whose full name was Abū Marwān ʿAbd al-Malik b. Abī' l-ʿAlā' Zuhr, died in 1162 AD, worked as physician for the Almoravids, then the Almohads who succeeded them. He moved to Morocco, and later became vizier to ʿAbd al-Mu'min (1130–63), for whom he wrote his *Kitāb al-aghdhiya*. His best known work is *Kitāb al-taysīr fi'l-mudāwāt wa 'l-tadbīr*, the 'facilitator in therapy and diet', from which Ibn Qayyim quotes twice, on the toothbrush (*siwāk*) and narcissus (*narjis*). (Ullman, *Medizin*, 162–63).

****

The translator would like to express her gratitude to all who have helped in various ways to bring this translation to completion with advice, encouragement, corrections and amendments. In particular she thanks the library of the Oriental Institute, Oxford, for the extensive loan of their copy of *al-Ṭibb al-Nabawī*, and Muhsin Najjar for his painstaking extraction of the *Ḥadīth* references.

MEDICINE OF THE PROPHET

PART ONE

CHAPTER

1

Introduction and general considerations[1]

Praise be to God, the Lord of the Worlds, and His blessings on the noblest of Messengers, Muḥammad, Seal of the Prophets, and his family and Companions, on them all.

THESE are some useful chapters on the guidance of the Prophet ﷺ, concerning the medicine which he used, was treated with, or recommended for others. We shall elucidate what it contains of wisdom which is not accessible to the intellects of the greatest of physicians.

We ask help from God, and from Him we draw strength and power.

(a) *The two types of sickness*

We begin by declaring that sickness is of two kinds: sickness of the heart, and sickness of the body, both mentioned in the Qur'ān.

Sickness of the heart is of two kinds: Sickness of uncertainty and doubt, and sickness of desire and temptation, and these both appear in the Qur'ān. Concerning sickness of uncertainty, the Most High has said: *'In their hearts is a disease; and Allāh has increased their disease'* (II:10).

Again, He said:

'That those in whose hearts is a disease, and the unbelievers, may say: What does Allāh mean by this as a parable?' (LXXIV:31).

1 In Ibn Qayyim's opinion, the Prophet is a better source of guidance than are the physicians, and so he categorises sickness in accordance with the Qur'ān's pronouncements. Sickness of the heart (*qalb*) is of two kinds: uncertainty and doubt (*shubha wa-shakk*) and desire and temptation (*shahwa wa-ghayy*). Bodily medicine he considers under two headings: there is medicine which is treatment by simple opposites (*aʿḍād*) and medicine requiring thought. An illness may be a disturbance of the temperament (*mizāj*) which upsets the equilibrium or mean (*iʿtidāl*); it may be material, from an internal cause (*māddiyya*), qualitative, upsetting the constitution (*kayfiyya*), or organic, in one or other of the limbs or organs (*āliyya*).

Sickness of the body is dealt with under certain principles: preservation of health (*ḥifẓ*

And concerning anyone called to accept judgement in accordance with the Qur'ān and *Sunna*, but who refused and turned away, He said: *'When they are summoned to come to Allāh and His Messenger so that He may judge between them, behold some of them decline. But if the right is on their side, they come to him in submission. Is it that there is a disease in their hearts? Or do they doubt, or are they in fear, that Allāh and His Messenger might treat them unjustly? But it is they who do wrong?'* (XXIV:48–50). This is the sickness of uncertainties and doubts.

Concerning the sickness of desires, He has spoken: *'O wives of the Prophet! You are not like any other women. If you fear God, do not be too complaisant in your speech, lest one in whose heart there is sickness should desire you'* (XXXIII:32).

That is the sickness of the desire of adultery. And God knows best.

(b) *Principles of bodily illness*

On bodily sickness, He has spoken: *'There is no blame upon the blind, nor one born lame, nor on the one who is sick . . .'* (XXIV:61). He mentioned bodily sickness in connection with pilgrimage, fasting and ablution, for an amazing reason that indicates the glory of the Qur'ān, and how sufficient it is for the one who truly comprehends it. The rules of bodily medicine are three: preservation of health, expulsion of harmful substances, and protection from harm. Thus the Most High has mentioned these three principles in these three most relevant places: In the verse on fasting He said: *'If any of you is ill, or on a journey, (then fasting should be made up from) a set number of other days'* (II:184). For He permitted a sick person to break the fast because of illness; and the traveller in order to preserve his health and strength, as fasting while travelling might cause injury to health through the combination of vigorous movement and the consumption of the vital bodily energy which often is not properly replaced due to lack of food. So He permitted the traveller to break his fast.

In the verse of the Pilgrimage, He said: *'If any of you is sick, or has an ailment in his head, then (he can make) compensation of fasting or almsgiving or sacrifice'* (II:196). He gave permission to the sick, and to anyone with some ailment in his head, such as lice or itching, to shave his head, while in a state of *iḥrām*. This was to evacuate the substance of harmful vapours that brought about the ailment on his head through being congested beneath the hair. When the head is shaved, the pores are opened up, and these vapours make their way out. This kind of evacuation is used to draw an analogy for all other kinds of evacuation, where congestion of the matter would cause harm.

---

al-ṣiḥḥa), protection from harm (*al-ḥimya ʿan al-mu'dhi*) and expulsion of corrupt substances (*istifrāgh al-mawādd al-fāsida*). In a medical textbook the chief divisions were of the 'preservation of health, and its restoration when disturbed'.

There are ten things which if blocked or restrained cause harm: blood when it is agitated, semen when it is moving, urine, faeces, wind, vomiting, sneezing, sleep, hunger, thirst. Each of these ten, if repressed, bring about some kind of malady. The Most High drew attention to the least significant—the vapour congested in the head—to indicate the importance of evacuating what is more serious. Such is the method of the Qur'ān: to give instruction about the greater, through mentioning the lesser.

In the verse of ablution the Most High referred to the protection from harm: *'If you are sick, or on a journey, or one of you comes from the privy, or you have been in contact with women, and you can find no water, then take for yourselves clean sand or earth'* (IV: 43). He permitted the sick person to desist from using water and to use earth instead, in order to protect the body against harm. There again the attention is drawn to take the necessary precautionary measures against anything which could harm the body, internally or externally.

The Most High has thus guided His servants to the three main principles of medicine, and the total sum of its numerous rules. We shall mention the guidance of the Messenger of God concerning these, and shall elucidate how his guidance is the most perfect.

(c) *Medicine of the heart*

As for Medicine of the Heart, this has been entrusted to the Messengers, God's blessings and peace upon them; there is no means of obtaining this, except through their teaching and at their hands. For the tranquillity of the heart is obtained through recognition of its Lord and Creator, His Names and Attributes, His actions and judgements; and it should prefer what He approves of and loves, and should avoid what He forbids and dislikes. Only thus can true health and life be found, and there is no path to acquire these save through the Messengers. Any idea that health of the heart can be achieved except by following them is an error on the part of the one who so thinks unless he only means the life and health of his animal soul and its desires, while the life of his heart, its health and strength, are totally ignored. If anyone does not distinguish between the one and the other, he should weep over the life of his heart, as it should be counted among the dead, and over its light, for it is submerged in the seas of darkness.

(d) *Medicine of the body*

Medicine of the body is of two kinds:

(1) The first kind is in accordance with God's creation of the animals, both rational beings and dumb animals, and it does not require the intervention of a physician. Treatment of hunger and thirst, cold, weariness, and suchlike is by their opposites and by that which will put an end to these states.

(2) The second kind is that which requires thought and reflection: such as repelling 'similar' illnesses, occurring in the temperament, thus unbalancing the equilibrium, whether erring towards heat or cold, dryness or moisture, or a combination of two of these. This is itself of two kinds: either material or qualitative, that is, either through the secretion of a matter, or the appearance of a condition. The difference between them is that illness of condition appears when the matters which actually caused it have ceased to exist, for while these matters abate, their effects remain as a condition within the temperament. But illnesses of matter are reinforced by their own causes; and when the cause of an illness remains along with it, then one must first pay attention to the cause, secondly to the illness itself, and thirdly to the medicine for it.[2]

Then there are illnesses of the organs, which cause the organ to depart from its normal state. This may affect it in form, or in cavity, or vessel; affecting texture or proximity; or glands, or bones, or position. For when these organs are put together to constitute the body, their composition is called: conjunction; and any departure from this equilibrium in this respect is called: disjunction.[3]

Or there are the general diseases, which comprise the 'similar' and the organic. The similar are those whereby the temperament departs from a balanced state, and this departure is named sickness, once it has caused actual perceptible damage. It is of eight types: four simple, and four compound. The simple are: hot, cold, moist and dry. The compound are: hot and moist, hot and dry, cold and moist, cold and dry. These occur either with or without the secretion of some matter. If the sickness causes no actual damage it is called 'departure from the mean', yet being within the limits of a healthy balance.

The body has three states: (1) natural state, (2) abnormal state, (3) a state midway between the two. The first is that in which the body is healthy; the second is that in which it is sick; while the third state is that which is intermediate between these two states. For nothing transfers to its opposite except by an intermediate.

The departure of the body from its natural state may be from an internal cause, since it is composed from hot and cold, moist and dry; or it may be due to an external cause, because whatever the body encounters may be either suitable or unsuitable.

Harm that occurs to a human being may be caused by disorder of the temperament, through its departure from the mean; or it may be caused by corruption of an organ; or it may be caused by weakness in the faculties or in the spirits which convey them. This harm can be traced back to an increase of something, which in the balanced state should not be in excess; or deficiency of

2 When there is an external cause to an illness, the removal of the cause will end or alleviate the illness. But illnesses of 'matter', with an internal cause, indicate a disturbance of bodily substances which must first be rectified. 'Material' illness is described in more detail in section (h) below.

3 Conjunction (*ittiṣāl*) and its opposite, disjunction (*tafarruq al-ittiṣāl*).

what the balanced state requires in order not to be deficient; or separation of what the balance requires to be separate; or expansion of what the balance requires to be contracted; or finally through a change in shape or location of an organ from its original customary one that causes it to deviate from its equilibrium.

The physician is the one who disperses that which harms the human being when it is congested, or concentrates that which harms him by being separated; he decreases that which, if increased, causes him harm, or increases that which harms by its decrease. Thus he restores lost health, or he preserves it by form and likeness and repels the illness which is present, through its opposite and antithesis; and he confronts illness by that which prevents its occurrence, through precautionary measures. And you will see how these principles are reflected in the guidance of the Messenger of God ﷺ, bringing healing and sufficiency, through the power and strength of God, His bounty and assistance.

(e) *Principles of medication*

Among his guidance, we include the medication he used on himself, or prescribed to the sick among his family and Companions. But neither his guidance, nor that of his Companions, includes the use of those medicines known in general as compounds (*aqrābādhīn*).[4] On the contrary, most of their medicines are simples, though they often add to the simple that which will reinforce it or temper its strength. This forms the major part of the medicine of all the different nations, Arabs, Turks and people of the deserts, without exception. The only people to be concerned with compounds were the Byzantines and the Greeks, while most of the medicine of the Indians consists of simples.

Physicians are agreed that when treatment is possible through diet, there should be no recourse to medicine; and when treatment is possible through a simple, there should not be recourse to a compound. It is said: Whenever it is possible to heal an illness by diet and precautions, there should be no attempt to heal it with medicines. Also, the physician must not be enthusiastic for the administration of medicines; for when a medicine does not find any illness in the body to dissolve, or when it finds an illness for which it is not the appropriate treatment, or finds one which is appropriate, but for which its amount or quality is too great, it clings to the healthy state and impairs it.

As for the experienced physicians, their medicine consists mostly of simples. These people represent one of the three categories of medicine. The confirmation of this is that the classification of medicines is strongly related to that of

4 *Aqrābādhīn*, medical formulary, giving the composition of drugs and medications; from the Greek *graphidion*, through Syriac. Such compounds would include theriac (*tiryāq*), electuaries (*maʿājīn*, sing. *maʿjūn*), compound oils (*adhān*, sing. *duhn*) and medications for internal and external complaints. See EI^2, s.v. 'Akrabadhin', (B. Lewin), and Levey, *Pharmacology*, 72 f.

foodstuffs. Those of the population who keep mostly to simple food suffer from very few illnesses, and their medication is by simples. But the city dwellers, whose food is mostly composite, need compound medicines, the reason being that their illnesses are mostly complex ones, for which compound medicines are most useful. Bedouin and desert dwellers suffer from simple illnesses, so for their medication simple drugs suffice. This has been proved in accordance with the medical tradition.[5]

We would say that the connection between the medicine of the Messengers and that of physicians is as tenuous as its connection with the medicine of village healers.[6] This is acknowledged by the skilled and leading men among both the physicians and village healers. Concerning the knowledge they have of medicine, some say: it is a matter of analogy; some say: it is empiricism; some say: it is by inspiration and dreams, fortuitous conjecture and intuition. Still others say: much of it is taken from the dumb animals, as when we see cats who have eaten any poisonous creature find a lamp and lick up some of the oil in order to treat themselves with that. Likewise it is seen that serpents, when they come forth from the depth of the earth, at which time their sight is dim, go to find leaves of fennel and rub their eyes against them. And it is known that some birds give themselves an enema with sea water when they suffer from an obstruction. (There are similar stories, mentioned in books about the origins of medicine.)[7]

(f) *Religion and medicine*

Where does the medical knowledge of the physicians stand in relation to the Revelation which God revealed to His Messenger as to what would benefit or harm him? The relationship of the physicians' medicine to this Revelation is similar to the relationship of their sciences to what the prophets taught. Religious and prophetic medicines heal certain illnesses that even the minds of great physicians cannot grasp, and which their science, experiments and analogical deductions cannot reach. Such are the medicines of heart and soul, which promote the strength of the heart and its reliance upon God; its complete trust in Him, and taking refuge with Him; dejectedness and submission in His presence; humility towards Him; almsgiving and supplication, repentance and seeking forgiveness; beneficence towards humankind, and giving succour to the troubled and relief to the distressed. All humanity has tested these remedies, and despite their differences of creed and religion, they have found them to have

5 Ibn Khaldūn says that medicine is needed only by those who dwell in cities, since their life is less healthy than that of bedouin. *Muqaddima*, II. 373 and III. 149. See also Chapters 10 and 24.

6 Medicine of itinerants: practitioners who were not part of the local community but wandered from place to place and whose knowledge of medicine could not be guaranteed as reliable. Old women: *ʿajā'iz* (sing. *ʿajūz*), the traditional village healers.

7 Theories on the origins of medicine are found in more detail in Ibn Abī Uṣaybiʿa, *ʿUyūn*, Introduction.

a great influence in healing such as cannot be attained by the medicine of the most learned of physicians, nor by their experiments or deductions.

We and others have tested a great many of these prophetic medicines. We have seen them effect that which physical medicines cannot; and by comparison they are rather like the medicine of village healers when compared to that of the physicians. This follows the course of the law of divine wisdom, and is not outside it. But the causes are varied. For when the heart turns toward the Lord of the Worlds, the Creator of both illness and medicine, the One Who regulates nature and disposes of it as He wishes, it responds to other medicines, different from those which are the concern of one whose heart is turned away and far from Him.

It is known that when spirits are strong, and soul and nature are strong, they help one another to repel and conquer the illness. We can hardly deny the overwhelming strength and the all-healing powers accessible to the soul and nature through experiencing the delight of love, intimacy and being nigh to the Creator; the joy of invoking Him, the annihilation of all faculties in Him, union with Him and complete trust and reliance on Him. Only the most ignorant, the most veiled one whose soul is so dense that he becomes the furthest from God, and thereby the nature and reality of man, would deny this. We shall mention, if God wills, the reason whereby reciting the *Fātiḥa* as an incantation puts an end to the painful ailment of a bite.[8]

These are the two types of the medicine of the Prophet. With God's support, we shall speak about them both, to the best of our ability and capacity, and according to our knowledge and learning which are scarcely adequate, and we shall present our unworthy offering. But we make our request of the One in Whose hand is all good, and ask support from His bounty. For He is the Noble, the One Who gives.

(g) Ḥadīth *Concerning medicine*

Muslim relates in his *Ṣaḥīḥ*, from the *ḥadīth* of Abū' l-Zubayr, from Jābir b. ʿAbd-Allāh, from the Prophet ﷺ: 'To every disease (*dā'*) there is a remedy (*dawā'*), and when the remedy to the disease is found, he is cured, by the permission of God, the Glorious One.'[1]

In the two books of the *Ṣaḥīḥ*, from Abū Hurayra it is related that the Prophet ﷺ said: 'God did not send down (*anzala*) any illness without sending down healing (*shifā'*) for it.'[2]

In the *Musnad* of Imām Aḥmad, from *ḥadīth* of Ziyād b. ʿAlāqa from Usāma b. Sharīk it says: I was with the Prophet ﷺ, when some bedouin came and asked: 'O Messenger of God, should we treat the sick (*natadāwā*)?' He replied:

8 The *Fātiḥa* is the opening chapter, Sura 1, of the Qur'ān; it is recited in the *ṣalāt* (ritual prayer) five times a day, and often as a prayer, or even incantation. For its use in the latter sense, see Chapter 31.

'Yes, O servants of God, treat your sick. For indeed God, the Glorious One, did not make any disease without making healing for it, except for one disease.' 'What is that?' they asked. 'Old age,' he replied. In another wording: 'God did not send down any illness without sending down any healing for it; the one who knows it, knows it, and the one who is ignorant does not.'[3]

In the *Musnad* from *ḥadīth* of Ibn Masᶜūd, (*marfūᶜ*): 'God the Most Glorious did not send down an illness without sending down healing for it; the one who knows it, knows it, and the one who does not is ignorant thereof.'[4]

In the *Musnad* and the *Sunan*, from Abū Khuzāma: I said: 'O Messenger of God, do you consider incantations to which we have recourse a suitable means of treatment, and are they useful in protection? Do they turn back anything from God's decree?' He replied: 'They are part of God's decree.'[5]

These *ḥadīth* have both confirmed the reality of such causes and effects, and invalidated the words of anyone who denies them.

It is also possible that his actual words were: 'For every disease there is a remedy', to be taken in a general sense, so as to encompass fatal illnesses and those which no physician can cure. In that case, God the Most Glorious has appointed remedies to cure them but has concealed the knowledge of such remedies from humankind, and has not given man the means to find out. For created beings have no knowledge except that which God has taught them.

Therefore the Prophet ﷺ indicated that healing is dependent on the concurrence of the medicine with the illness. For every created entity has an opposite, thus every disease has an opposite as a remedy by which it can be treated. The Prophet ﷺ also indicated that cure is dependent on the suitability of the remedy to the disease, in addition to its mere existence. For when a medicine is too potent for the illness or is administrated in excess, then it transforms the original illness into another. When it is insufficient for the illness then it does not fully combat it, and the treatment is defective; and when the healer is unable to identify the right medicine, healing does not result. When the time is not suitable for a particular remedy, it does not take effect. Likewise when the body is not receptive, or the faculty is incapable of bearing it, or there is some other factor preventing its influence, a cure will not be obtained, because of the lack of compatibility. But when there is complete compatibility, a cure must inevitably occur. This is the best of the two assumptions in the *ḥadīth*.

The second is that, within the general meaning, it is the particular which is intended, especially seeing that what is contained within an expression is much greater than what comes out from it, and this is common usage in every language. So the meaning would be: God has not made any disease that can be treated without making a remedy for it. So this does not include those diseases which are not receptive to medicine.

This is similar to the words of the Most High concerning the wind which He imposed upon the people of ᶜĀd: *Everything will it destroy, by the command of its Lord!* (XLVI : 25), meaning everything that can be destroyed and all that wind can destroy. And there are many other parallels to this throughout the Qur'ān.

If anyone reflects on the creation of opposites in this world, and the way they oppose, repel, and conquer one another, he will see clearly the complete power and wisdom of the Lord Most High and how He has perfected His creation, and that He alone has all Lordship, Oneness and Power. All else has something which opposes and hinders it, but He alone is Self-sufficient, while every other being is essentially dependent.

These sound *ḥadīth* contain the command to carry out treatment, and this does not negate trust in God (*tawakkul*), any more than does the repelling of hunger, thirst, heat and cold by their opposites. Moreover, the reality of divine unity (*tawḥīd*) is only made complete by direct use of the means which God has appointed as being essential to bring about certain effects, according to the Decree and the religious Law.

Also, neglecting to use these means would cast doubt on the virtue of trust itself, just as it casts doubts on the Command and Wisdom, and weakens trust, insofar as the one neglecting these means considers that to disregard them is a greater degree of trust. But in fact disregarding them is incapacity, which negates trust, whose reality is reliance of the heart on God, in the acquisition of what is beneficial to the servant in this world and the next, and repels what harms him in either sphere. This reliance must be accompanied by pursuit of the available means; otherwise, the servant is negating both the divine wisdom and the religious Law. Thus the servant should not turn his incapacity into trust, nor his trust into incapacity.

Now these *ḥadīth* contain the reply to anyone who denies medical treatment saying that if healing has been decreed, then medical treatment is not useful, and if it has not been decreed, then the case is the same; or again, that illness arrives by God's Decree, and God's Decree can neither be repelled nor resisted.

This is the question which the bedouin brought to the Messenger of God ﷺ. But the very best of the Companions had better knowledge of God and His Wisdom and Attributes than to ask such questions.

The Prophet ﷺ answered them, with that which healed and was sufficient, saying: 'These medicines, incantations and talismans are all part of God's Decree, for there is nothing outside His Decree; rather, His Decree is resisted by His Decree, and this resistance is from His Decree. There is absolutely no way to escape from His Decree. This is similar to resisting the Decree of hunger, thirst, heat and cold by their opposites, and like resisting the Decree of the enemy by personal effort (*jihād*); all are from God's Decree: the one who resists, the one resisted, and the act of resistance.'

The person asking this question can be told: This would oblige you not to make use of any of the means whereby you would obtain benefit or repel harm. For benefit and harm, if they are decreed, must inevitably occur, and if they are not decreed, they cannot possibly occur. Therein lies the ruin of religion and worldly affairs, and corruption of the world. But this is only stated by someone who resists and opposes the truth, who mentions the Decree so as to evade confronting the truth. Likewise, the polytheists said: *'Had Allāh wished, we should not have been polytheists, nor our fathers'* (VI:148), and *'If Allāh had wished, we should not have worshipped aught but Him, neither we nor our fathers'* (XVI : 35). They said this in defiance of the proof that God established against them through the Messengers.

The reply to this questioner is to say: There remains a third division you have not mentioned, that God decreed such things by such a cause, so that if you produce the cause the effect will occur, otherwise it will not.

Then he may say: If He has decreed the cause for me, I shall do it, but if He has not decreed it for me, I shall not be able to do it.

The reply is: Do you accept this argument from your slave, your son or your hired man, when one of them argues in this way concerning what you have ordered or forbidden him, and then he opposes you? If you accept it, then do not blame one who disobeys you and takes your money, slanders your honour and denies you your rights. But if you do not accept it, how then can it be acceptable from you in fulfilment of God's rights over you!

It is related in an Israelite tradition that Abraham, the Friend of God, said: 'O Lord, from whom comes illness?' He replied: 'From Me.' So he asked: 'And from whom comes the remedy?' 'From Me.' He asked: 'And what is the business of the physician?' The Lord replied: 'Someone by whose hands I send the remedy.'

The words of the Prophet ﷺ: 'For every illness a remedy' contain strengthening for the soul of the sick man and for the physician, and encouragement to seek and investigate that remedy. For when the sick person is aware that for his illness there is a remedy which will make it cease, his heart clings to the spirit of hope, so he is cooled from the heat of despair, and the door of hope is opened to him. When his soul is strong, his innate heat is sent forth, and that is a cause of strength for the spirits, animal, vital and constitutional. When these spirits are strong, so are the powers which convey them, thus they conquer and repel the illness. Similarly, when the physician knows that this illness has a remedy, he is encouraged to seek and investigate it.

Illnesses of the body follow the pattern of illnesses of the heart. God did not allow any illness for the heart without making healing for it, through its opposite. If the sick person knows and uses it, and it concurs with the illness of his heart, it cures him, by the permission of God the Most High.

(h) *Precautions against indigestion and general rules to be observed concerning food and drink*

In the *Musnad* and elsewhere it is reported that the Prophet ﷺ said: 'The human being can fill no container worse than his belly. Sufficient for the son of

Adam are so many morsels as will keep his spine upright. But if he must eat more, then a third for his food, a third for his drink and a third for his breath.'[6]

Illnesses are of two types. Material illnesses arise from an increase of matter which comes to a point of excess in the body where it harms its natural functions. And these are the most common illnesses. They are caused by consuming more food before the previous meal has been properly digested; by eating in excess of the amount needed by the body; by taking in food which is of little nutritional value and slow to digest; and by indulging in different foods which are complex in their composition. When a human being fills his belly with these foods and it becomes a habit, they cause him various diseases, some of which come to an end slowly, some swiftly. When he is moderate in his eating and takes only so much of it as he needs, keeping a balance of quantity and quality, the body benefits more from this than it does from a large amount of food.

There are three degrees of eating: (1) out of need; (2) in moderation; and (3) in excess. The Prophet ﷺ has made it known that he found sufficient such morsels as would keep his spine upright, with which his strength would not be lowered nor weakened; but if one goes beyond that, then let him eat to fill a third of his belly, and leave another third for water and a third for breath. This is most useful for both body and heart. For if the belly is filled with food, it has not enough space for drink, and when the drink is added to it, this leaves little space for the breath. Thus it is afflicted by distress and fatigue, and it bears this like one carrying a heavy burden. This state will also lead to heart trouble; the limbs become too lazy to perform the obligatory rituals, and conversely they move swiftly in submission to desires brought about by satiety.

Eating to repletion, continually and in excess damages heart and body. Occasionally, there is no harm. Abū Hurayra drank milk in the presence of the Prophet ﷺ until he said: 'By the One Who sent you with the truth, I cannot find any more space for it!' And the Companions often ate, in his presence, until they were sated. Excessive satiety, however, weakens the faculties and the body, even though it is fattening. The body only becomes strong in accordance with the quality of the food it accepts, not its quantity.

(i) *Components of the body*

It is because the human body is made up of parts of earth, air, and water that the Prophet ﷺ spoke of food, drink, and breath.

Someone may ask: 'What about the share for the component of fire?' The reply is: 'This is a question which has been discussed by physicians, who have said: "There is, in fact, a component of fire in the body for it is one of its constituents (*arkān*) and elements".[9]

9 Fire (*nār*), one of the four elements(*isṭiqsāt*), which together compose material substances, including the human body. The argument is whether or not this latter contains the element of

But they have been opposed in that by learned men, physicians and others, who say there is no component of fire in the body. They deduce this in various ways:

1. It could be claimed that the fiery component descended from the ether and mixed in with the earthy and watery components; or it could be said that it was generated and took form in them.

The first is unlikely on two counts: (1) fire by nature rises, and if it were to descend it would be through some force which compelled it from its own place to this world; (2) those fiery components must inevitably, in such a descent, pass through the sphere of intense cold (*zamharīr*) which is in the highest degree of coldness. We observe in this world that even a mighty fire is extinguished by a relatively small amount of water. So those small portions, in passing through the sphere of intense cold—since this is in the highest degree of cold, and so immense in size—would most likely be quenched.

The second theory, that they came into being here, is even more unlikely. For if a body is transformed into fire, never having been so previously, then before this process of transformation it was either Earth, Water or Air, because the basic elements (*arkān*) are restricted to these four. This means that the component which becomes fire originally was mixed with one of these elements and joined to it, while we know when the body which is not fire is mixed with mighty bodies none of which is fire, it will not turn into fire. For in itself it is not fire, and the bodies which are mingled with it are cold. So how could it possibly turn into fire?

You may ask: why can there not be fiery components which mingle with these bodies and turn them into fire? We would reply that the argument on the acquisition of fire into these bodies is similar to the argument on the first point.

You may say: When water is poured onto extinguished lime (*nūra*), we see fire issuing from it; if the sun's rays fall upon a crystal, fire comes forth from it; and if we strike a stone onto iron, fire appears; all of this fieriness comes about in the process of mixing. That disproves your conclusions in the first section also.

Those who deny this will reply: We do not deny that a hard striking may produce fire as with the blow of stone upon iron, or that the power of the sun's heat may produce fire as in the crystal. But we consider that most unlikely in the case of plants and animals, because their bodies do not contain such force of friction as would bring about the production of fire; nor are they sufficiently pure or refined to reach the extent of the crystal; the sun's rays fall on their exterior, and no fire is produced. So how could rays which reach their interior produce fire?

---

fire. The difficulty as perceived by IQ is how the fire could have descended from the upper spheres, or could have come into being within the body; for his reasoning shows that any fiery components would have been transformed by the greater quantity of watery components. But the over-riding argument is Qur'ānic: mankind is created from clay, whereas Iblīs is created from fire. Therefore, warmth of the body is introduced from external sources and is not an essential component.

2. Physicians are agreed that old wine by its nature is in the highest degree of heat; if the heat were by reason of fiery components, that would be impossible. Since those fiery components are so small, how can it be imagined that they would remain within the predominating watery components for such a long while without being extinguished, despite the fact that we see that a great fire can be extinguished by a relatively small amount of water?

3. If indeed plants and animals contained a fiery component, this would be dominated by the watery component that it contains. The predominance of one of the natures and elements over another requires the transformation of the nature of the one conquered into the nature of the one which is dominant. By necessity this would imply the transformation of those very few fiery components into the nature of water which is the opposite of fire.

4. God the Most High, exalted and praised be He, spoke of the creation of humankind in numerous places in His Book. In some He specifically said that He created them of water (XXXII: 8), and in some that He created them of earth (III: 59, XVIII: 37), and in others that He created them of a mixture of the two, which is clay (VII: 12). In some again, that He created them from a sounding clay like pottery (LV: 14). This means a clay that has been beaten by the sun and wind, until it has become sounding clay like earthenware. In no place did He say that He had created them from fire, but He specified that of Iblīs (XXXVIII: 76).

It is confirmed in the *Ṣaḥīḥ* of Muslim, from the Prophet ﷺ, that 'the angels were created from light', and Iblīs from a *fire free of smoke* (LV: 15), and Adam was created from 'that which was described for you.'[7] This clearly shows that man was created only from what Allāh described in His Book. For God, praised be He, did not tell us that He created Adam from fire, nor that his substance contained any fire whatsoever.

5. Their most effective source of deduction is such heat as they see in the bodies of animals, as an indication of fiery components. But this is not a proof; for heat can be caused by things other than fire. Sometimes it comes from fire, at other times from motion, and from the reflection of rays, from heat of the air and from the proximity of fire, and this happens even through the medium of the air. There are still further causes, since heat is not always connected with fire.

Those who support the fire theory say that it is a well-known fact that when earth and water mix there must be heat to bring about their cooking and mixing; otherwise, neither one of them will mingle with the other nor unite with it. Similarly, if we cast seed into the earth, in such a way as both the air and the sun do not reach it, it decays. Either some new body that by its nature brings about germination and maturity is formulated in the mixture, or it is not. If it formulates, this is the fiery component, and if it does not, then the compound substance is not able to generate heat by its nature. Rather, if it becomes hot, the heating process is accidental. If the accidental heating ceases, then the compound substance is not hot in its nature, nor in its quality, but will be cold absolutely. But we already know that certain foods and drugs are hot by nature, therefore we can establish that their heat is only because they contain a fiery essence.

Moreover, if the body contained no heating particles, it would have to be exceedingly cold. For if the matter is naturally disposed to coldness, and meets no impediment or opposition, the coldness would reach its furthest limit. If this were so, it would not produce the sensation of cold, because the cold reaching the body, if at the furthest limit, would be like it, and nothing is affected by its like. If it is not affected by it, it does not feel it, and if it does not feel it, it is not pained thereby. Equally if it is a lesser degree of coldness, then absence of any effect is more likely. As the body did not contain any heating component by nature, thus it would not be affected by cold nor feel pain from it.

They say that our proofs negate the words of those who declare that the fiery components in these compounds retain their condition and fiery nature. We do not say that, rather we mean that their specific nature will be corrupted by any admixture.

Others ask: Why is it not possible to say that when Earth, Water and Air are mixed together, the heat which matures and cooks them is the heat of the sun and the other planets? Then that compound, when completely matured, is prepared to receive the composite form (*hay'a*) through the intermediacy of warmth, whether it be plant, animal, or mineral. Is it not as possible that the warmth and heat which exist in the compounds are generated through specific properties and powers which God the Most High creates at the moment the mixing takes place, not through actual fiery components? You cannot refute this possibility. This has been acknowledged by many of the most excellent physicians.

Concerning the question of the body's sensation of cold, we say that this shows that the body contains heat and a heating power, and who will deny that? But then what is the proof that the heating power should be restricted to fire? For even if 'all fire generates heating', this statement cannot be completely true when reversed, but its antithesis is true: 'Only a category of heat is generated by fire'.

As for your statement about the destruction of the specific form of fire, most physicians are agreed upon the continuation of its specific form. The claim that it is destroyed is not valid, as is acknowledged by the best of your recent scholars, in his book entitled *al-Shifā'* (Healing);[10] he has proved that the basic elements retain their natures in the compounds. And God gives success.

10 *Kitāb al-shifā'*, Ibn Sīnā's 'masterpiece of Peripatetic philosophy', with considerable material on natural science and philosophy. See Nasr, *Introduction*, 179–81.

CHAPTER

2

Natural and divine treatment[1]

TREATMENT of illness by the Prophet ﷺ was of three types: (1) with natural medicines; (2) with divine medicines; and (3) with a combination of the two. We shall speak of the three types of his guidance, beginning with the natural medicines which he prescribed and used, then the divine medicines, then the combined.

We shall merely give an indication of all this, for the Messenger of God ﷺ was sent as a guide to call people to God and His Paradise, and to give knowledge of God, making clear to the Community what pleases Him and commanding them accordingly, and what angers Him and forbidding them accordingly; to teach them about the prophets and messengers, and their lives within their respective communities, and about the creation of the world, about the beginning and the end, and that which causes suffering or happiness for mankind.

As for the guidance of the Prophet ﷺ on physical medicine, it came as a completion of his religious law (*sharīʿa*), and equally to be used when needed. When it is not needed, one's concern and energy should be directed to the treatment of heart and soul, the preservation of health, treating illnesses, and protection against harm. That is its first purpose. Restoration of the body without restoration of the heart is of no benefit, whereas damage to the body while the spirit is restored brings limited harm, for it is a temporary damage which will be followed by a permanent and complete cure. And from God comes success.

1 In this short section IQ sets out the principles upon which his work is based and organised. He points out that he is chiefly concerned with treatment of the heart and spirits, without which bodily health is of little benefit and may not, according to his viewpoint, even be possible.

CHAPTER

3

Treatment of fever by natural medicines

IT IS confirmed in the two books of the *Ṣaḥīḥ*, by Nāfiᶜ from Ibn ᶜUmar, that the Prophet ﷺ said: 'Fever is from the boiling of hell, so cool it down with water.'[8] This *ḥadīth* has caused confusion to many ignorant physicians, who have seen it as a prohibition of medication and treatment for fever. So, with God's help, we shall make clear the meaning and true significance of this *ḥadīth*.[1]

The Prophet's statements are of two kinds: general, for all people on earth, and particular, for some of them. The *ḥadīth* quoted demonstrates the general category of his preaching. An example of the second is his saying: 'You must not face south (towards the *qibla*) when relieving nature, nor should you turn your back directly to it; rather face to the east or the west.'[9] Now these words are not intended for the people of the Eastern region, nor of the Maghrib, nor Iraq; but for the people of Madīna and others in the same longitude, such as Syria. Another example can be found in his words: 'Between the east and the west lies the *qibla*.'[10]

Once this is understood, we see that his words in this *ḥadīth* are addressed specifically to the people of the Ḥijāz and the neighbouring regions; for the most common type of fevers from which they suffer is quotidian contingent fever (*yawmiyya ᶜaraḍiyya*), arising from the fierceness of the sun's heat. For such fever cold water is beneficial, whether to drink or to bathe the body. For fever is a strange heat which flares up in the heart, and thence is spread throughout the body by means of the vital spirit (*rūḥ*) and the blood in the arteries and veins, burning in such a way as to harm all the natural functions.

There are two types of fever: (1) contingent (*ᶜaraḍiyya*), which is caused

1 IQ realises that fevers are of different kinds. Thus it may be that the *ḥadīth*, concerned with the external symptoms, is meant for the contingent (*ᶜaraḍiyya*) type, whose cause can be excessive heat; in this case the opposite, extreme cold, could remove the symptoms and the cause together. In support, he quotes recommendations by Galen and al-Rāzī. Arab doctors recognised numerous kinds of fever, often classified according to duration: eg. tertian or quotidian (*yaumiyya*), or nature: putrid (*ᶜafaniyya*). Cf. Isaac Isrāʾīlī's (c. 855–950 AD) work on *Fevers*.

either by inflammation or by movement, or by sunstroke or by fierce noon heat, and similar causes; (2) pathological fever (*maraḍiyya*), of three kinds. It is formed in a particular location, and thence it spreads to affect the whole body. If at first it afflicts the vital spirit, it is called tertian or quotidian fever (*ḥummā yawm*) for it generally ceases within one day, and its limit is three days.

If it primarily afflicts the humours, it is called putrid fever (*ʿafaniyya*), and is of four kinds: bilious, atrabilious, phlegmy, or sanguineous, while if it afflicts mainly the primary organs, it is called hectic fever (*ḥummā diqq*). In these kinds there are many sub-categories.

The body can in fact gain great advantage from fever, an advantage which cannot be achieved by medication. It often happens that a quotidian or putrid fever can cause the coction of thick matters which could not otherwise reach a state of coction, or it can cause the opening of some obstruction which desobstruant medicines could not achieve. As for ophthalmia (*ramad*), recent or at an advanced stage, fever can cure most kinds, speedily and in an amazing way. It is useful in the treatment of palsy (*fālij*), facial paralysis (*luqwa*), and convulsions (*tashannuj*) from a plethora of humours, and many of the diseases which are caused by thick superfluities.

An eminent physician has told me: In many diseases, we take fever as an auspicious sign, just as the patient is gladdened by the return of health. Fever can be far more beneficial than taking medicaments, when it brings about the coction of those humours and corrupt matters which harm the body. When their coction has been effected, and these matters are ready for expulsion from the body, medicine completes the process and expels them. Thus, fever can be seen as a cause of healing.

With this in mind, it is possible that the *ḥadīth* in question is concerned with a division of contingent fevers. For it can be calmed on the spot by immersion in cold water and by drinking iced water, and the sufferer needs no further treatment. It is simply a condition of excessive heat which attaches to the vital spirit, needing for its removal only the onset of a condition of cold, which quietens it and extinguishes its burning. There is no need for the evacuation of matter nor waiting for coction to occur. However, it is also possible that all kinds of fevers are intended by this *ḥadīth*.

That most excellent physician, Galen, recognised that cold water is beneficial in fever. He says in Chapter Ten of his work *The Stratagem of Healing* (*Ḥīlat al-Bur'*) that if the patient is a young man, of sound body, well-covered—and this is in the noon heat, and when the fever nears its end—if he has no inflammation in the intestines, he should bathe or swim in cold water, and he will benefit from this. He also said: We prescribe this treatment continually.

Rāzī in his great work (*al-Ḥāwī fi'l-Ṭibb*) said: 'When the patient is strong and the fever is very severe—and coction is evident, and there is no inflammation in the abdomen, nor rupture—to drink cold water is beneficial. If the patient is of sound flesh, and the season is hot, and he is accustomed to the use of cold water externally, then this should be permitted.'

The saying of the Prophet ﷺ 'Fever is of the boiling of hell' refers to the fierceness of its heat and its spreading. Similar is his saying that 'the fierceness of heat is the boiling of hell.' In this there are two aspects:

Firstly, it is like a sample and a part taken from hell, so that the servants of God may become aware of the intensity of its heat and receive warnings from it. The Almighty decreed the outbreak of fever through causes which would logically bring it about. Likewise, the delight, joy, happiness, and pleasure are among the bounties of Paradise, which God the Almighty has allowed to appear in this abode, as a lesson and an example; He decreed its appearance in this world through causes which entailed it.

Secondly, his intention might simply have been to establish a similarity between the boiling heat of fever and the fierceness and intensity of both hell and heat likewise. This comparison is an admonition to mankind concerning the fierceness of the punishment of the fire, and that this scorching heat of fever is similar to its burning flames. And it is the burning that afflicts the one who approaches it.

His words 'cool it with water' are taken in two senses: First, the correct meaning, that this means any water; second, that it is water of Zamzam. Those who support the second reading rely on the narrative of al-Bukhārī in his *Ṣaḥīḥ* from Abū Jamra Naṣr b. ʿImrān al-Ḍubāʿī: I was sitting in the company of Ibn ʿAbbās in Mecca, when I was seized by fever. He said: 'Cool yourself from it with the water of Zamzam, for the Messenger of God has said: "Fever is of the boiling of hell, so cool it with water; "or, he said: "with water of Zamzam".'[11] The one who related this was in some doubt. Had he been certain about it, this would have been a command for the people of Mecca to use the water of Zamzam, since they could easily obtain it; and for others, whatever water they had.

Those who claim that it was meant generally differ as to two possible readings, whether the meaning was 'water given as alms' or 'its use'. The true one is 'its use'. My opinion is that the person who related the saying that almsgiving is meant found (the idea of) the use of cold water for fever difficult, and did not understand its intention. Nevertheless, his interpretation has a pleasing aspect, which is that the reward is commensurate with the action. For as the burning thirst of the parched man is quenched by cold water, so does God quench the burning of his fever as an appropriate reward. However, this is derived from the Fiqh and the symbolic expression of the *ḥadīth*; the plain intention is the use of water.

Abū Nuʿaym and others have said, from the *ḥadīth* of Anas (*marfūʿ*): 'When one of you is fevered, let him be sprinkled with cold water, on three consecutive days in the early morning.'

2 Zamzam: the well within the sanctuary (*ḥaram*) of Mecca, that sprang up to provide Hagar with water in the wilderness.

In the *Sunan* of Ibn Māja, from Abū Hurayra, (*marfūʿ*) it says: 'Fever is the bellows of hell, so keep it off you with cold water'.[12]

In the *Musnad,* and other works, among the *ḥadīth* of al-Ḥasan, from Samura, (*marfūʿ*): 'Fever is a portion of the fire, so cool it and keep it from you with cold water.'[13]

When the Messenger of God ﷺ was fevered, he used to call for a water skin, empty it over his head, and wash himself completely.

In the *Sunan,* from the *ḥadīth* of Abū Hurayra it says: 'Someone spoke of fever in the presence of the Messenger of God, and one man cursed it; but the Messenger of God said: "Curse it not, for indeed it wipes out sins, just as fire purges the dross out of iron".'[14]

For fever entails the avoidance of harmful foods, the taking of useful foods and medicines, which is all most helpful for the body's cleansing, and expulsion of its impurities and superfluities, and purification of its harmful substances. It has the same effect as fire has on iron, in removing its dross, and purifying its essence; of all things it is most like the fire from the bellows, which purifies the essence of iron. This much is known to physicians of physical medicine.

Regarding the fact that it purifies the heart from its dirt and uncleanness and expelling all its dross: this is something known to the physicians of hearts, and they find it to be just as their Prophet, the Messenger of God ﷺ, told them. But when sickness of the heart reaches a desperate stage, this treatment cannot help it.

For fever benefits the body and the heart. Anything of this kind one should not curse; to do so is a transgression, and unjust. Once when I was fevered, I recalled the words of a poet who cursed the fever:

'The expiator of sins [fever] visited me, and then said farewell.
" May it perish!" I said, both when visiting and departing.
It said—already preparing to leave "What do you desire?"
I replied, "That you should not return."'

My comment was: May he [the poet] perish! For he cursed what the Messenger of God forbade to be cursed. Had he but said:

'The one who expiates sins [fever] visited me, the one who ardently loves her.
I said, "Welcome!" both when a visitor and departing.
It said—while preparing to leave, "What do you desire?"
I replied, "That you should not depart."

That would have been more appropriate, and the fever would have left him as it swiftly departed in my case.'

It has been related—I do not know how correctly—that 'A day's fever is expiation for a year.'[15] This could be understood in two different ways: (1) that fever enters all the organs and the joints, which number three hundred and sixty joints, and makes expiation for each one of them, each joint corresponding to the sins of one day; (2) that it has an effect on the body which does not completely wear off for a year.

This is similar to the report that the Messenger of God ﷺ said: 'If anyone drinks wine, his prayer (*ṣalāt*) will not be accepted for forty days,'[16] as the residue of wine remains in his veins and organs for forty days. And God knows best.

Abū Hurayra said: No disease which afflicts me is more welcome to me than fever; for it enters each one of my organs, and God the Most High gives each organ its share of reward.

Al-Tirmidhī reports in his *Jāmiᶜ* from a *ḥadīth* of Rāfiᶜ b. Khadīj, (*marfūᶜ*): When fever afflicts one of you—and fever is nought but a piece of the fire—let him extinguish it with cold water. Let him go out to a flowing river, and meet the rush of the water after dawn and before sunrise. Let him say: 'In the Name of God, O my Lord, heal Your servant, and prove Your messenger true.' Then he shall plunge into it three times, on three consecutive days. And if he is cured, well and good; if not, then for five days; if not in five, then for seven days; for fever scarcely ever passes seven days, by God's command.[17]

I say: Indeed this action is beneficial during summer and in hot countries, under the conditions mentioned. Water at that time of day is at its coldest, it has not been exposed to the sun for the longest time, and one is at one's strongest at that time because of the benefit given by sleep, rest, and the coolness of the air. For the strength of the natural powers joins forces with the strength of the medication, which here is cold water, against the heat of the contingent fever. Or it may be the simple tertian fever (*ḥummā al-ghibb*); that is to say, it is not accompanied by inflammation nor any serious symptoms or corrupt matters. Water extinguishes it, with God's permission, especially on one of those days mentioned in the *ḥadīth*; these are the days on which occur the crises of the very severe diseases. This is especially so in the countries mentioned, because of the fineness of humours of their inhabitants and the speed with which they respond to beneficial medicine.

CHAPTER

4

Treatment of diarrhoea and the benefits of honey

IN THE two books of the *Ṣaḥīḥ* it is related, from the *ḥadīth* of Abū al-Mutawakkil, from Abū Saʿīd al-Khudrī: A man came to the Prophet ﷺ and said: 'My brother is suffering in his belly' [or, according to another version: 'his belly is loose', ie. he has diarrohoea].[1] He replied: 'Give him honey to drink.' The man went away, but returned saying: 'I have dosed him, but it has done him no good' [in another version: 'It has only increased his diarrhoea']. This took place two or three times, and the Prophet said each time: 'Give him honey.' On the third or fourth occasion, he said: 'God has spoken the truth, but your brother's belly has lied.'[18]

In the *Ṣaḥīḥ* of Muslim we read: Your brother's belly is in a disordered state (*ʿariba*), meaning that his digestion was corrupt and his stomach was weak. The noun is *al-ʿarabu* or also *al-dharabu*.

Honey contains great benefits: it removes the impurities from the veins, the intestines and elsewhere, and it dissolves the moistures when it is eaten or used as an embrocation. It is beneficial for old people and those with excess phlegm, and those of cold and moist temperament; it is nutritious and is an emollient to the constitution. It preserves the strength of ointments and anything of which it is an ingredient; it dispels the unpleasant properties of medicines; it cleanses the liver and the chest; it is a diuretic; and it is appropriate for a cough arising from the phlegm. When drunk hot with rose oil, it is beneficial against the bite of poisonous vermin or the effects of opium. Alone and mixed with water it is beneficial against the bite of a mad dog or the results of eating deadly fungus (*fuṭur*). When fresh meat is put in honey, it preserves its freshness for three months; the same applies to squash, cucumber, gourd and aubergine. Honey

1 Diarrhoea, or 'looseness of the belly' (*istiṭlāq al-baṭn*); in a variant the complaint is described thus: 'he is suffering, or complaining of his belly' (*yashtakī baṭnahu*). Another variant term, *ʿariba*, signifies that the belly is 'disordered'. Honey is recommended, see also Chapter 33 for its use as a drink.

preserves most fruit for six months. It can also preserve dead bodies. It is known as the 'trustworthy preserver'.

When the affected skin of the body and the hair are anointed with honey, it kills any lice or nits. It can lengthen, enhance and soften the hair. Used as an eye salve, it clears dimness of the sight. Used as a dentifrice it whitens and polishes the teeth, and preserves the health of teeth and gums; it opens the mouths of veins, and is an emmenagogue. If taken as an electuary[2] on an empty stomach it removes phlegm and washes the surface of the stomach, and repels superfluities from it; it warms the stomach to a moderate degree and opens its obstructions, and it does the same for the liver, kidneys and bladder. It contributes the least to the obstructions of the kidney and the spleen, compared with all other sweet substances.

Along with all this, it is guaranteed to be free of side effects and can do very little damage. It can accidentally harm those of a bilious temperament, but this can be averted by the use of vinegar or something similar, whereupon it is again of great benefit.

It is to be classed among both foods and medicines, and among drinks; it is regarded as a sweetmeat, and as an embrocation, and as one of the delights of life. Nothing of this kind has been created for us which is more excellent, nor even similar or near to it in quality. The Ancients placed all their confidence in it. Hardly any of the books of the Ancients mention sugar, nor did they know it, for it is of a fairly recent date.

The Prophet ﷺ used to drink honey with water, on an empty stomach; herein lies a most notable secret for the preservation of health that is only to be grasped by the astute and the discerning. This we shall mention, if God wills, under his guidance for the Preservation of Health.

In the *Sunan* of Ibn Māja (*marfūʿ*), from the *ḥadīth* of Abū Hurayra it says: 'If someone takes an electuary on three mornings in every month, he will not be touched by a major affliction.'[19]

Another *ḥadīth* says: 'You must use the two sources of healing, honey and the Qur'ān.'[20] For it combines human and divine medicine, the medicine of the body and of the spirit, the earthly and the heavenly remedy.

Bearing these unique properties of honey in mind we see why the Prophet ﷺ prescribed it. The man's diarrhoea was caused by indigestion which afflicted him because of repletion, so he ordered him to drink honey to repel the superfluities congested in both the stomach and intestines, as honey can cleanse and repel superfluities. His stomach had become afflicted by viscid humours, which through their stickiness prevented the food from settling down. The stomach has a fibrous surface like that of a towel, and when the viscid humours attach themselves to it, they corrupt both the stomach and the food. The appropriate medication is that which will cleanse it of these

2 'Take an electuary', *laʿaqa*, lit. to lick, hence *laʿūq*, electuary.

humours. Now honey is a cleanser and is one of the best ways of treating this complaint, especially when it is mixed with hot water.

In giving repeated doses of honey there is an excellent medical concept, namely that the medicine must be of a measure and quantity in accordance with the state of the illness. If insufficient it will not completely eliminate it; and if in excess it will weaken the strength and cause some other harm. When the Prophet ﷺ ordered the man to give his brother honey, he did not give enough to combat the disease nor attain the objective. Then when the man told him, he knew that the dose given did not reach the required amount. When the request was repeated, the Prophet ﷺ confirmed the repetition of the dose so that it would reach the amount required to combat the illness. So when successive doses have been given in accordance with the substance of the disease, the cure is manifest, by God's permission. Thus carefully calculating the measures and qualities of medicines, and the extent of the power of the illness and the strength of the patient, are among the major rules of Medicine.

The saying of the Prophet ﷺ: 'God has spoken truly but your brother's belly has lied'[21] confirms that this remedy is useful and that the persistence of the illness is not due to a defect of the medicine in itself, but rather due to the belly's unreliability and the amount of corrupt matter within it. Therefore he ordered a repetition of the dosage according to the quantity of putrid matter.

The medicine of the Prophet ﷺ is not like that of the physicians. For the medicine of the Prophet ﷺ is certain, definitive, and divine; it originates in Revelation, the niche of prophecy and the perfection of intellect. The medicine of others consists for the most part of conjecture, suppositions and experiments. It is not denied that in many cases sick people do not benefit from the medicine of the Prophet. For those who can benefit from it are only those who are ready to accept it, and who believe in its healing powers, and perfectly trust it through faith and obedience. Even the Qur'ān, which certainly heals the illness of hearts, if not accepted in this way, will not cause any healing. As for the hypocrites it will but increase their uncleanness and add to their previous illness; and to what possible extent could physical medicine be applied here? For the Medicine of the Prophet is only suitable for pure bodies, and in the same way the healing of the Qur'ān is only suitable for pure spirits and hearts that are alive. People's aversion to the Medicine of the Prophet is like their aversion to seeking healing through the Qur'ān, which is effective healing. This is not because of any defect in the medicine, rather it is due to their evil nature, distorted physique and ultimately their reluctance to accept such healing.

May God grant us success.

The following Qur'anic verse has been interpreted differently: *There comes forth from their bellies a drink, varying in its colours; and in it is healing for the people* (XVI:69), concerning whether the pronoun of *in it* refers to the drink or to the Qur'ān. There are two opinions, the correct one being that it refers to the drink, and this is the opinion of Ibn Masʿūd, Ibn ʿAbbās, al-Ḥasan, Qutāda, and the majority of commentators. Honey is what is actually being referred to in the verse, and it is what the statement is about. On the other hand there is no mention of the Qur'ān in the verse. Furthermore the sound *ḥadīth,* with the words of the Prophet 'God has spoken the truth', confirms this beyond doubt.

God the Most High knows best.

CHAPTER

5

Treatment of plague (*ṭāʿūn*) and precautions against it[1]

IT IS related in the two books of the *Ṣaḥīḥ*, from ʿĀmir b. Saʿd b. Abī Waqqāṣ, who heard his father ask Usāma b. Zayd: 'What did you hear from the Messenger of God ﷺ concerning the plague?' Usāma replied: 'The Messenger of God ﷺ said: "The plague is a punishment which was sent upon a group of children of Israel, or upon those before them." So if you hear of it occurring in any land, do not enter there and if it breaks out in any land while you are there do not leave it in flight.'[22]

Also in the two books of the *Ṣaḥīḥ*, from Ḥafṣa bint Sīrīn: Anas b. Mālik said: The Prophet ﷺ said: 'The plague is a martyrdom for every Muslim.'[23]

As to the linguistic aspect, plague (*ṭāʿūn*) is a type of pestilence (*wabā'*), says the author of the *Ṣiḥāḥ*. According to the medical people it is an evil inflammation, fatal in outcome, accompanied by a very fierce and painful burning that exceeds the norm; most of the surrounding area of inflammation becomes black, green or of a dusky colour, and the condition quickly turns to ulceration. Mostly this appears in three places: under the arm in the armpit, behind the ear and on the tip of the nose, and in the soft flesh.

It is quoted in a tradition from ʿĀ'isha that she said to the Prophet ﷺ: '*Ṭaʿn* we know, but what is *ṭāʿūn*?' He replied: '*Ṭāʿūn* is the swelling of a gland like that of the camel, which affects the soft places and the armpit.'[24]

Physicians say that when this abscess occurs in the soft flesh, the groin and armpit, behind the ear and the tip of the nose, and it is of a corrupt and poisoned nature, it is called plague (*ṭāʿūn*). It is caused by bad blood which tends to putrefaction and corruption, and transforms into a poisonous substance. It corrupts the organ and changes what is adjacent to it; sometimes it allows blood

1 Plague, *ṭāʿūn*, is a more specific term than *wabā'*, pestilential illness or epidemic in general. The causes are variously explained, and IQ takes the opportunity to discourse upon the effect of evil spirits and unseen influences upon the human constitution, and the way in which they can be repelled by religious means. He acknowledges that 'corruption of the air' (*fasād al-hawā'*) is one of the effective causes of plague. See however Chapter 27 on Contagion. See Dols, *Medicine* (Ibn Riḍwān).

and pus to leak out; and it produces an unhealthy condition in the heart. It causes vomiting, palpitation and fainting.

Even though this name is used in general for every inflammation which produces in the heart a malignant fatal quality, it is used specifically to describe the inflammation that occurs in the glandular flesh; and because of its malignancy only organs that are weak by nature accept it. The worst kind is that which occurs in the armpit and behind the ear, because these places are near to the principal organs. The least harmful are the red inflammations, then the yellow; while the black allows no one to escape.

Because the plague is a frequently occurring pestilence and is common in the non-Muslim lands, it is referred to as 'epidemic'. As al-Khalīl says:[2] An epidemic (*wabā'*) is a plague (*ṭāʿūn*). It has been said that plague is every illness which becomes epidemic. But the truth of the matter is that *wabā'* and *ṭāʿūn* differ, one representing the general, the other the particular; every plague is a pestilence, but not every pestilence is a plague. Likewise, infectious diseases are more general than plague, for plague is but one of them. *Ṭawāʿīn* (the plural form) indicates abscesses, ulcers, and evil inflammations occuring in the places already mentioned.

To sum up: these ulcers, inflammations and abscesses are symptoms of the plague, but they are not the disease itself. However, since the physicians have only properly understood its external symptoms, they have considered them to be the plague itself.

Plague is designated by three factors: (1) the external symptoms as mentioned by the physicians; (2) the resulting death, and this is the meaning of the sound *ḥadīth*: 'Plague is a martyrdom for every Muslim'; and (3) the cause that activates this disease.

In the sound *ḥadīth* it is related that this disease is the remainder of a punishment sent upon the Children of Israel, or 'the wounding of the Jinn,'[25] and in a third narration it is in answer to the supplication (*daʿwa*) of a prophet.'[26]

The physicians have nothing whereby to repel these illnesses and their causes, any more than they have anything to explain them.

The prophets give information about hidden matters. On the other hand the physicians have no reason to deny that these symptoms which they understand about the plague should be caused through the mediation of spiritual beings. For the influence of spirits upon the body's constitution, its illnesses, and its eventual destruction, is only denied by people who are quite ignorant of spirits and their influences and the reaction they produce in bodies and constitutions. God, praised be He, can give to these spirits power over the bodies of the sons of Adam, during the occurrence of infection and through corruption of the air. In

2 al-Khalīl b. Aḥmad, grammarian and philologist, a native of Oman who died in Basra between 786–91 AD. Of his dictonary, *Kitāb al-ʿayn*, only an abridged version now remains. (EI^2, 4, 962–64)

the same way, He gives them power to act in the predominance of unhealthy substances, which produce an evil condition for souls, especially in the disturbance of blood, black bile, or semen.

Now the satanic spirits have a power of working upon the person who is affected by these conditions in a way which they cannot regarding others. Their power continues so long as they are not repelled by some defence stronger than their causes, such as *dhikr* and prayer, supplication and entreaty, almsgiving and recitation of the Qur'ān. These deeds will invoke the angelic spirits who can conquer the evil spirits, make void their evil and repel their influence. Now we, and others, have experienced this, as often as only God can reckon, and we have seen that the invocation of these blessed spirits and summoning them to come near yields an overwhelming improvement in the strengthening of the constitution and repelling of evil substances, before they have become strong and dominant. This can hardly be denied. The one whom God assists, as soon as he feels the approach of causes of evil, hastens to seek those things that will defend him against evil. This is a most beneficial remedy for him.

When God, the Exalted, wishes to put His decree and command into effect, He causes the heart of the servant to neglect knowledge of these angelic spirits and to cease to imagine or seek them. Thus he is not aware of them and does not want them, so that God may accomplish in him some deed already decreed. We shall clarify and explain this concept further, if God wills, when we deal with medication by incantation, the Prophet's way of taking refuge with God, remembrance of God (*dhikr*), supplications, and performing good deeds.

We must make clear that the relationship of the medicine practised by physicians to the medicine of the Prophet is like the relationship of medicine practised by village healers to the physicians' medicine, and this is acknowledged by most experts and leaders among physicians. It should be clearly seen that human nature is the most susceptible of all to the influence of spirits and that the powers contained in the formulas of taking refuge and in spells and supplications are superior to the powers of medicines, even counteracting the force of deadly poisons.

In short, corruption of the air is one part of the overall effective causes of plague, and corruption of the essence of the air is the prerequisite to the occurrence of pestilence. Its pollution comes about because its essence changes into an unhealthy state; one of the negative qualities predominates over it, such as putrefaction, decay or poison. It is true at any season of the year, although it occurs mostly in the latter part of the summer and most frequently in the autumn. The reason is that the sharp, bilious superfluities and others collect during the summer season, and they are not dissolved at the end of summer. In autumn, the miasma occurs because the air is cold, and the vapours and superfluities which were wont to dissolve freely during the summer now become thick and murky. Thus they are constricted, become heated, and putrefy, bringing about the putrid diseases. This is especially so when the body which they encounter is susceptible to them by being flaccid, sedentary and replete; such bodies can hardly hope to escape unharmed.

The most healthy season in this respect is the spring. Hippocrates has said: In the autumn occur the fiercest and most deadly of sicknesses, while spring is the most healthy of all the seasons, when the fewest deaths occur.[3] It is customary for pharmacists and those who prepare dead bodies to fall into debt and borrow money in the spring and summer, while autumn is their springtime. They anticipate it eagerly and are most pleased when it arrives.

A *ḥadīth* relates: 'When the Star rises, then malady disappears from every land' this being interpreted to indicate the rising of the Pleiades, or the growth of herbage in spring. The latter refers to *the herbage and the trees prostrate themselves* (LV: 6) (i.e. *najm*, usually 'star', here is taken to mean 'herbage'). The herbage completes and finishes its rising in the spring, the season in which epidemics disappear.

Regarding the constellation of the Pleiades, illnesses are frequent at the time when they rise and set with the dawn. Al-Tamīmī said, in the book *Māddat al-Baqā'*:[4] 'There are two periods of the year which are the most polluted, and which inflict the greatest trial on the human body: firstly the period when the Pleiades set below the horizon at the rising of dawn, and secondly the period when they rise from the east before sunrise, in one of the mansions of the moon. This is the time when spring wanes and comes to an end. However, pollution which comes about when they rise is less harmful than that which comes about at their setting.'

Abū Muḥammad b. Qutayba said:[5] 'It is said that whenever the Pleiades rise or depart, some affliction falls upon people and camels; their setting causes more affliction than their rising.'

Among the *ḥadīth* there is a third saying, and it may in fact be the most appropriate: *najm* means the Pleiades, and affliction means the disaster which befalls agricultural land and crops in the season of winter and the beginning of spring. It is only secure when the Pleiades rise in the period mentioned. Therefore the Prophet ﷺ forbade the selling and buying of agricultural produce before its fruits are ripe. The intention is still to show what he advised in the occurrence of plague.

In forbidding the Community to enter a land where the plague had occurred and forbidding them to depart thence after its occurrence, the Prophet ﷺ

3 See Hippocrates, *Airs Waters Places*, Loeb I. 99 f.

4 Abū ʿAbd-Allāh Muḥammad b. Aḥmad b. Saʿīd al-Tamīmī of Jerusalem specialised in pharmacy and plant drugs. He wrote *Māddat al-baqā' bi-iṣlāḥ fasād al-hawā' wa-l-taḥarruz min ḍarar al-awbā'* (Material of survival, by remedying the corruption of the air and taking precautions from the harm of pestilences) towards the end of the 4th/10th century. GAL I. 272–73. Sezgin, *Geschichte*, III. 317–18, Ullmann, *Medizin*, 270.

5 Abū Muḥammad b. Qutayba, theologian and writer on literature, 828–89 AD, probably best known for his *Book of Poetry and Poets*, wrote *Kitāb al-anwā'* on astronomy and meteorology. (EI², 3, 844–47)

combined all precautionary measures. For in entering a land where it is present, one is exposing oneself to the danger of being affected through communication with the plague in the very land where it is most powerful, and thus acting against one's own interests. This behaviour is contrary to the religious law and to common sense. Whereas to avoid entering a plague-stricken land is a protection to which the Almighty has guided, as we are guided to protect ourselves from harmful airs and places.

His prohibition of leaving a plague-stricken land has two meanings: (1) this prohibition brings one to have complete trust and confidence in God and to endure patience and accept with contentment His decrees; (2) as the authorities in medicine have said, everyone who takes precautions against pestilence must expel from his body the superfluous moistures, must take little food, and incline towards a drying regime in every way except for exercise and bath, for these two should be avoided. For the body is not generally free of hidden corrupt superfluity, which exercise and bath stir up and mix with the good chyme, and this mixing brings on a severe illness. When plague occurs, it is necessary to rest quietly and to quieten the disturbance of the humours. It is possible to travel away from a land where there is pestilence only with a great deal of activity, and this can have a damaging effect. This is the opinion of the most excellent of physicians and of modern writers. This latter medical opinion corroborates the same concept which is contained in the prophetic *ḥadīth* and its concern with treatment and welfare of heart and body.

It may be claimed that the saying of the Prophet ﷺ 'Do not flee from it' does not necessarily suggest the conclusion discussed above, namely that preventing departure in an emergency, nor preventing all travellers from their journeys. The reply is that no one, physician or not, has said that poeple should leave their occupations during times of plague and fall into a state of lethargy. It is simply necessary to undertake as little movement as possible under the circumstances. The one who flees from it is not under compulsion to undertake this activity, but he is simply in flight; whereas to be quiet and at rest is more beneficial for his heart and his body, and is more likely to bring him to trust in the Almighty and surrender to His decree. Those who cannot avoid activity—such as craftsmen, hired labourers, travellers, metal-workers, and others—are not told to leave their occupations entirely, although they are ordered to leave aside what is not essential for them; and such is the movement of the traveller who is fleeing. God the Most High knows best.

The ban on entering a land where plague has occurred demonstrates many wise principles: (1) avoiding harmful causes and distancing oneself from them; (2) preserving health, which is the very essence of life here and hereafter; (3) avoiding intake of air which is putrefied and polluted causing disease; (4) avoiding of proximity to the sick who have fallen ill of plague, for by such proximity infection is inevitable. In the *Sunan* of Abū Dāwūd (*marfūʿ*) it says: from *ʿirq* comes destruction.[27] Ibn Qutayba explains *ʿirq* as: coming close to the pestilence and to the sick; (5) protection of persons from evil portents and contagion, for one can be affected by these factors, and the evil portent is harmful to whoever believes in it.

In short, the prohibition of entering a land where there is plague commands caution and self-protection, and prohibits exposing oneself to the causes of destruction; this is a matter of discipline and education. The prohibition of flight from it commands reliance on God, and lays stress on acceptance and submission.

In the *Ṣaḥīḥ*, it is related that ʿUmar b. al-Khaṭṭāb set out for Syria, and when he reached Sargh he was met by Abū ʿUbaydah b. al-Jarrāh and his companions who told ʿUmar that plague had broken out in Syria. There was a difference of opinion, so he said to Ibn ʿAbbās: 'Bring to me the earliest Emigrants [*muhājirīn*].' So I summoned them, and ʿUmar asked their advice, and told them that pestilence had broken out in Syria. They disputed, some telling him: 'You have set forth for a purpose, and we do not consider that you should turn back from it.' Others said: 'You have with you the remainder of the people and the Companions of the Prophet ﷺ, so we do not consider that you should expose them to the risk of this plague.' ʿUmar said: 'Leave me for now,' and he asked me to summon the Helpers (*anṣār*) and I did so. When he asked their advice, they followed the path of the Emigrants, disagreeing in the same way. Said he: 'Leave me.' Then 'Summon to me those shaykhs of Quraysh, from the Emigration of the victory who are present.' So I summoned them for him, and they were unanimous in their advice: 'We think that you should take the people back and not expose them to this plague.' So ʿUmar proclaimed: ' We are turning back.'

Abū ʿUbaydah b. al-Jarrāh exclaimed: 'O Commander of the Faithful! Are you fleeing from God's decree?' He replied: 'Had anyone else but you said this, Abū ʿUbaydah . . .! Yes, we are fleeing from the Almighty's decree, to His decree. Imagine if you had camels which went down into a valley with two embankments, one of them fertile and the other barren. If you pasture them on the fertile side, would you not do so according to God's decree? Equally if you pastured them on the barren side, it would still be God's decree.'

Then there came ʿAbd al-Raḥmān b. ʿAwf, who had been absent on some business, and said: 'I have precise knowledge regarding this matter. I heard the Messenger of God saying: 'If it occurs in a land while you are there, then do not leave in flight; if you hear of it in another land, then do not venture to go there.'[28]

CHAPTER

6

Treatment of dropsy (*istisqā'*) and the benefits of camel's milk[1]

IN THE two books of the *Ṣaḥīḥ* there is a *ḥadīth* from Anas b. Mālik: A group of people from ʿUrayna and ʿUkal came to the Prophet ﷺ, for they were becoming ill in Madīna, and they complained of that to him. He replied: 'Go out to the camels of the alms tax, and drink of their urine and their milk', and they did that. In the morning, they set upon the herdsmen, killed them and drove off the camels; they fought against God and His Messenger. So he sent after them, and they were captured. He ordered their hands and feet to be cut off, and their eyes gouged out, and they were thrown out in the sun to die.[29]

The indication that their illness was dropsy is given in Muslim's narrative of this *ḥadīth*, where they said: 'We have become sick in Madīna, for our bellies have swollen up and our limbs are trembling.'[30] Then he related the whole *ḥadīth*.

Jawā (the term used in the quotation above) is one of the maladies of the abdomen. Dropsy is an illness of congested matter. Its cause is a cold foreign 'matter' which permeates the limbs so that they increase in size: either all the external members or the empty places from the areas which contain the digestive system and the humours. It is of three sorts: in the flesh, which is the most severe; in the skin; and in the membranes.

The medicines needed for its treatment are the 'drawing' medicines which contain a moderate loosening power and produce a flow according to need. These qualities are present in the urine and milk of camels.[2] Therefore the Prophet ﷺ ordered them to drink these substances. For the milk of the camel contains power to cleanse and soften, it is diuretic and emollient and opens

1 Dropsy (*istisqā'*) is seen as an illness of excess matter which permeates through the limbs. Camel's milk is discussed at some length; the use of urine, and its lawfulness, are important. For 'forbidden substances', see chapter 28.

2 'Drawing' medicines, *adwiya jāliba*, those which draw or attract the superfluities needing to be evacuated.

obstructions, especially when the camels pasture mostly on artemisia and achillea, camomile, anthemis, and lemon-grass, and other plant drugs useful for dropsy.

This illness is inevitably accompanied by damage to the liver in particular, or to other organs as well, most of this being caused by obstruction. Milk of Arabian camels is beneficial for obstruction, for it contains a desobstruant power as well as the other qualities mentioned.

Al-Rāzī said: Milk of camels cures pains of the liver and corruption of the temperament.

Al-Isrā'īlī said: Milk of camels is the thinnest of all milk and contains the most liquid and sharpness and the least nutriment. Therefore it is the most effective for softening superfluities, releasing the belly and opening obstructions. The indication of that is its slight saltiness, caused by the excess of animal heat which it has by nature. Therefore when fresh it is the most appropriate milk for moistening the liver, for opening its obstructions and dissolving foods that are difficult to digest. It is especially beneficial for dropsy when it is used while still warm, straight from the udder, together with the urine of the newly weaned camel that is still warm, as it issues from the animal. That is one of the factors which increases its saltiness, its breaking up of superfluities, and its loosening of the stomach. If this mixture is unable to descend and to release the belly, this must be effected by a laxative medicine.

Ibn Sīnā does not pay attention to a point which has been made, that the nature of milk is opposed to the treatment of dropsy. He said: 'Know then that the milk of the camel is a beneficial medicine, for it contains gentle power to cleanse and special characteristics. This milk is of extreme benefit; if a man were to live on it instead of water and food, he would be cured. This has been tested on a group of people, for they were obliged to go to the land of the Arabs and were forced to this by circumstances, and they regained health. The most beneficial type of urine is that of the Arabian camel, which is of noble breeding.'

This story contains a number of important legal issues which we shall list here:

1. The permission of seeking medication and treatment.

2. The legal purity of the urine of animals which are lawful to eat. Medication with forbidden substances is not permitted. The people from ʿUrayna and ʿUkal were not ordered to wash their mouths, although they had just recently become Muslims, nor to wash any of their clothes which might have come into contact with camels' urine, before prayer. On this matter it was not possible for the Prophet to delay clarification at the time when it was needed.

3. The transgressor's requital with the like of his own deed. For these people had killed the herdsman and gouged out his eyes; this is confirmed in the *Ṣaḥīḥ* of Muslim.

4. The legality of killing a group and cutting off their extremities, in requital

for one man; it shows that when both a legal punishment (*ḥadd*) and a retaliation (*qiṣāṣ*) are applicable, both are exacted. The Prophet ﷺ had their hands and feet cut off, which was God's ordinance (*ḥadd*) for their transgression, and he killed them in retaliation for their killing the herdsman.

5. It shows that when the warrior has taken property and has killed, his hand and foot are cut off at the same time, and he is killed.

6. When crimes are multiple, their punishments are made harsher. These men had apostasised after they had entered Islam; they had killed and maimed a man, taken property, and showed open hostility.

7. The judgement of apostasy of those fighting is the judgement of whoever of them actually committed the deed; for it is a recognised fact that not every one of them took part directly in the killing, and the Prophet ﷺ did not enquire about that. Assassination makes obligatory the killing of the murderer as legal punishment; no pardon can waive this nor can blood money be allowed instead. This is the practice of the people of Madīna; it is one of the two alternatives allowed by the practice of Aḥmad; it was chosen by our shaykh, who gave this as a legal opinion (*fatwā*).

CHAPTER

7

Treatment for wounds

IN THE two books of the *Ṣaḥīḥ*, from Abū Ḥāzim, it says: 'He heard Sahl b. Sa ʿd ask about the treatment for the Prophet's ﷺ wound on the day of Uḥud. His face was wounded, his incisor tooth was broken and the helmet on his head was crushed. Fāṭima his daughter washed the blood away, and ʿAlī b. Abī Ṭālib brought water to her in his shield. When Fāṭima saw that the blood was only increasing, she took a piece of matting and burnt it to ashes which she applied to the wound, and the blood dried up.'[31] This was effected through ashes of matting made from papyrus. This material has a powerful effect in staunching blood, for it contains a strong drying slightly caustic property. Medicines with a strong drying power, if they are somewhat caustic, stir up and draw the blood.

When these ashes are applied, alone or mixed with vinegar, into the nose of one suffering a nosebleed, it ceases.

Ibn Sīnā said: 'Papyrus is beneficial for haemorrhage and makes it cease; when sprinkled on fresh wounds, it causes them to scar over. Egyptian writing paper (*qirṭās*) was formerly made of it. Its consitution is cold and dry, and its ashes are beneficial for sores of the mouth. It restrains spitting of blood and prevents foul ulcers from spreading.'

CHAPTER

8

Drinking honey, cupping and cautery[1]

IT IS reported in Bukhārī's *Ṣaḥīḥ* from Sa ʿd b. Jubayr, from Ibn ʿAbbās that the Prophet ﷺ said: Healing lies in three things: drinking honey, the incision of the cupping glass, and cautery by fire. I forbid my community to practise cautery.[32]

Abū ʿAbd-Allāh al-Māzarī said: 'The diseases from repletion are either sanguineous, bilious, caused by phlegm, or atrabilious. If sanguineous they are cured by letting blood; if they are of the other three kinds then by purging as appropriate for each particular humour.' It seems that the Prophet ﷺ pointed to the superiority of honey over laxative drugs, and to cupping as preferable to venesection. For some have said that venesection is included in his words: 'the incision of the cupping glass,' and when medicine has no effect, then the final resort of medical skill is cautery. The Prophet ﷺ mentioned it among medical means, because it is used where the unbalanced nature is stronger than the powers of the medicines, and where medicine taken by mouth is of no use. In his words: 'I forbid cautery to my community,' and in the other *ḥadīth*: 'I do not like to be cauterised,'[33] are indications that one should postpone this form of treatment until compelled to it by necessity, and should never hasten to use it. For it will bring about great pain, in warding off a pain which might be less than that of the cautery itself.

One physician has said: The temperamental illnesses[2] are either accom-

1 Cupping (*ḥijāma*) and cautery (*kayy* or *kawy*) are both practices of considerable antiquity, the use of which lasted in some places until the nineteenth century and can still be occasionally seen in the Middle East today. Cupping consisted generally in heating a small vessel, usually of glass, which was placed over the skin of back or chest; the loss of heat and resultant vacuum would draw congestion to the surface. The practice of cautery is clearly more dangerous. The standard process was the appliction of a red hot nail or other sharp piece of iron to specified areas of the body to relieve pain. Its use is still described for sciatica and for certain stomach pains. The Prophet's attitude is here discussed; the interpretation of cautery as a 'final remedy' at least shows that it is only to be considered as a last resort. For cupping as a remedy for poisoning, see Chapter 24b.

2 Temperamental illnesses, *amrāḍ mizājiyya*, ie. where it is the constitution or temperament (*mizāj*) which is itself disturbed and thus causes the illness.

panied by 'matter', or not. If they are, this is either hot, cold, moist or dry, or a combination of them. Of these four qualities, two are active, heat and cold and two are passive, moisture and dryness. Wherever one of the active qualities is predominant, it must be accompanied by a passive quality. Equally each of the humours which exists in the body and in other compound forms possesses two qualities: one active and one passive.

The result is that the cause of the temperamental illnesses is largely attributed to the predominance of the qualities of either of the two active humours, heat or cold. The prophetic saying about the underlying principles for the treatment of diseases, caused by excessive heat and cold—ie. treatment by opposites—is in harmony with this opinion. If the disease is hot, we treat it by drawing out blood, whether by venesection or cupping; this means an evacuation of the 'matter' and a cooling of the temperament. If it is cold we treat it by warming, a property which is present in honey. If besides that there is need for evacuation of the cold 'matter', honey also works on that because it has a power of coction, of cutting, and alleviation, and can cleanse and soften. Thus there comes about the evacuation of that 'matter', gently, and safe from the harm caused by strong laxative drugs.

Concerning cautery, each of the physical diseases will either be acute—and then it will be swift to reach one of the two extremes and there is no need for cautery—or will be chronic, and then the most excellent treatment, after evacuation, is cautery on those limbs whenever applicable. It is chronic only because of some thick cold 'matter' which has rooted itself in the limb and corrupted its constitution, and has transformed neighbouring areas into the same substance as itself. Consequently an inflammation flares up within that limb. That 'matter' can be extracted by means of cautery from the place where it has lodged, by destroying the fiery element which is present through cauterising that 'matter'.

We have learnt from this excellent *ḥadīth* how to treat all physical diseases, just as we have deduced the treatment of the simple disease from the saying of the Prophet ﷺ: The fierceness of fever is from the boiling of hell, so cool it down with water.[34]

(a) *On Cupping*

It is related in the *Sunan* of Ibn Māja from the *ḥadīth* of Jubāra b. al-Mughallis (weak), from Kathīr b. Salīm: I heard Anas b. Mālik report that the Prophet ﷺ said: 'On the night of my Journey to heaven I did not pass by any group of people but they said: "O Muḥammad! Order your community to practise cupping!"'[3][35] Tirmidhī in his *Jāmiᶜ* relates this from a *ḥadīth* of Ibn ᶜAbbās as 'O Muḥammad, practise cupping!'[36]

3 The Night Journey of the Prophet, *isrā'* or *miᶜrāj*, hinted at in Sūra XVII:1 and much elaborated in *ḥadīth*.

Likewise, in the two books of the *Ṣaḥīḥ*, we read from the *ḥadīth* of Ṭāws, from Ibn ʿAbbās, that the Prophet ﷺ was cupped, and gave the cupper his fee.[37]

Again in the two books of the *Ṣaḥīḥ* it is related from Ḥumayd al-Ṭawīl, from Anas: The Prophet ﷺ was cupped by Abū Ṭayba. He ordered him to be given two measures of food, and he asked his masters (for he was a slave) to reduce the levy they usually demanded. He said: 'The best treatment you have is cupping.'[38]

From the *Jāmiʿ* of al-Tirmidhī from ʿAbbād b. Manṣūr, who said: I heard ʿIkrima say: Ibn ʿAbbās had three young slaves who were cuppers, two of whom used to work to earn money for Ibn ʿAbbās and his family, while one used to carry out cupping on them. And Ibn ʿAbbās said: The Prophet of God ﷺ said: 'Good is the slave who practises cupping, for this expels the blood, dries the backbone, and makes the sight clear.' And he said: When the Messenger of God ﷺ went on his journey to Heaven every group of angels he passed by said to him: 'Practise cupping!' He said: 'The best times for being cupped are the seventeenth day, the nineteenth day and the twenty-first day of the month.' And: 'The best forms of treatment you can use are the sternutatory, the *ladūd* (medicine poured in at the side of the mouth), cupping, and the laxative.'[4] The Messenger of God ﷺ was given a *ladūd* and asked: 'Who gave it to me?' But they all kept silent. He said: 'All of you should have *ladūd* done to you, except al-ʿAbbās.'[39] Said the narrator: This is a strange *ḥadīth*, but Ibn Māja related it.

The benefits of cupping are that it cleanses the surface of the body more than does venesection, though the latter is preferable for the deeper parts of the body. Cupping extracts the blood from the areas nearer to the skin.

My comment concerning most authoritative opinion on cupping and venesection is that they both vary according to the season and locality, and the age and temperament of the patient. As for hot countries, hot seasons, and hot temperaments, the blood of whose people is in a high state of coction: for these cupping is far more beneficial than venesection, because the blood is ripe and clear, and goes outwards to the inner surface of the body. Therefore, cupping expels that which venesection does not. For this reason it is the more beneficial for young people, and for anyone who is not strong enough for venesection.

Physicians have also specified that in hot countries cupping is more beneficial and preferable to venesection. The best time for it is in, and after, the middle of the month, and generally the third quarter of the month. In the early part of the month the blood has not yet become stirred up and risen, and in the last part it has already settled. But in the middle and shortly after, it is at the furthest point of agitation.

4 *Ladūd*: a type of medicine given at the side of the mouth, see also Chapter 13.
Saʿūṭ, sternutatory, a medicament, usually powder, inserted in the nostrils to produce sneezing and thereby clear the head and the nasal passages. See also Chapter 18b. *Mashiy*, — laxative, from *mashā* to walk, probably because the one so treated has to take frequent walks to relieve himself. See also Chapter 11 and Chapter 25 n. 5

Ibn Sīnā prescribes the use of cupping, but not in the beginning of the month, for the humours have not yet moved nor been stirred up; nor at the end, for then they have decreased. But rather in the middle of the month, the time when the humours are stirred up and are greatly increasing due to the increase of light in the body of the moon. It has been related that the Prophet ﷺ said: 'The best forms of treatment you can carry out are cupping and venesection'. And in a *ḥadīth*: 'The best medicines are cupping and venesection.'

When the Prophet ﷺ said: 'The best treatment . . . is with cupping' this was guidance addressed to the people of the Ḥijāz and other hot countries; for their blood is thin and flows closer to the surface of the body, because the external heat attracts it, and it collects in the areas near the skin; also it is because the pores of their bodies are wide, and the physical strength of those people easily disintegrates. Thus venesection would be dangerous for them, whereas cupping is a disjunction which is continuous and voluntary, followed by a complete evacuation of the veins, especially the veins which are not often treated by venesection. In the treating of each of these veins, there is special advantage.

Venesection of the basilic vein is beneficial for heat of the liver and spleen, and for inflammation occurring in them caused by the blood. It is also beneficial for inflammation of the lung, pleurisy, pain in the side, and all sanguineous illnesses which manifest themselves from below the knee to the hip. Venesection of the medial arm vein (*akḥal*) is beneficial for repletion which occurs in any part of the body, when this is sanguineous in origin, or when the blood has putrefied throughout the body. Venesection of the cephalic vein is useful for ailments which occur in the head and neck from plethora or corruption of the blood. Venesection of the jugular vein is beneficial for pain in the spleen, asthma, pain in the rib cage, and pain of the forehead. Cupping on the upper part of the back (*kāhil*) is beneficial for pain of the shoulders and throat. Cupping of the occipital veins (*akhdaʿayn*) is beneficial for illnesses of the head and parts of it such as the face, teeth, ears, eyes, nose and throat, when these have arisen from excess or corruption of the blood, or from both causes combined. According to Anas, the Messenger of God ﷺ used to be cupped on the occipital veins and the upper part of the back.[40] It is reported in the two books of *Ṣaḥīḥ*, from Anas that the Messenger of God ﷺ would be cupped three times: once on the upper part of his back, and twice on the occipital veins.[41]

In the *Ṣaḥīḥ* (from Anas) it says: He was cupped, while in a state of *iḥrām* (ritual consecration for pilgrimage), on his head to relieve him of a headache.[42]

In the *Sunan* of Ibn Māja, from ʿAlī: Jibrīl gave the Prophet ﷺ instructions about cupping on the occipital veins and the upper back.[43]

In the *Sunan* of Abū Dāwūd: from a *ḥadīth* of Jābir: the Prophet ﷺ was cupped on his hip (*wark*) for a state of fatigue.[44]

(b) *Cupping on the nape of the neck*

The physicians dispute about cupping at the furrow of the nape of the neck (*qafā*): the *qamaḥduwa*. Abū Nuʿaym recalled, in his *Book of the Prophet's Medicine*, a *ḥadīth* (*marfūʿ*): 'You must carry out cupping at the point of the nape of the neck, for indeed it can cure five illnesses' among which he mentioned leprosy. Another *ḥadīth*: You must carry out cupping at the point of the *qamaḥduwa*, for it is a cure for seventy-two illnesses.

Some physicians have entirely approved of it, saying: It is beneficial for protruberance of the eyes, and for any protrusion which occurs in them, and for many eye diseases, for heaviness of eyebrows and eyelids, and it is beneficial for trachoma.[5]

It is related that Aḥmad b. Ḥanbal was in need of this treatment, so he was cupped at the side of the nape of the neck, not at the centre point (*nuqra*).

One who disapproved of it was Ibn Sīnā, for he said: 'It leads in truth to forgetfulness, as Muḥammad our leader, master and the founder of our *sharīʿa* (religious law), has said; the back of the brain is the place of memory, and cupping may disperse it.'

Some commentators have rejected Ibn Sīnā's view, saying that the *ḥadīth* is not confirmed; and if it were, cupping weakens the back of the brain only when it is applied unnecessarily. When it is performed because of the excess of blood there, then it is beneficial both medically and according to the *sharīʿa*. For it is confirmed that the Prophet ﷺ was cupped in a number of places on the nape of the neck, as his condition required, and he was cupped in other places according to need.

Cupping beneath the chin is beneficial for toothache and pain of the face and throat, when it is used at the right time, and it cleanses the head and palms of the hands. Cupping at the back of the foot is an alternative to the venesection of the foot (*ṣāfin*). This is a large vein at the ankle. It is useful for ulcers of the thighs and legs, for amenorrhea and for itching in the testicles. Cupping at the lower part of the chest is beneficial for boils on the thigh, and for scabs and pustules there; also for gout, haemorrhoids, elephantiasis, and itching of the back.

(c) *On times of cupping*

It is related by Tirmidhī, in the *Jāmiʿ*, from a *ḥadīth* of Ibn ʿAbbās, (*marfūʿ*): 'The best day on which you can be cupped is the seventeenth, or the nineteenth, or on the twenty-first day.'[45] In the *Jāmiʿ*, from Anas: The Messenger of God ﷺ would be cupped on the occipital veins and the upper back, and he would be cupped on the seventeenth, nineteenth and twenty-first day.[46]

In the *Sunan* of Ibn Māja, from Anas, (*marfūʿ*) it says: Whoever wishes to be

5 *Jarab* generally means scab or psoriasis, but in the context, 'its *jarab*' (ie. of the eye lid), refers to a localised condition, hence 'trachoma'.

cupped, let him do this precisely on the seventeenth, or nineteenth, or twenty-first day; let not the blood of any of you be agitated,[6] lest this destroy him.[47] From the *Sunan* of Abū Dāwūd, from a *ḥadīth* of Abū Hurayra (*marfūᶜ*): Whoever is cupped on the seventeenth, nineteenth or twenty-first day, that is healing for every illness[48] (which means, any illness caused by excess of blood).

These *ḥadīth* are in accordance with the physicians' unanimous agreement that cupping in the second half of the month or the nearby days of the third quarter is more beneficial than at the beginning or end of the month, but when it is carried out in a case of need, it is useful at any time, whether at the first beginning or last part of the month.

Al-Khallāl said: ᶜUṣma b. ᶜIṣām told me: Ḥanbal told us that Abū ᶜAbd-Allāh Aḥmad b. Ḥanbal used to be cupped whenever his blood was agitated at whatever time that might be.

Ibn Sīnā said: The times for cupping during the day are the second or the third hour, and its timing should be after the bath, except for those whose blood is thick; they must take a bath, then keep warm for an hour, then be cupped.

Physicians disapprove of cupping when the patient is replete, for it can sometimes bring about an obstruction and a severe illness, especially when the food is poor and heavy.

A tradition relates that 'While cupping, on an empty stomach, is a medicine, in repletion it causes disease, and on the seventeenth of the month, it is a cure.'

The choice of these times is restricted for when cupping is undertaken as a precaution against any harm, and in order to preserve health, while when needed as a medical treatment of illnesses, it may be undertaken whenever the need arises. We have seen that the Imām Aḥmad used to be cupped at whatever time of the month it was necessary.

As for the choice of days of the week for cupping, Al-Khallāl says in his *Jāmiᶜ*: Ḥarb b. Ismāᶜīl told us: I asked Aḥmad: 'Do you dislike cupping on any particular day?' He said: 'This applies to Wednesday and Saturday.' On this subject it is related from al-Ḥusayn b. Ḥassān: He asked Abū ᶜAbd-Allāh about cupping: 'What time do you dislike?' and he replied: 'Saturday and Wednesday. And they say on Friday, too.' Al-Khallāl related, from Abū Salma and Abū Saᶜīd al-Muqbirī, from Abū Hurayra (*marfūᶜ*): 'Whoever is cupped on Wednesday or on Saturday and becomes afflicted by leprosy or leucoma will have no one to blame but himself.'[49] Al-Khallāl said: Muḥammad b. ᶜAlī b. Jaᶜfar told us that Yaᶜqūb b. Bakhtān told them: Aḥmad was asked about lime (*nūra*) and about cupping on Saturday and on Wednesday. He disapproved of this, saying: 'I have heard about a certain man, who used lime and was cupped (ie. on a Wednesday) and was

6 Blood should not 'become agitated' (*lā yatabayyagh*). This is an indirect command using the *jazm*, which IQ explains as being equal to the *naṣab* after *li-allā*, i.e. 'that it should not be agitated' but the particle having been omitted. IQ explains *tabayyugh* itself as *hījān* 'disturbance', from *bghy* but with inversion of the last two letters.

afflicted by leprosy. I said to him: it seems that he was heedless of the *ḥadīth*, and he replied: Yes.'

In the book of *al-Afrād* by Dāraquṭnī we find among the *ḥadīth* of Nāfiʿ: ʿAbd-Allāh b. ʿUmar told me: My blood is in an agitated state, so summon a cupper for me. Let him not be a youth, nor a very old man. For I have heard the Messenger of God ﷺ say: 'Cupping increases the mindful in memory, and the intelligent in intelligence; so undergo cupping in the name of the Almighty, but do not do so on a Thursday, Friday, Saturday or Sunday, but on a Monday. For every case of leprosy and vitiligo comes down on a Wednesday.'[50] Dāraquṭnī commented that this was only related by Ziyād b. Yaḥyā, but we have found that Ayyūb related it from Nāfiʿ with a variant saying: 'So be cupped on a Monday or Tuesday, and never on Wednesday.'

Abū Dāwūd relates in his *Sunan*, from *ḥadīth* of Abū Bakr, that he used to dislike cupping on Tuesday. He said, the Messenger of God ﷺ said: 'Tuesday, the day of blood! In it there is one hour when the blood does not clot.'[51]

(d) *Cupping and fasting*

In all these *ḥadīth* we have mentioned, we find approval of medical treatment, and of cupping; it should be undertaken in the locality where it is required, and it is permissible even in the state of *iḥrām*. Even if it resulted in the cutting of some hair, it is permitted; concerning the obligation to make expiation for it, opinions differ. There is not much support of its obligation.

And it is permitted to be cupped when fasting. In the *Ṣaḥīḥ* of Bukhārī we read that 'the Messenger of God ﷺ was cupped, while fasting';[52] but whether he thereby broke his fast is a different issue. The truth is that cupping does break the fast, as is shown from the Messenger of God ﷺ, without any contradiction. The most reliable opposition to this is the *ḥadīth* of his being cupped while fasting. But it does not demonstrate that breaking of the fast did not occur, except after four points: (1) that the fast was obligatory; (2) that he was not travelling; (3) that he was not suffering from any illness which required cupping; and (4) that this *ḥadīth* is later than the words: 'the one cupping and the one being cupped have broken their fast'.[53] When these four premisses are confirmed, then his action can be used as proof that the fast was not broken even after cupping. Otherwise, what prevents fasting from being a voluntary action which one can break by cupping or in some other way; or being a fast during Ramaḍān when one is on a journey, or while one is not travelling, but some need requires an interruption of the fast, just as necessity summons anyone who is ill to break it; or that it should be an obligation of Ramaḍān while one is not travelling and without any need to break the fast. Yet the primary fact remains that the Prophet ﷺ practised cupping while fasting. His words: 'the cupper and the one cupped have broken their fast' are handed down, and thus subsequent textual reference should be restricted to it. On the other hand there is no way to establish any one of the four premisses, so how could one establish them all?

There is an indication, too, of the remuneration of physicians and others, without any fixed contract of hire, but he is to be given the standard remuneration, or whatever he is satisfied with.

There is also an indication of the permissibility of earning through the practice of cupping, as it is not feasible that the free man should deny paying the cupper his fee without falling into any prohibition. For the Prophet ﷺ gave him his fee, and he did not prevent him from using it. But for him to name the fee as impure would be like calling garlic and onion impure; yet it did not entail their prohibition.

It also indicates the permissibility of a man's requiring revenue of his slave, every day: a sum, agreed according to his ability; and the slave may have the right to dispose of whatever is in excess of this sum. If he were prevented from disposing of it, then all he earned would be paid to his master, and there would be no benefit in fixing a sum in the first place. But what is over and above these fixed payments is conceded to him from his master, and he may dispose of these payments as he wishes.

God knows best!

(e) *On cutting of veins, and cautery*

It is established in the *Ṣaḥīḥ*—from the *ḥadīth* of Jābir b. ʿAbd-Allāh—that the Prophet ﷺ sent a physician to Ubayy b. Kaʿb who cut one of his veins and cauterised the place.[54]

When Saʿd b. Muʿādh was wounded on the medial arm vein, 'the Prophet ﷺ cut this (*ḥasamahu*); then it became inflamed, and he cut it again'. Cutting (*ḥasm*) means cautery (*kayy*). In another line of narrative it says: 'The Prophet ﷺ cauterised (*kawā*) Saʿd b. Muʿādh on his medial arm vein, with an arrow head. Then Saʿd b. Muʿādh, or one of his companions, cut the place.'[55] In another version: 'A man of the Anṣār was hit on his medial arm vein with an arrow head, and the Prophet ﷺ ordered that this should be cauterised.'[56]

Abū ʿUbayd said: 'A man was brought to the Prophet ﷺ, for whom cautery had been prescribed. He said: 'Cauterise him, and use hot stones' (*irḍifūhu*).[57] Abū ʿUbayda explained: *raḍf* means a stone which is heated and then used as a hot poultice.

Al-Faḍl b. Dukayn said: Sufyān related to us, from Abī'l-Zubayr, from Jābir, that the Prophet ﷺ cauterised him on his medial arm vein.[58]

In the *Ṣaḥiḥ* of al-Bukhārī, from the *ḥadīth* of Anas it says that he was cauterised for pleurisy during the lifetime of the Prophet ﷺ.'[59]

Al-Tirmidhī's book, from Anas, quotes that the Prophet ﷺ cauterised Asʿad b. Zurāra for a thorn.[60]

But we have already mentioned a *ḥadīth* on which there is agreement: 'And I do not wish to be cauterised',[61] or in another version: 'I forbid cautery for my community.'[62]

In the *Jāmi*ᶜ of al-Tirmidhī, and elsewhere, from ᶜImrān b. Ḥaṣīn it says: the Prophet ﷺ forbade cautery.'[63] He said: 'We have been afflicted, we have been cauterised; we have been successful.' In another version: 'We have neither gained any benefit nor forbidden cautery,' and he said: 'We have neither gained any benefit nor been cured.'

Al-Khaṭṭābī said: He cauterised Saᶜd only in order that the blood from his wound should be clotted, for he feared he might have a fatal haemorrhage. Cautery is used for this kind of case, just as a person is cauterised when his hand or foot is amputated. The prohibition of cautery concerned its use in search of a cure. People used to believe that unless a person was cauterised he would die. The Prophet ﷺ forbade cautery to those with this intention. It has been said: he forbade it only in the case of ᶜImrān b. Ḥaṣīn, in particular, because he had a fistula in a dangerous place, so he forbade its cauterisation. It is most likely that the prohibition was particularly concerned with the place about which there was some anxiety. And the Almighty knows best.

Ibn Qutayba said: Cautery is of two kinds: (1) Cautery of the healthy person, so that he will not fall ill; this is the sort of which it was said: 'The person who performs cautery does not have trust in God, because he wishes to ward off the Decree from himself;' (2) cautery of a wound which festers and a limb which is cut off; in this there is healing. Now when cautery is used as medical treatment, which may or may not succeed, it comes closer to the class of actions which are disliked.

It is established in the *Ṣaḥīḥ* from the *ḥadīth* about the seventy thousand who will enter Paradise without a reckoning that 'they are those who have never stolen, nor practised cautery, nor consulted omens, and who have had complete trust in their Lord.'[64]

The *ḥadīth* about cautery comprise four categories: (1) its practice; (2) that it is not greatly liked; (3) praise of those who do not practise it; and (4) its prohibition. There is no mutual contradiction between them, praise be to God the Most High. Its practice shows that it is permitted, while dislike of it does not indicate that it is prohibited. The praise of one not carrying it out shows that its avoidance is preferred and praised. Its prohibition is in the way of choice and disapproval, or concerning the sort of case where it is not needed, while it can be performed as a precaution against the onset of sickness. And God knows best.

CHAPTER

9

Treatment of epilepsy (*ṣarᶜ*)[1]

IN THE two books of the *Ṣaḥīḥ* we find, from the *ḥadīth* of ᶜAṭā' b. Abī Rabāḥ, that Ibn ᶜAbbās said: 'Shall I show you a woman who is one of the people of Paradise?' 'Yes indeed,' I said. So he continued: 'This black woman came to the Prophet ﷺ and said: "I am an epileptic, and when I have a seizure I get uncovered and my body becomes exposed. So will you make supplication to God on my behalf?" He replied: "If you wish, you may persevere patiently and be assured of Paradise, but if you wish, I shall beseech God to heal you." She replied: "I shall be patient. But as for being uncovered, will you pray to God that this may not happen." So he prayed for her.'[65]

My comment on this is: Epilepsy is of two kinds: (1) epilepsy from evil, earthly spirits; and (2) epilepsy from bad humours. The second is that of whose cause and treatment the physicians speak. As for epilepsy of spirits, the most learned and intelligent among physicians do recognise it, but they do not know how to cure it. They admit that its treatment is in the confrontation of those wicked evil spirits by noble, good, lofty spirits, for these ward off their influences and oppose and make void their actions. Hippocrates specified this in one of his books, and he spoke of some of the treatments for epilepsy, saying: 'This treatment is useful only for epilepsy that is caused by humours and matter; but for epilepsy from spirits, this treatment is of no use.'

In the case of the ignorant, base, and worthless physicians and those who consider that atheism is a virtue, those people deny the type of epilepsy caused by spirits and will not confirm that they have an effect on the body of the epileptic. They are simply ignorant. There is nothing within medical science which can refute it, for both sensory perception and experience are evidence that confirm it. The fact that they attribute it instead to the predominance of one of the humours is true in some types, but not in all of them.

1 On epilepsy (*ṣarᶜ*) of which there are two kinds: (1) caused by evil earthly spirits, (2) caused by bad humours (*akhlāṭ*). IQ takes epilepsy also as a metaphor of the 'greatest epilepsy' (*al-ṣarᶜ al-aᶜẓam*) or madness, the harm wrought by evil spirits who seduce humankind from the true path. It was called by the Ancients 'the Sacred Disease', though Hippocrates does not consider it a suitable name (Loeb, II. 139 f.)

The ancient physicians used to call this type of epilepsy the Divine Illness, and they said that it was from the spirits. Galen and others disagreed with them in their interpretation of this name, saying that they only named it the Divine Illness because it occurs in the head and damages the outward divine part of man, which dwells in the brain.

This interpretation grew up among those physicians because of their ignorance of these spirits, their influence, and the conditions governing them. Then came the atheist physicians, and they confirmed only the epilepsy caused by the humours.[2] Whoever has intelligence and knowledge of these spirits and their influence can laugh at the ignorance of these people and the weakness of their minds.

The treatment of this kind takes place in two ways: one concerning the epileptic, and one concerning the person treating him. With regard to the epileptic, the treatment is through the power of his own soul by the genuine attention he pays to the Maker and Creator of these spirits and by truly taking refuge with God, as expressed by his tongue and confirmed in his heart. This is a kind of warfare, and the fighter can completely vanquish his foe by force of arms only under two conditions: that the weapon should be true and good in itself and that the user himself be strong. When one of these fails, the weapon itself is not of much avail. How can it be when both elements are missing? If the heart has lost its belief in the unity of God, its trust in Him, and its piety and attention, then he has no weapons!

Secondly, concerning the one carrying out the treatment: he must possess these two factors as well. There are some healers who need only to say: 'Depart from him!' Or he may say: 'In the name of God!' or 'There is no power and no strength but with God!'

The Prophet ﷺ used to say: 'Depart, enemy of God, I am His Messenger.'[66]

I have seen our shaykh send to the epileptic someone who would speak to the spirit within him, saying: 'The Shaykh says to you: Depart! Your presence with this person is not lawful.' And the epileptic would recover. Sometimes he would speak himself to the spirit. Sometimes the spirit would be rebellious, and he would expel it with blows, and the epileptic would recover feeling no pain. We, and others, have often witnessed this kind of thing from him. Often the shaykh would recite into the ear of the epileptic: *'Do you think that We created you in sport and that you will not be summoned back to Us?'* (XXIII:115).

The shaykh told me that he once recited this verse into the ear of an epileptic, and the spirit said: 'Yes,' and its voice reached him. He said: 'So I took a stick to it, and I beat the patient with it on the veins of his neck until my hands grew tired from the beating. The people present had no doubt that he would die from the blows. During this beating the spirit said: "I love him." So I said to it: "He

2 *zanādiqa*, pl. of *zindīq*, free thinker or heretic.

does not love you. "Then it said: "I wish to accompany him." I replied: "He does not want your company." It said then: "I will leave him, out of respect for you." I replied: "No, rather in obedience to God and His Messenger." And it said: "I am departing from him." Then the epileptic sat up, looked around to right and left, and asked: "What brought me to the shaykh?" They asked if the beating had wearied him, and he asked: "For what reason should the shaykh beat me, as I have done no wrong?" He had not felt any of the blows that had fallen upon him.'

The shaykh also used to treat patients by reciting the verse of *Āyat al-Kursī*, and he would order both the epileptic and the person treating him to recite this verse frequently and to recite the two *sūras* of 'Seeking Refuge' (the *Muʿawwid hatayn*).[3]

In short, this type of epilepsy and its treatment are denied only by those who have but little learning, intelligence and knowledge. Most of the dominance which evil spirits have over sufferers is caused by their lack of religion and the fact that their hearts and tongues are far from the truths of remembering God and from taking refuge with Him, and from the various means of protection afforded by prophethood and faith. Thus an evil spirit may meet a man isolated with no defence and he may be quite unprotected, so the evil spirit can influence him.

If the veil could be removed, you would find that most human souls are afflicted by these evil spirits, and they are their captives and prisoners. The spirits drive them where they wish, and they cannot prevent them nor oppose them. This torment is the greatest type of epilepsy, from which the sufferer can only escape when these evil spirits are driven away while being watched by others. Only then can it be confirmed to him that he was truly possessed. We ask help from God.

The treatment for this epilepsy is by joining the healthy correct understanding with faith in what the Messengers brought, which will result in a fine awareness of both Paradise and the fire of Hell that will make him always keep them before his eyes and make them the direction of his heart. He should call to mind the people of this world and the examples, wrath, punishment and affliction which befall them during their earthly existence, just as the rain befalls them. Yet they are epileptic and unaware.

How strong are the means to repel the madness caused by this evil spirit! Yet the affliction has become so common that wherever one looks one sees only a possessed human being. It no longer seems strange nor out of place. Because of the great number of afflicted people, what was strange and outlandish has become quite the opposite.

When God intends good for one of His servants, he recovers from this

3 Throne Verse: Sura II:255. The *Muʿawwidhatayn: Sūras* 113 and 114, the two final *sūras* of the Qur'ān.

demented state and considers the people of this world; all around him are people possessed by these evil spirits, to the right and to the left, in different degrees. Among them are those who have completely lost control of their minds and become totally mad; some who recover for short periods and then return to their madness; and some who are mad at one time and sane at another. When they are awake, they do the works of people who are awake and intelligent, then their epilepsy comes upon them again and they fall into insanity.

Epilepsy caused by the humours is an illness which partially prevents the principal parts of the body from action, movement and remaining upright. The cause is a thick sticky humour, which partially obstructs the openings of the inner parts of the brain; thus, the effectiveness of senses and movement are hindered, there and in the limbs, though the effectiveness is not completely cut off. There may be other causes also: a dense wind, trapped in the openings of the breath, or an evil vapour, or an acrid quality rising up to the brain from one of the organs. Then the brain contracts to repel the harmful agent, and there follows trembling in all the limbs; the person cannot remain upright but falls down, and usually foam appears in the mouth.

This illness is considered to be one of the episodic diseases,[4] because its occurence is particularly painful. It is sometimes considered to be one of the chronic diseases because it remains a long time and is difficult to cure, especially so when the patient is more than twenty-five years old. This illness occurs in the brain and especially in its essence. So epilepsy in these people will persist. Hippocrates has said: 'In these people, epilepsy continues until they die.'

In view of this the woman whom the *ḥadīth* says was an epileptic and would be uncovered was possibly suffering from epilepsy of this kind. So the Prophet ﷺ promised her Paradise in recompense for her patience with this disease, and he prayed for her that she should not be uncovered. He gave her the choice between endurance and Paradise, or prayer for her healing without any guarantee; she chose endurance with Paradise.

This account indicates that it is permissible to leave aside treatment and medication; treatment of spirits with prayers and turning to God achieves what cannot be obtained by the treatment given by physicians; and its influence and action, and the way the nature is effected and reacts, are greater than the influence of bodily medicines and the body's reaction to them. We and others have witnessed this often.

The intelligent physicians admit that the action of the soul's powers and their reactions can do wonders in curing illnesses. Nothing is more harmful to the medical art than the unbelieving, foolish, or ignorant physician.

4 Episodic diseases, *amrāḍ ḥāditha*, as opposed to chronic diseases, *amrāḍ muzmina*. This disease has two aspects: its sudden attacks, and its long-term persistance as a latent condition, which warrant its description both as recurring at intervals and as being chronic.

It is clear that the epilepsy of this woman was of this type. It is possible that it was from spirits, and the Messenger of God ﷺ gave her the choice between bearing it patiently with the reward of Paradise, or prayer for her healing. So she chose patience and not being uncovered during her fits.

God knows best.

CHAPTER

10

Treatment of sciatica (*ʿirq al-nasā*)[1]

IBN MĀJA relates in his *Sunan*, from a *ḥadīth* of Muḥammad b. Sīrīn from Anas b. Mālik: I heard the Messenger of God ﷺ say: 'The cure for sciatica is the tail fat of an Arabian sheep, melted, then divided into three portions, one to be taken, on an empty stomach, on each day.'[67]

ʿIrq al-nasā is a pain which begins at the joint of the hip and descends from behind to the thigh and sometimes extends to the ankle. The longer it persists, the more it spreads, and with that the foot and the thigh become emaciated.

This *ḥadīth* has a philological and a medical meaning: The philological aspect shows that this illness may rightly be given the name of *ʿirq al-nasā*. This is contradicted by those who do not allow this name, saying: *nasā* is the vein itself, so it would be grammatically a kind of *iḍāfa* of something to itself, and is not permitted. The reply to this argument is twofold: (1) *ʿirq* is more general than *nasā*, so it is a type of *iḍāfa* [adding] of the general to the particular, like 'all the *dirhams* and some of them'; (2) *nasā* is the disease which is located in the vein (*ʿirq*), so the *iḍāfa* here is a type of *iḍāfa* of the thing to its location and place. It has been said that it was so called because the pain makes one forget (*nasiya*) everything else. This vein extends from the hip joint to the end of the foot behind the ankle, from the outer side in between the bone of the leg and the tendon.

As for the medical interpretation, it has already been stated that the words of the Messenger of God ﷺ are of two types: (1) general, conditioned by time and place, persons and circumstances; (2) particular, depending on one of these matters or all of them together.

This saying is of the latter category, for it is addressed to the Arabs and people of the Ḥijāz and nearby regions, and most especially the Arabs of the desert. This treatment is of the most beneficial kind for them, for this illness arises from dryness and may also arise from thick sticky matter. Its treatment is by evacuation. The tail fat contains two special properties, coction and dissolution,

1 Sciatica, *ʿirq al-nasā*. The name, says IQ, could be 'vein of the sciatic vein', an *iḍāfa* (construct or genitive) which he explains as either 'general to the particular', as a specificative, or describing location, as one might say 'the vein of the jugular'.

for it contains the cocting and expulsive powers. The treatment for this illness requires these two actions.

The Arabian sheep is specified because its superfluities are slight, it is small, its essence subtle, and its pasture special. The sheep feeds upon the hot herbage of the land, such as artemisia, achillea, and similar plants. When animals feed on these plants, their meat acquires some of the properties of these plants, only more subtle and with a milder temperament because of having been digested. This is especially so in the case of the tail. The action of these plants in the milk comes out more strongly than it does in the meat. But the cocting and emollient property in the tail fat is not found in the milk. This is connected with what has already been stated: the medication of most of the desert peoples is by simple medicines, as the physicians of India say.

However, the Byzantines and Greeks were concerned with compound medicines. All of these men agree that it is more auspicious for the physician to carry out treatment through diet, and if this is not possible, then with simple medicines; if these are not effective, then with the least complex compounds.

It has already been stated that the Arabs and people of the desert suffer mostly from simple illnesses, for which simple drugs are suitable; this is because the majority of their food is simple. As for compound diseases, these are generally caused by the composite and varied nature of foodstuffs; for them, the compound medicines are chosen.[2]

God the Most High knows best.

2 As in Chapter I e, and Chapter 24.

CHAPTER

11

Treatment of constipation and the benefits of senna[1]

AL-TIRMIDHĪ'S *Jāmiʿ* and Ibn Māja' in his *Sunan* relate a *ḥadīth* from Asmā' bint ʿUmays: The Messenger of God ﷺ asked: 'What did you use as a purgative?' She replied: 'Euphorbia'. And he exclaimed: 'Hot, drawing!' (*ḥārr jārr*). Then she said: I have used senna as a purgative,' and he remarked: 'If there were anything which could cure the pains of death, it would be senna!'[68]

In Ibn Māja's *Sunan*, from Ibrāhīm b. Abī ʿAbla it says: 'I heard ʿAbd-Allāh b. Umm Ḥirām—one of those who prayed with the Messenger of God ﷺ at Qiblatayn mosque—say: I heard the Messenger of God ﷺ say: 'You must use senna and *sannūt*, for indeed they contain healing for every illness except the fatal one (*sāmm*).' Someone asked: 'O Messenger of God, what is the fatal one?'[2] He replied: 'Death.'[69]

When he asked: 'What do you use as a purgative?' this word means loosening of the constitution (*ṭabʿ*) until it moves and is not in any way static. The retention of excrement would cause harm. Thus the laxative medicine is called the 'mover' (*mashiyya*).[3] It is also said that this name refers to the fact that one who has taken a laxative walks about frequently to relieve his needs.

It is related also: 'With what do you seek a remedy?' (*istashfā*), and she replied: 'With euphorbia.' That is one of the medicines from the Euphorbiaceae, and it is the bark of the root of a shrub. It is hot and dry in the fourth degree. The best is that which inclines to red, light, and thin, resembling wrapped-up leather. In short, it is one of the medicines which physicians recommend should not be used because of its danger and its excessive purgative power.

Concerning the remark of the Prophet ﷺ: *ḥārr jārr*, which is also narrated

1 Dryness of the constitution, or the nature, *yubs al-tabʿ*, here indicates constipation, but includes any retention of humour or matter which needs to be moved or evacuated.

2 *Ḥadīth* which mentions and explains the term 'the fatal one' (*al-sāmm*) is narrated by Bukhārī, but this refers to *ḥabba sawdā'*, nigella.

3 *Mashiy*, laxitive, see Chapter 8 n. 4 and Chapter 25 n. 5

as *ḥārr yārr*, Abū ʿUbayd said: Mostly they relate it with a *yā'*. My comment is: There are two versions here, one being that *ḥārr jārr* means 'with great purgative power', so he described it as having heat and a powerful purgative effect; and this is said also by Abū Ḥanīfa al-Dīnawarī. The second—which is correct—is that this is a case of intensification through repetition (*itbāʿ*), where the second term serves to emphasise the first, a combination of verbal and semantic emphasis. So people observe this intensification with most of the letters, as when they say: *ḥasan basan*, meaning exceedingly good, or *ḥasan qasan*, with a *qāf*. There is also *shayṭān layṭān*, and *ḥārr jārr*. However, in *jārr*, there is another meaning: that which draws anything it comes into contact with, by the strength of its heat and its power of attraction to it, as if it overcomes and strips it. *Yārr* is either a variant of *jārr*—as when people say *ṣahrā* and *ṣahrīj*, and *ṣahāra* and *ṣahārīj*—or an independent intensifier.

Senna has two pronunciations, long or short.[4] It is a Ḥijāzī plant, the best kind of which is Makkan, and it is a noble, trusted, excellent medicine. It is near to the mean, hot and dry in the first degree, which purges the yellow and the black bile and strengthens the heart. This is one of its excellent qualities. Its speciality is to benefit cases of melancholic delusion and any fissures which occur in the body. It opens the muscles, helps the spreading of the hair and is good for lice and chronic headache, for scabies and pustules and for itching and epilepsy. A draught of its cooked juice is preferable to a draught of the crushed plant. The dosage is up to three *dirhams*, and of its juice up to five *dirhams*. If it is cooked with a little flower of violet and stoned red raisins, it is even better.

Al-Rāzī said: Senna and fumitory both purge the burned humours, and they are beneficial for scabies and itching. The dosage for each is from four to seven *dirhams*.[5]

Sannūt has eight explanations:[6] (1) honey; (2) *rubb* concentrate of the skin of fat, which comes out in black lines on the fat—both of these opinions are from ʿUmar b. Bakr al-Saksakiyy; (3) a grain similar to cumin but is not cumin, according to Ibn al-Aʿrābī; (4) Kirmānī cumin; (5) fennel, both according to Abū Ḥanīfa al-Dīnawarī from certain bedouin; (6) dill (7) dates, both according to Abū Bakr b. al-Sunnī the Qur'ān reader; and (8) honey which is in the containers of fat, according to ʿAbd al-Laṭīf al-Baghdādī. Certain physicians have said: This is the most appropriate and the nearest to what is correct: that crushed senna is mixed with honey which is mixed with fat; then it is taken as an electuary. This is better than taking it alone, because honey and fat contain substances that rectify the senna and assist its purgative properties. God knows best.

4 Pronounced *sennā* or *senna*.

5 One *dirham* = ca.312g.

6 Various explanations include: (2) *rubb* of the skin of fat, which is, according to Lane, *Arabic – English Lexicon*, p. 1002, inspissated date juice which imparts a good odour to [skin for clarified butter]; (8) honey kept with *samn*. *Sannūt*, according to IQ, is senna mixed with honey and *samn*, thus being rectified, so that any excessive qualities are moderated.

Al-Tirmidhī and others have related, from *ḥadīth* of Ibn ʿAbbās (*marfūʿ*), 'that the best treatment you can give is by the sternutatory, *ladūd*, cupping, and laxative';[70] the word *mashiy* means what moves and loosens the constitution and eases the movement of evacuation.

CHAPTER

12

Itching (*ḥikka*) of the body and the causes of lice

IN THE two books of *Ṣaḥīḥ*, the *ḥadīth* of Qatāda, from Anas b. Mālik, says: The Messenger of God ﷺ allowed ʿAbd al-Raḥmān b. ʿAwf and al-Zubayr b. al-ʿAwwām to wear silk on account of itching that affected them. In another narrative: 'ʿAbd al-Raḥmān b. ʿAwf and al-Zubayr b. al-ʿAwwām complained to the Prophet ﷺ of lice during a raid they went on, so he allowed them to wear silk shirts, which I saw them wearing'.[1][71]

This *ḥadīth* has two salient points, one legal, the other medical. The legal point is that the *Sunna* of the Prophet ﷺ has given permission for women to wear silk without exception and has made it prohibited for men except for a definite need or an established benefit. Need might arise from intense cold, when nothing else is available, or when there is no other material one can use to cover what should not be exposed. These include the use of silk in war or during sickness, or in a case of itching or infestation with lice, as is indicated by this sound *ḥadīth* from Anas. Its authorisation has validated the two narratives from Imām Aḥmad and the two sayings of al-Shāfiʿī. The general juristic principle is that rules cannot be confined nor restricted to a particular situation or group of people. When permission is confirmed concerning a section of the community for some significant reason, it is extended to everyone in whom is found that significant reason. The rule becomes general when the reason for it becomes general.

Anyone objecting to that would say: the *ḥadīth* of prohibition are general; the *ḥadīth* of permission are specifically applicable to ʿAbd al-Raḥmān b. ʿAwf and al-Zubayr, and it is possible they may extend to others. When the two possibilities exist, then to take the general sense is more appropriate. For this

1 The *ḥadīth* concerning the wearing of silk is taken as an example to show that where permission is given for a specific reason, any other occurrence of the same circumstances is a reason for the same permission. Although the law in general prohibits silk for men, the concession to these two is considered to extend to others in their particular situation. There is a warning however against any 'pretext', *dharīʿa*, taking any concession further than is intended.

reason, one of the narrators said of this *ḥadīth*: I do not know whether or not the permission applies to others.

The correct view is that the concession is general; it is customary for the law to speak in that way, so long as it does not declare its specific nature nor state that it cannot apply to anyone who was not given this permission at the beginning. An instance is when the Prophet ﷺ said to Abū Burda: 'It is sufficient for you, but will not be sufficient for anyone else after you.' Or when the Most High said to His Prophet ﷺ, concerning marriage with the woman who gave herself to him: *'Solely for thee, and not for the believers in general'* (XXXIII: 50). Banning of silk was part of the juristic principle blocking off the means to harm (*sadd al-dharā'iʿ*), and therefore it was allowed for women, and in cases of need and for special benefit. This is the purport of this juristic principle, i.e. what is banned to prevent pretexts is allowed in cases of need or benefit. Similarly looking at women (that are lawful to marry) was prohibited as part of preventing pretext—yet is not prohibited in case of need or benefit. Likewise any extra prayers were banned before sunset or sunrise, thus preventing the pretext of the superficial resemblance to the sun-worshippers; nevertheless prayers are allowed for a greater benefit.[2] Also, usury on surplus was banned, preventing the excuse for usury of credit, but it was permitted when need required, as in the case of stripped date trees. We have spoken at length on this subject in the book *Composition on Silk Clothing which is Lawful or Prohibited.*

The medical point is that silk is one of the drugs of animal origin, and therefore it is reckoned among the animal drugs because it is extracted from an animal. It is very useful and important. Among its special properties, it strengthens and brings joy to the heart and is beneficial for many of its diseases; it overcomes the black bile and illnesses which it generates. It sharpens the sight when used as an eye salve. Raw silk (*khām*)—which is used medicinally—is hot and dry in the first degree; it is also said to be hot and moist in the first degree; and it is said to be moderate in medicinal use. Clothing made from silk is of moderate heat in its constitution, warming to the body; and sometimes the body is cooled by it causing it to be fattened.

Al- Rāzī said: Raw silk (*ibrīsim*) is warmer than flax but cooler than cotton; it nourishes the flesh. Every coarse clothing makes the body lean and the skin firm, and so the reverse is true.

My comment: Clothing is of three kinds: one kind that heats and warms the body, one kind that warms it but does not heat it, and one kind that neither heats nor warms it. There is none that heats but does not warm it, for whatever heats it is even more likely to warm it. Clothing of hair and woollen material heats and warms, while clothing of linen, silk and cotton warms but does not heat. For garments of linen are cold and dry, those of wool are warm and dry,

2 Prayers, i.e. supererogatory additional prayers.

those of cotton are of moderate warmth, and those of silk are softer and have less heat than cotton.

The author of the *Minhāj* said: Clothing from silk does not heat as cotton does, but it is moderate. All soft and smooth clothing is less heating to the body, gives less aid to the dissolving of such matters as are to be dissolved, and is more suitable for wearing in summer and in hot lands.

Since silken garments are of this nature and contain no dryness nor harshness—qualities which are found in others—they are beneficial for itching, because itching is only from heat, dryness and harshness. For this reason the Messenger of God ﷺ allowed al-Zubayr and ʿAbd al-Raḥmān to wear silk to relieve their itching. Garments of silk are the least likely to allow the generation of lice in them, because their temperament is opposite to the sort where the generation of lice would occur.

The kind which neither warms nor heats is that made from iron, lead, wood, earth and suchlike.

It may be asked: If silk clothing is the most moderate and the most suitable for the body, why has it been banned by the *sharīʿa*, which is outstanding in its perfection and has permitted good things and banned evil? The reply is that this question has been answered by every group of Muslims. Those who deny the importance of finding the underlying wisdom and justification for divine injunctions say: the whole affair is unfounded, therefore the question needs no answer.

Among those who confirm justification and reasons—and these are in the majority—are some who reply that the law has banned it so that people's souls may learn to endure thereby, refraining from the use of it for the sake of God, and get rewarded for that, especially when they are compensated for it by something else. Others reply that silk was originally created for women, like adornment with gold, and was forbidden to men because of its evil effect of making men resemble women. Some say that it was forbidden because it gives rise to conceit, pride, and vainglory.

Still others say that it was forbidden because touching it can give rise to such weaknesses as effeminacy, and to the opposite of energy and manliness. Wearing it gives the heart a certain characteristic of the female. Therefore, you will find hardly anyone who frequently wears it who has not some qualities of effeminacy and weakness, which cannot be concealed, even if he were one of the most energetic, manly, and bold. Inevitably, the wearing of silk would decrease these qualities, if it did not remove them entirely. If anyone's temperament is too thick and heavy to understand that, let him submit himself to the wisdom of the Lawgiver. Thus, the more correct of the two opinions is that it was forbidden to the guardian to dress the young lad in it because it could produce in him certain effeminate characteristics.

Al-Nisāʾī has related, from *ḥadīth* of Abū Mūsā al-Ashʿarī, from the Prophet ﷺ who said: Indeed God has made silk and gold lawful for the women of my Community and unlawful for the men.[72] In another version: Silken clothing and gold have been forbidden to the men of my Community, but permitted for their women.

In the *Ṣaḥiḥ* of Bukhārī, from Ḥudhayfa: The Messenger of God ﷺ forbade the wearing of silk and brocade, or sitting upon it. He said: It is for them in this world, and for you in the hereafter.[73]

CHAPTER

13

The treatment of pleurisy (*dhāt al-janb*)

AL-TIRMIDHĪ relates in his *Jāmiʿ*, from *ḥadīth* of Zayd b. Arqam, that the Prophet ﷺ said: 'Treat pleurisy with sea costus and oil.'[74]

According to physicians, pleurisy is of two kinds: authentic and false. The authentic kind is a hot inflammation occuring in the areas of the rib cage in the membrane deep within the ribs. The false variety is a similar pain, occurring in the area of the side, arising from dense harmful winds trapped within the dermis. This causes a pain very similar to the pain of true pleurisy, except that the pain from this kind is widespread, and in the authentic kind it is an acute stabbing pain.

Ibn Sīnā said: In the side and the dermis and the muscles which are in the chest and ribs and surrounding area there may occur painful and very harmful inflammations which are called pleurisy (*shawṣa*, *birsām* and *dhāt al-janb*). There may also be pains in these members which are not from inflammation but from dense winds. They are thought to be caused by this illness, but they are not. Know then, that every pain in the side can be called *dhāt al-janb*, derived from the location of the pain. The meaning of *dhāt al-janb* is that belonging to the side (*janb*), so what is intended here is pain of the side. When a pain occurs in the side, from whatever cause, it is attributed to it. Here Hippocrates' words are relevant: Sufferers from *dhāt al-janb* benefit from bathing.

It is said that the meaning here is pain in the side, or pain of the lung arising from an upset of the constitution, or from thick or burning humours, yet without either inflammation or fever.

Certain physicians have said: The meaning of *dhāt al-janb* in the Greek language is hot inflammation of the side; likewise, inflammation of any one of the internal organs. Inflammation of an organ is called *dhāt al-janb* simply when it is a hot inflammation. True *dhāt al-janb* has five symptoms: fever, cough, sharp pain, shortness of breath and irregular pulse.

The treatment found in the *ḥadīth* is not for this division but for the second division that is caused by dense wind. Sea costus—which is Indian aloe, according to the commentaries on other *ḥadīth*—is a type of costus. When it is pounded very fine and mixed with warm oil and rubbed onto the place affected, or when it is swallowed, it is a medicine suitable and beneficial for that trouble, able to dissolve and disperse its matters; it strengthens the internal organs and is desobstruant. Aloe, mentioned above, has similar benefits.

Al-Masīḥī has said: 'Aloe is hot, dry, astringent, restrains the belly, strengthening the internal organs, expelling wind; it is desobstruant, beneficial for *dhāt al-janb*, and disperses superfluity of moisture. The same aloe is good for the brain'. It is possible that costus may benefit the true *dhāt al-janb* also, when its origin is from phlegmy matter, especially at the time when the illness is on the decline.

God knows best.

Dhāt al-janb is one of the dangerous illnesses. In the sound *ḥadīth*, Umm Salma said: The last illness of the Messenger of God ﷺ began in the house of Maymūna, and whenever it abated he would go out and lead the people in prayer. Every time he found this burdensome, he would say: 'Command Abū Bakr to lead the prayer.' His distress intensified until he was overcome by the severity of the pain. His wives gathered round him, together with his uncle al-ʿAbbās, and Umm al-Faḍl bint al-Ḥārith and Asmā' bint ʿUmays. They took counsel about administering to him a *ladūd*. So they dosed him while he was unconscious. When he recovered, he asked: 'Who did this to me? This is the work of women who have come from that direction'—and he pointed with his hand towards the land of Ethiopia. It was Umm Salma and Asmā' who had dosed him, so they said: 'O Messenger of God, we feared lest you might have *dhāt al-janb*'. He asked: 'And with what did you dose me?' They replied: 'With Indian aloe, a little false saffron, and some oil pitch.' He said: 'God is not going to afflict me with that illness.' Then he said: 'I strictly order that everyone in the house should be dosed, except for my uncle al-ʿAbbās.'[75]

In the two books of the *Ṣaḥiḥ*, from ʿĀ'isha it says: We dosed the Messenger of God ﷺ with a *ladūd*, and he indicated that we should not do so. We said: This is just the patient's aversion to medicine. When he woke, he asked: 'Did I not forbid you to dose me? Not one of you remains but will be dosed, except for my uncle al-ʿAbbās, for indeed he did not take part in it.'[76]

Abū ʿUbayd said, from al-Aṣmaʿī: *Ladūd* is that which is given to a man to drink in one side of the mouth, and the word is taken from the two embankments (*ladīd*) of a valley, that is, its two sides. The *wajūr* is that which is put into the centre of the mouth. My comment: the *ladūd* is the medicine by which one is thus dosed. *Saʿūṭ* (sternutatory) is what is instilled into the patient's nose.

The legal aspect of this *ḥadīth* is the punishment of the offender by the like of what he has done, when what he has done is not prohibited by God's law. This is the correct answer which is declared in some ten indications which we have mentioned elsewhere; it is the confirmed judgement of Aḥmad (b. Ḥanbal) and established by the Rightly-Guided Caliphs. The further interpretation of the question is requital concerning blows and striking. In this matter there are numerous *ḥadīth* which are not opposed in any way, therefore judgement should be made accordingly.

CHAPTER

14

On the treatment of headache (*ṣudāʿ*) and migraine (*shaqīqa*)[1]

IBN MĀJA related in his *Sunan* a *ḥadīth*, whose authenticity has been questioned: When the Prophet ﷺ suffered from headache he would cover his head with henna, for he said: 'It is beneficial for headache, by God's permission.'[77]

Headache is a pain in certain parts of the head or throughout it. Pain that persists in one of the two sides of the head is called migraine (hemicrania). If it persists in the whole of the head it is called *bayḍa* or *khūdha*, a simile with the helmet (*bayḍa*) which covers the entire head. Sometimes it is in the back of the head or the front of it, and there are many kinds from a variety of causes. The correct description of headache is a warmth and feverishness of the head which is a result of vapours, which, circulating the head in seeking to escape and not finding a way, cause a headache, just as a container is broken when its contents are heated and seek a way out. Everything moist, when heated, seeks a wider area than the one which it occupies. When this vapour occurs throughout the head, so that it cannot spread about and dissolve, it moves around in the head and is called vertigo (*sadar*).

Headaches can have numerous causes: (1)–(4) the predominance of one of the four temperaments; (5) ulcers in the stomach, so that the head is pained by that inflammation through the conjunction of the nerve that descends from the head to the stomach; (6) dense wind located in the stomach, which rises to the head and afflicts it with headache; (7) an inflammation in the veins of the stomach which in turn will cause inflammation in the head because they are linked; (8) the repletion of the stomach with food; then the food descends, and part of it remains undigested, so that it afflicts the head and makes it heavy; (9)

1 Headache (*ṣudāʿ*), from *ṣadaʿa*; migraine (*shaqīqa*), from *shaqqa*, both meaning to split. *Shaqīqa* generally indicates migraine (hemicrania) explained as being in one of the two sides (*shaqqayn*) of the head. Both terms are connected with the concept of the causes of headache, one of which is seen here as the accumulation of vapours in the head, which then seek to escape and cause severe pain (as 'splitting') in the process. See Chapter 19 n.1.

subsequent to intercourse, because of the body being somewhat disordered, so more heat arrives there from the air than is appropriate for the head; (10) emesis or evacuation, either from predominance of dryness or from the rising of vapours from the stomach to the head; (11) the intensity of heat and warmth of the air; (12) intensity of cold, when vapours thicken in the head and do not dissolve; (13) lack or suppression of sleep; (14) pressure on the head, or carrying something heavy on it; (15) speaking too much, for the power of the brain is impaired thereby; (16) excessive movement and exercise; (17) psychological causes, such as worries and anxieties, griefs, stress and evil thoughts; (17) melancholic delusion; (18) intense hunger, for then the vapours do not find anything to work upon, so they continually rise to the brain and cause it pain; (19) inflammation in the membranes of the brain; the patient feels as though he is being beaten on the head with hammers; (20) fever, because its heat is kindled in the head which then feels pain.

God knows best.

Hemicrania or migraine (*shaqīqa*) can be caused by matter in the arteries of the head alone, being produced there, or by matter rising up to the brain, so that the weaker of the two sides of the head accepts it. That matter is vaporous or consists of hot or cold humours. Its particular symptom is the throbbing of the arteries and especially those full of blood; when you apply bandages and prevent the throbbing, then the pain is quietened.

Abū Nuʿaym said, in his book on the *Medicine of the Prophet*, that this type of headache used to afflict the Prophet ﷺ, who would stay indoors for a day or two and not go out. On the same subject, Ibn ʿAbbās said: The Messenger of God ﷺ preached to us, after having wrapped his head in a bandage.[78]

It is related in the *Ṣaḥīḥ*: He said, in his last illness: 'O my head!' and he used to bandage his head during his illness.[79]

Bandaging for the head is beneficial for the pain of migraine and for other pains of the head.

Treatment varies according to its various types and causes. These treatments include: evacuation, diet, rest and quiet, dressings, cooling or warming, and avoiding listening to noises and avoiding movement. Having said this, we can see that the treatment by henna, as it applies only to a specific type of headache, in the *ḥadīth*, is seen to be particular, not general, because it is a treatment for one type.

When headache is from burning heat and is not from some substance which must be evacuated, henna has a very evident benefit. When it is pounded and applied to the forehead as a dressing with vinegar, it calms the headache. It contains a power which is appropriate to the nerves; when it is applied as a poultice it calms these pains. This is not specifically for pain in the head but is generally for all the limbs. It has a constringent property whereby the limbs are strengthened, and when applied as a dressing to the site of the burning inflammation, it calms it.

Al-Bukhārī relates, in his *History*, and Abū Dāwūd in his *Sunan*, that the Messenger of God ﷺ, if anyone ever complained to him of a pain in the head, would say: 'Have yourself cupped.' If anyone complained to him of a pain in the legs, he told them: 'Anoint yourself with henna.'[80]

Al-Tirmidhī relates from Salma Umm Rāfiᶜ, servant of the Prophet ﷺ, who said: 'If ever the Prophet ﷺ was afflicted by ulceration or thorns, he would apply henna to them.'[81]

Henna is cold in the first degree and dry in the second. The power of the henna plant and branches is composite, from a dissoluent power which it acquires from a water, moderately hot essence and from a costive power which it acquires from an earthy cold essence in it.

Among its advantages is that it is a useful dissoluent for burns by fire. When used as a poultice, it has a power appropriate for the nerves; when chewed, it is beneficial for ulcers of the mouth and any blisters which occur in it. It heals thrush which occurs in the mouths of children. Bandaging with it is beneficial for hot inflammations, and its effect on abscesses is similar to that of dragon's blood plant.[2] When its flowers are mixed with warm wax and rose oil, it is good for pains of the side.

Among its special usages is that when applied to the feet of children during the early stages of smallpox, it prevents the disease from reaching the eyes. This is a tried and true formula. When its flowers are put between the folds of woollen clothing, they scent it and keep moths away. When its leaves are soaked in sweet water, thoroughly immersed and then squeezed and the clear liquid drunk over a period of forty days (twenty *dirhams* per day mixed with ten *dirhams* of sugar), followed by a meal of baby lamb's meat, this is beneficial against the start of leprosy(*judhām*), through a remarkable property of the leaves.

It is said that a certain man's finger-nails were splitting, and he spent much money seeking a cure without success. Then a woman prescribed for him drinking henna for ten days. At first he refused. But then he soaked the henna in the water and drank it. He was cured, and his finger-nails returned to their former good state.

When finger-nails are smeared with henna paste, it improves and benefits them. When made into a dough with ghee, it can be used as a dressing for the vestiges of hot inflammation which exude yellow liquid, and it is beneficial for them. It has an excellent effect on ulcerated chronic scabies. It causes the hair to grow, strengthens and beautifies it, and strengthens the head. It is good for blisters and pustules occurring on the legs and feet and the rest of the body.

2 Dragon's blood, *dam al-akhawayn*, a red gum from *Dracaena draco* L. or D. *cinnabari* L., recommended in mediaeval times for disorders of the blood. The substance sold today in the *sūqs* as *dam al-akhawayn* is not a gum but tubipora, a hard coral-like substance.

CHAPTER

15

Treatment of the sick by excluding food and drink which they dislike[1]

AL-TIRMIDHĪ relates in his *Jāmiᶜ*, and Ibn Māja from ᶜUqba b. ᶜĀmir al-Juhnī: The Messenger of God ﷺ said: 'Do not compel your sick to take food and drink, for indeed God, the Exalted, will feed them and give them water.'[82]

Certain physicians have commented: 'How abundantly useful is this saying of the Prophet ﷺ, full of divine wisdom, especially for physicians and those who treat the sick. For when the sick person has an aversion to food or drink, it is because his constitution is busied with fighting the disease, or else this is due to the decrease or loss of appetite, because of the decline of the innate heat. Whatever may be the case, at such a time it is not permitted to give food.'

Know then that hunger is merely the organs' seeking for food, so that the constitution may thereby be reinforced, to replace what has been dissolved; the further organs draw it from the nearer organs, until this drawing effect finally reaches the stomach, so that the person feels hunger and seeks food. When sickness is present, the constitution is concerned with its matter, to coct it and expel it, and is not concerned to seek food or drink. When the patient is compelled to take something, the constitution is thereby hindered from its activity, is busied with digesting it and disposing of it, and is distracted from cocting and repelling the matter of the illness. This is one cause of harm to the patient, especially at the times of crisis or weakness or decline of the innate heat.

1 Foods for the sick are to conform with the patient's inclination, since this will prove more beneficial. The theory here is that the constitution (*ṭabīᶜa*) should not be distracted from its chief task of counteracting illness, and therefore if it has no desire for food this should not be forced upon it. For the body can be distracted by psychological factors, whether friendly or hostile, to the extent of not noticing hunger and thirst. The 'coction' or cooking process will break down the phlegm already in the body and supply sufficient blood (ie. for nourishment). IQ gives twenty causes in all, beginning with those connected with the humours and including the influence of the stomach and various kinds of stress.

Then that would increase the affliction and hasten the feared consequences. At such a time and under these conditions, only those means should be used which will preserve and fortify his strength, without using anything at all which would upset the constitution. That must be with such food and drink of which the texture is simple and the temperament moderate, such as drinks made of waterlily and apple and moist rose, and similar things; and of foods, only broth of chickens, moderate and flavoured. The restoration of his faculties will be by spiced and appropriate scents and by being in a stress-free and positive atmosphere. For the physician is the servant and assistant of the innate nature, not one who impedes it.

Know then that it is the good blood which nourishes the body and that phlegm is unripe blood, which has cocted to a certain extent. Now if a patient's body contains a great deal of phlegm and food is lacking, the constitution turns towards it, cooks and cocts it, and turns it into blood, on which the members feed and find this sufficient on its own. The innate nature is the power which God, praised be He, has entrusted with managing the affairs of the body, its preservation and its health, and guarding it for the whole length of its life.

Know then that it is very seldom necessary to force a patient to eat and drink. This only happens in the diseases which are accompanied by disturbances of the mind.

On this point, the *ḥadīth* is both general and at the same time specific or absolute with an indication of its restriction. The *ḥadīth* means that a sick person may live without food for some days, in a way that would not be feasible for a healthy person.

The words of the Prophet ﷺ: 'For God will feed them and give them water' have a subtle meaning, in addition to what physicians have said. This is known only to those whose concern is for the judgements of heart and spirit, their influence on the constitution of the body and the constitution's reactions to them, just as they react to the constitution. When the soul is touched by something which distracts it, whether it is something it likes, dislikes or fears, it is kept from seeking food and drink, feeling neither hunger nor thirst, nor even heat or cold, and thereby is even left unaware of the sensation of severe pain. There is no one who has not experienced this in one way or another.

When the soul is distracted by something unexpectedly, then it does not feel the pain of hunger. If something should occur which arouses great joy, this takes the place of food, and the soul is thereby sated, and its faculties are restored and increased. The blood supply flows in the body until it appears on its surface, causing the face to light up, and making its sanguine nature apparent. For joy causes an expansion of the heart's blood, so that it is sent coursing through the veins, which are filled with it. Thus the organs ignore their accustomed need for food, as they are fulfilled through what is more pleasing to them and to the constitution, namely blood. When the constitution has successfully acquired what it likes, then it prefers this above all else.

If something happens which causes pain, distress or fear in the soul, the constitution becomes engaged in fighting, opposing and repelling this, and is thus distracted from seeking food. When engaged in a fight, it is not able to seek food and drink. If it is successful in its struggle, its strength is restored and it compensates this loss of food and drink with an equivalent amount. Then if it is vanquished, its faculties decline accordingly. If the struggle between the soul and its adversary is an even match, then the strength is sometimes apparent and sometimes hidden. In short, the fight is similar to the external fight between two opponents with victory going to the dominant force, and the one defeated slain, wounded, or taken prisoner.

The sick person has help from God the Most High, which comes in the form of nourishment, in addition to what physicians have mentioned concerning nourishment from the blood. This help is in accordance with his weakness and humility, and his total submission of his affairs to the hands of his most exalted Lord. This will qualify him for nearness to his Lord. For the servant is nearest to his Lord when he attains humility in his heart, and then his Lord's mercy is close to him. If he is close to Him, he acquires food of the heart from which the faculties of his constitution are restored; this is far greater than the restoration brought about by bodily food. So long as his faith, love, intimacy and joy for his Lord increase, and his certainty intensifies, and his longing for Him, his contentment with Him and for Him multiply, then he shall find in his soul a mighty strength which cannot be expressed nor perceived nor attained by any physician.

If anyone's nature is too dense and his soul too heavy to understand and believe this, let him regard the condition of those who love superficial things, whose hearts are full of affection for what they love, whether objects, honour, wealth, or knowledge. People have seen remarkable examples of this in themselves and in others.

It is confirmed in the *Ṣaḥīḥ*, regarding the Prophet ﷺ, that he used to make his fasting continuous over many days, but he forbade his Companions to do the same, saying: 'I am not like you, for I continue fasting and my Lord supplies me with food and drink.'[83] It is clear that this food and drink are not the sort of food a man takes by mouth; for then the fast would not have been continuous and there would not be a true distinction, but rather he would not have been fasting. For he said: 'I continue fasting, and my Lord supplies me with food and drink.' Also he made the distinction between himself and them in the same situation; and he could undertake fasting such as they could not. If he had been taking food and drink by mouth, he would not have said: 'I am not like you'. That would be understood from the *ḥadīth* only by the one whose share of nourishment of the Spirit and heart is minimal. For its influence on the faculty and its restoration and nourishment thereby are above the influence of physical food.

God gives success.

CHAPTER

16

Pain in the fauces (*ᶜudhra*) and the use of sternutatory (*saᶜūṭ*)[1]

IT IS confirmed in the two books of the *Ṣaḥīḥ* that the Prophet ﷺ said: 'The best forms of treatment you can employ are cupping and sea costus. Do not afflict your children by palpation for pain in the fauces (*ᶜudhra*).[84] In the *Sunan* and *Musnad*, from *ḥadīth* of Jābir b. ᶜAbd-Allāh it says: The Messenger of God ﷺ entered ᶜĀ'isha's room, where there was a small boy with blood pouring from his nose. He asked: 'What is this?' and they replied: 'He has fauces, or pain in his head.' He said: 'Woe on you! Do not kill your children! If any woman's child is afflicted with fauces or a pain in his head, she should take Indian costus, crush it with water and give it to him to sniff.' So ᶜĀ'isha gave instructions, and this was done for the boy, who was cured.[85]

Abū ᶜUbayd reported, from Abū ᶜUbayda, that fauces is an agitation of blood in the throat. When one is treated for this, people say: 'He has been treated for fauces.' It is also said that fauces is an ulcer which erupts between the ear and the throat, and it occurs chiefly in young children.

The benefit of the sternutatory in this case with crushed costus is because the substance of fauces is blood in which phlegm predominates, but it is generated in the bodies of children. Costus contains a dessicative power which strengthens the uvula and pulls it to its proper place. Its benefit in this illness is attributed to its special property. It can be beneficial for the treatment of hot diseases also when mixed with hot medicaments either through its special or accidental properties. Ibn Sīnā has recommended costus with Yemeni alum and seeds of origanum for the treatment of slipping of the uvula.

1 *ᶜUdhra*: pain in the fauces (cavity at the back of the mouth, from which open out pharynx and larynx). The word *ᶜudhra* refers to the specific area of the head, but from IQ's comment it appears that the term was also applied to the ailment, when it was thought to be caused by an ulcer in that region. *Saᶜūṭ*, the sternutatory: powder inserted in the nose (see Chapter 8 n.5). Bleeding from the nose is taken as an indication that the bleeding is caused through the excess of phlegm which has been produced.

Sea costus as mentioned in the *ḥadīth* is Indian aloes, which is the white variety. It is sweet and has many benefits. People used to treat their children by palpation of the uvula, and by an *ʿilāq*, which is something they hang round the children's necks.[2] The Prophet ﷺ forbade them that, and guided them to something which is more beneficial and easier for the children.

The sternutatory is a medicine put into the nose, and it can be of simple or compound drugs. They are pounded, sieved, kneaded and dried, then dissolved as required. This is then put into a person's nose to be sniffed up, while he is lying on his back, with something between his shoulders to lift him up so that his head is lowered and the sternutatory can thus reach his brain and expel the illness through sneezing.

The Prophet ﷺ praised medication with the sternutatory in cases where it was required. Abū Dāwūd mentioned in his *Sunan* that 'the Prophet ﷺ used the sternutatory.'[86]

2 *ʿIlāq*, some kind of amulet, so called from the verb *ʿallaqa* to suspend. This evidently was seen to be verging on the forbidden use of spells, and anyway contravening the principle of *tawakkul*. For the use of *ʿallaqa* for *ʿudhra*: Bukhāri, *Ṭibb* 21, VII. 410–11.

CHAPTER

17

Treatment for cardiac pain (*al-maf' ūd*)

(a) *Various Treatments*

ABD DĀWŪD relates in his *Sunan*, from *ḥadīth* of Mujāhid, from Saʿd (b. Abī Waqqāṣ): Once when I fell sick, the Messenger of God ﷺ came to visit me and placed his hand upon the centre of my chest, until I felt its coldness penetrate to my heart. Then he said to me: 'You have heart trouble. Go to Ḥārith b. Kalada of the tribe of Thaqīf, a man who practises medicine; let him take seven pressed dates (ʿ*ajwa*), of the Madīnan variety, and crush them with their stones, and give them to you as a dose (*ladūd*).'[1][87]

The one with cardiac pain (*maf'ūd*) is the one whose heart is affected to the extent that he complains of it. Similarly, the *mabṭūn* is one troubled by his belly (*baṭn*). *Ladūd* is medicine administered to a person at one side of his mouth. Dates possess a marvellous property in this illness, especially dates from Madīna, and in particular the ʿ*ajwa* variety. In choosing seven of them, there is another property, known through revelation.

It is related in the two books of the *Ṣaḥīḥ*, from *ḥadīth* of ʿĀmir b. Saʿd b. Abī Waqqāṣ, from his father that the Messenger of God ﷺ said: 'Whoever starts the day with seven dates from al-ʿĀliya will not be harmed that day by poison nor by magic.'[2] In another version: 'If anyone eats seven dates from between the city limits of Madīna (between their two tracts of stony ground), when he rises in the morning, no poison will harm him before the evening.'[88]

(b) *Dates*

Dates (*tamr*) are hot in the second degree, dry in the first. Others say that they are moist in the first, while others say moderate. They are an excellent food,

1 Treatment for the *maf'ūd*, ie. one whose heart (*fu'ād*) is afflicted. *Ladūd*: Cf. Chapter 8 n.5. The use of dates: *tamr*, dried dates; ʿ*ajwa*, dates dried and pressed into a kind of paste.

2 The treatment with seven dates, elaborated by IQ, seems to owe its claim to effectiveness solely to the number seven. However, he backs up his affirmation by an analysis of their properties. Al-ʿĀliya: the villages near Madīna.

which preserve health, especially if one makes a habit of eating them, as do the people of Madīna and elsewhere. They are among the most excellent foods in cold countries and in those hot countries where the heat is of the second degree. They are more useful for the people of these latter areas than for people in the cold countries because their temperaments are cold, while the temperaments of the inhabitants of cold countries are hot. For this reason, people of Ḥijāz, Yemen, and Ṭā'if and neighbouring countries and those with similar climates eat a great deal of hot foods which others find difficult, such as dates and honey. We have seen them put ten times the amount of pepper or ginger into their food as others or even more, and eat ginger as others eat sweetmeats. I have seen some who used to add it even to dried fruit. It is appropriate for them and does not harm them because of the coldness of their internal organs and because the heat makes its way to the outside of the body. Similarly, one finds that well water becomes cold in summer and warm in winter; in the same way the stomach can coct heavy foods in winter to an extent it cannot do in summer.

The people of Madīna use dates almost as other people use wheat, and dates are their food and a main ingredient of their diet. Dates of al-ʿĀliya are among their best kinds of dates, for they are solid in substance, delicious in taste and truly sweet.

Dates are included among foods, medicines and fruit; they are suitable for most constitutions; they strengthen the innate heat, and no harmful superfluities are generated from them such as arise from other foods and fruit. Rather, to one accustomed to eating them, they prevent any putrefaction or corruption of the humours.

This *ḥadīth* is one of those sayings that has a specific meaning, in this case, for the people of Madīna and its surrounding area. There is no doubt that certain locations have a specific quality that assists many drugs in that place, not found in other places. Thus the drug that is grown here is beneficial for the illness, but the benefit is not found in it when it grows somewhere else. This difference is due to the influence of the soil, the air, or their combination. Each land has its properties and natures, which differ from those of other lands in the same way that humans differ in nature; many plants are edible food in one land and deadly poison in another. Often what is a drug for one people is food for others. Similarly, a drug for some people for some illnesses when used by others is for different illnesses, while drugs for the inhabitants of one country are not appropriate for others and are of no benefit to them.

(c) *The number seven*

As for the special properties of the number seven, this is something which occurs in accordance with the decree and the religious law. For God the Exalted One created the heavens as seven, the earths seven, the days seven, and man's creation was completed in seven stages.

God made incumbent on His servants the circumambulation of the Kaʿba (*ṭawāf*) seven times, and the runnings (*saʿy*) between al-Ṣafā and al-Marwa seven times,[3] and throwing stones at the *jamarāt* (post representing Satan) seven times each. The *takbīrs* (calling 'God is Great') of the two Feasts are seven at the first *rakʿa*. The Prophet ﷺ said: 'Order prayer at the age of seven.'[89] When a young boy reaches seven years, he can be given the choice between his parents (in case of separation). However, another tradition says: His father has more right to him than his mother. A third tradition states: His mother has more right to him. The Prophet ﷺ ordered, in his illness, that water should be poured over him from seven water-skins. God sent the wind against the people of ʿĀd for seven nights.[4] The Prophet ﷺ prayed that God would help him against his people, with seven different manifestations like the seven signs of Yūsuf. God, praised be He, compared the manifold increase He grants to the alms of those who spend for His sake to a grain which gives rise to seven ears, in each ear a hundred grains; the ears which Yūsuf's master saw were seven, and the years they sowed consecutively (XII:47) were seven. The alms increase seven hundred times, even many times more. Of the Community, those who will enter Paradise without reckoning will be seventy thousand.

There is no doubt that this number has a special property which no other possesses and that seven includes the meanings and special properties of numbers in their entirety. For the number is both even (*shafʿ*) and odd (*witr*); the even number is first and second, and so is the odd (and there are four classes: first and second even, as well as first and second odd); and these degrees cannot be comprised in any other number less than seven. It is a complete number because it includes the four classes of numbers. That is to say: the even and odd, the firsts and seconds; by the first odd we mean three, and by the second, five; by the first even, two, and by the second, four. As for physicians, they too have great concern for the number seven, especially in the matter of crises. Hippocrates has said: Everything in this world is preordained in seven divisions. The planets are seven, the days are seven, the ages of humankind are seven: first the child, up to seven years, then a lad up to fourteen, then an adolescent, then a young man, then mature, then an old man, then aged, until the end of his life. God the Most High is the One who knows best His wisdom, law, and decree in making this number so special; is it for this meaning, or another?

Now this number, of this kind of date, from this country and this region, is beneficial against poison and magic, inasmuch as it prevents evil from striking. The benefit comes from special properties which, had Hippocrates or Galen or

3 *Ṭawāf*: the 'circumambulation' of the Kaʿba at Mecca, one of the rites of *ḥajj* and *ʿumra* (greater and lesser pilgrimage). *Saʿy*: the 'running' between the hills of Ṣafā and Marwa, another of the rites of pilgrimage.

4 The people of ʿĀd are mentioned several times in the Qur'ān, so is the wind, sent upon them as punishment: LI:41–2; LIV:18–21.

some other medical expert spoken of them, would have been eagerly accepted and followed by physicians, even though the one who said this based it on conjecture, guesswork and opinion. It is more appropriate to accept with submission and without negation the utterance of one who speaks out of certainty, reason, precision and revelation.

Drugs for poisons sometimes have a specific property, like the properties of many of the stones, jewels and diamonds.

God knows best.

(d) *Faith in treatment*

The variety of date *ʿajwa* can be beneficial for some poisons. The *ḥadīth* is of the qualified class of general *ḥadīth*. It may be beneficial because of the special property of that land, and that particular soil, for every poison. There is however a point which must be clarified, namely that one of the conditions for the patient to benefit from medicine is that he should accept it and believe in its usefulness; then the constitution will accept the medicine and use its assistance to repel the illness.[5] Indeed, many treatments can be more beneficial if the patient believes and accepts them with complete trust. People have seen remarkable examples of this. This benefit is because the constitution has accepted the medicine enthusiastically, and the soul is gladdened thereby. The faculty is restored, and the sovereignty of the constitution is strengthened and the innate heat is sent forth, so that it assists in the repulsion of the harmful agent. Conversely, there are many medicines which are beneficial for an illness, but their action is hindered because the patient has no real confidence in them. The constitution fails to accept it, and no improvement is achieved.

Consider that in relation to the greatest of medicines and draughts, the most beneficial to hearts and bodies for this life and the return, and this world and the Hereafter: the Qur'ān, which is healing for every illness. Now it does not benefit hearts which do not trust that it contains healing and benefit; rather, it only increases their sickness. For the healing of hearts, there is no medicine whatever more beneficial than the Qur'ān. It is their complete and perfect healing, which leaves no sickness without cure, preserving for them their absolute health, and affording them complete protection against all harm or damage. Nevertheless, the aversion of most people's hearts to it, their lack of absolute belief in it, their failure to use it, their turning from it to medicines which have been compounded by people who work on conjecture—all this comes between them and healing from the Qur'ān. As habits predominate and aversion grows stronger, illnesses and chronic ailments are anchored in the hearts. Both the sick and the physicians become familiar with and can relate

5 In this section, IQ turns to the point which interests him: faith in the treatment is far more likely to produce good results. He extends this principle to support his belief in the efficacy of the Qur'ān; where this has no effect, the reason lies in the patient's lack of faith. He follows this with a rather disparaging view of the current state of medicine.

only to treatments prescribed by their priests and those whom they honour and hold in high esteem from within their own culture. So the affliction increases, and their illness becomes chronic, and diseases grow complex and the treatment becomes elusive. Whenever they apply these new treatments, the illness is but transformed, altered and greatly increased as if the situation repeats the words of the poet:

Of all the amazing things, how extraordinary, healing is near, and yet beyond reach;

Like the good camels in the desert, they die of thirst, carrying water on their backs.

CHAPTER

18

Prophetic guidance on diet

(a) *Rectifying food by opposites*

IT IS confirmed in the two books of the *Ṣaḥīḥ*, from *ḥadīth* of ʿAbd-Allāh b. Jaʿfar: 'I saw the Messenger of God ﷺ eating fresh dates (*ruṭab*) with cucumber (*qiththā'*)'.[90]

Ruṭab is hot and moist in the second degree; it strengthens and suits the cold stomach and is an aphrodisiac. But it is quick to decompose, causes thirst, disturbs the blood, causes headache, brings about obstruction and pain of the bladder, and is harmful to the teeth.

Cucumber is cold and moist in the second degree; it quenches thirst, restores the faculties because of its fragrance and extinguishes the heat of the inflamed stomach. When its seeds are dried and pounded, squeezed out with water and drunk, they quench thirst and are diuretic and beneficial for pain of the bladder. When pounded and sieved, used as a dentifrice, they clean the teeth. When the leaf is pounded and made into a dressing with cooked grape juice it is beneficial for the bite of a mad dog.

In short, the one is hot and the other cold.[1] Each of them contains rectification for the other and can prevent most of its ill effects. Each quality withstands its opposite and its fierceness is repelled by the other quality. This is the basis of all treatment, and a basis for the preservation of health; even more, the whole science of medicine makes use of this principle. The use of it and similar principles in foods and medicines contains their rectification and a moderating action, and it repels any harmful qualities they may contain, through what opposes them. In this medical principle there is assistance for the body's health, strength and well-being.

ʿĀ'isha said: 'They tried to fatten me with all sorts of things, but I did not put on weight. Then they gave me cucumber and dates and I did get plumper.'

In short, repelling harmful effects of the cold with the hot, the hot with the

1 The Prophet's use of cucumber (cold) and dates (hot) in combination is given as an example of the need to combine foods with opposite qualities, thus providing rectification and adjustment (*ṣalāḥ*) for each other. Cf. Chapter 34.

cold, of the moist with the dry and the dry with the moist—moderating one of them with the other—is one of the most effective means of treatment and preservation of health.

The near equivalent to that has already been mentioned, in the Prophet's ﷺ instruction for senna and *sannūt,* the latter being honey containing a little fat, whereby the senna is rectified and moderated.[2]

So, the blessing and peace of God upon him who was sent to bring prosperity to the hearts and bodies, and promote welfare for this world and the next.

(b) *Prophylaxis by diet* (ḥimya)[3]

Medicine in its entirety has two aspects: diet and the preservation of health. For when there is any sort of inappropriate mingling (*takhlīṭ*), there is need for appropriate evacuation. Thus medicine as a whole revolves around these three fundamental rules.

Prophylactic diet is of two sorts: precautions against what could bring on illness and precautions against what could increase it, so as to keep it within its present state. The first is diet for the healthy, the second is diet for the sick. When the sick person takes precautions in his diet, his illness stops increasing, and the faculties begin to repel it.

The principle for prophylaxis is found in the words of the Most High: *If you are ill, or on a journey, or one of you comes from the privy, or you have been in contact with women, or you do not find water, then cleanse yourselves with clean sand* (v : 6). Thus he protected the sick from the use of water which might harm them.

It is related in Ibn Māja's *Sunan,* and elsewhere, from Umm al-Mundhir bint Qays al-Anṣāriyya: The Messenger of God ﷺ came into my room accompanied by ʿAlī, who was then convalescing from an illness. Now we had some date clusters hanging there. The Messenger of God ﷺ got up to eat some of them, and so did ʿAlī. Then the Messenger of God ﷺ began to say to ʿAlī: 'You are convalescing', until he stopped. (Then, she continued): I made some barley and chard, and brought it; and the Prophet ﷺ said to ʿAlī: 'Take some of this, for it is more beneficial for you.' In another version, he said: 'Take from this, for it is more suitable for you'.[91]

Likewise in the *Sunan* of Ibn Māja, from Ṣuhayb, who said: I went up to the Prophet ﷺ when he had bread and dates before him, and he said: 'Come close, and eat.' So I took a date and ate it. He said: 'Are you eating dates when you have ophthalmia?' I replied: 'O Messenger of God I am chewing on the other side.' And he smiled.[92]

A well-known *ḥadīth* from the Prophet ﷺ says: Indeed when God loves a

2 *Sannūt*: See Chapter 11, n.4

3 Prophylaxis by diet: *ḥimya* implies precautionary measures, protection, from *ḥamā,* to defend or guard.

servant, He protects him (*ḥamāhu*) from this world, as one of you protects his patient from food and drink. In another version: Indeed God protects His believing servant from this world.[93]

There is a *ḥadīth* current on the tongues of many people: Diet is the chief part of medicine, and the stomach is the site of illness, so treat every body with what it is accustomed to. Now this *ḥadīth* is only from the words of al-Ḥārith b. Kalada, the Arab physician, and it is not correct to attribute it to the Prophet ﷺ. Several of the leading *ḥadīth* scholars have said this.

On the authority of the Prophet ﷺ it says: 'The stomach is the pool of the body, and the veins lead to it. When the stomach is healthy, the veins convey health from it; when the stomach is ill, the veins convey illness.'

Al-Ḥārith said: The chief part of medicine is taking precautions in diet. Among them, precautionary measures of diet for the healthy are considered harmful, at the same level as mixing foodstuffs for the sick and the convalescent.[4] The most beneficial sort of diet is for the one convalescing from illness. For his constitution has not returned to its full strength, the digestive faculty is weak, the constitution receptive and the organs susceptible to illness so mixing food causes a relapse, which at this stage is more serious than at the start of his illness.

Know that when the Prophet ﷺ prevented ʿAlī from eating date clusters while he was convalescent, this was an example of using good common sense in diet; for cluster dates are branches of fresh dates, hung up in the house to be eaten, after the manner of bunches of grapes. Fruit is harmful to one recuperating from an illness because it is quick to decompose, and the constitution is too weak to expel it, since its faculties have not yet regained full strength, and it is busy with repelling the effects of the illness and making it leave the body. In fresh dates there is especially a kind of heaviness upon the stomach; in being occupied with treating and rectifying this foodstuff, the constitution is distracted from its aim of putting an end to the remains of the illness and its effects, whether these remains are static or increasing. When the Prophet found before him chard and barley, he ordered ʿAlī to take from it. It is one of the most beneficial of foods for a convalescent: barley water contains qualities of cooling and nourishing, alleviation and softening, strengthening the constitution, such as is more suitable to the convalescent, especially when cooked with roots of chard. This is one of the most suitable of foods for anyone with weakness of the stomach, as no dangerous humours are generated from it.

Zayd b. Aslam said: ʿUmar fasted from food during an illness until, from the intensity of this abstinence, he was sucking at date stones.

To sum up: prophylaxis through diet is among the greatest of measures

4 A restricted diet for the healthy is considered as harmful as an unrestricted diet for the sick and the convalescent. The idea behind the restricted diet for the convalescent is that the constitution (*ṭabīʿa*) cannot muster the requisite strength to deal with more complex foods when it is already weakened and fully occupied with repelling the actual illness. Cf. Chapter 24.

before illness strikes, for it prevents its occurrence. If it does occur, this prevents it from developing and spreading.

(c) *Appropriate foods for the sick*

It should be known that much of what is forbidden to the sick, the convalescent and the healthy can in certain cases not cause damage, but rather can be of benefit.[5] This is when the appetite grows strong again and the constitution desires it, and a little is taken which the constitution is able to digest. The constitution and the stomach both accept it eagerly and with desire, and they rectify whatever harm had been feared from it. It may even be more useful than taking medicine which the constitution abhors and rejects.

Therefore the Prophet ﷺ agreed that Ṣuhayb, when suffering from ophthalmia, could take a few dates, and he knew that they would not harm him.

Of this type is the narrative concerning ʿAlī, when he had ophthalmia and entered the presence of the Messenger of God ﷺ who had before him dates which he was eating. He said: 'O ʿAlī, do you want some?' and threw him a date, then another until he had thrown seven to him. Then he said: 'Sufficient for you, O ʿAlī.'[94]

Similar, too, is the narrative of Ibn Māja in his *Sunan*, from a *ḥadīth* of ʿIkrima, from Ibn ʿAbbās, that the Prophet ﷺ visited a man, and said to him: 'What food do you desire?' He replied: 'I really want some wheat bread.' (In another version: 'I want some dry biscuit'). So the Prophet ﷺ said: 'Who has some wheat bread? Let him send it to his brother.' Then he said: 'When one of you has a patient who desires anything, give it to him to eat.'[95]

This *ḥadīth* contains a subtle medical secret. For if a sick person takes what he desires, from true natural hunger, even if this food has some potential harm, it is actually more beneficial and less harmful than something he does not want, even if this is beneficial in itself. For the true appetite and the desire of the constitution will repel the harm. But the constitution's aversion and dislike of something beneficial can harm it. In short, if anything is delicious and desired, the constitution will accept it eagerly and will digest it in the best way, especially when the soul reaches towards it with a true appetite and genuine vigour.

God knows best.

5 Here IQ reverts to an earlier discussion on the value of food which the patient desires, irrespective of its objective utility. See Chapter 15 and Chapter 33.

CHAPTER

19

Treatment of ophthalmia (*ramad*)[1]

IT HAS been related already how the Prophet ﷺ forbade Ṣuhayb dates, not allowing him to eat them while he was suffering from ophthalmia. And he forbade ʿAlī to eat fresh dates when ophthalmia had afflicted him.

Abū Nuʿaym said in his book, *The Medicine of the Prophet*, that when one of the wives of the Prophet ﷺ was suffering from ophthalmia, he did not have intercourse with her until her eye was healed.

Ophthalmia is a hot inflammation occurring in the conjunctival layer of the eye, which is its external whiteness. The cause is an effusion of one of the four humours; or a hot wind that increases in quantity in the head and the body, so that some of it is sent outwards to the substance of the eye; or a blow to the eye, so that the constitution sends to it a large amount of blood and essence, thereby seeking to heal it from this accident. For this reason, the member that has been struck becomes inflamed. As in all other similar cases this requires treatment by its opposite.

Just as two vapours rise from the earth into the air—one hot and dry, the other hot and moist—and come together as high clouds, they prevent us from seeing the sky; likewise, something similar rises from the lowest part of the stomach to its furthest limit, hindering the sight, and thence various ailments are generated. If the constitution overcomes the vapour, and pushes it to the nose, it causes a cold; if it pushes it to the uvula and nostrils, it causes choking; if to the rib area, pleurisy; if to the chest, catarrh; if it descends to the heart, it causes stroke; if to the eye, it causes ophthalmia. If it descends to the abdomen, it causes a discharge of liquid; if it pushes it to the regions of the brain, it causes loss of memory; if the vessels of the brain are moistened with it, filling its veins,

1 Ophthalmia (*ramad*), its treatment is by rest and refraining from any possible aggravation. IQ follows usual medical texts in describing *ramad* as a hot inflammation (*waram*) in the conjunctival layer (*al-ṭabaqa al-multaḥama*), explaining this latter as the external (*ẓāhir*) white area (*bayāḍ*). He gives several possible causes. He also describes how a single humour or vapour can cause widely differing ills according to the region or organ where it arrives, and here includes headache and migraine (see Chapter 14, n.1). Ophthalmia is mentioned in *ḥadīth*: Bukhārī, *Ṭibb* 18, VII. 408.

it causes deep sleep. Thus sleep is moist, and insomnia dry. If the vapour seeks to escape from the head, without being able to, this brings on headache and insomnia. If the vapour inclines to one of the two halves of the head, it brings on migraine. If it takes over the crown of the head and the centre of the very top of the head, the consequence is the illness called *bayḍa*. If the membrane dividing the brain is cooled, warmed or moistened by it, and from it winds are stirred up, this causes sneezing. If it stirs up the phlegmy moisture in it, until the innate heat is predominant, it causes fainting and attacks of unconsciousness. If it stirs up the black bile, darkening the atmosphere of the brain, it causes melancholic delusions. If vapour overflows into the nerve vessels, it causes constitutional epilepsy. If the entirety of the nerves of the brain are moistened and the moisture overflows into its vessels, the consequence is paralysis. If the vapour is from yellow bile, inflaming and heating the brain, it causes frenitis. If the chest is also involved, it will mean pleurisy. So you should understand this division.[2]

We see, then, that the humours of the body and head are agitated and stirred up in the condition of ophthalmia. Sexual intercourse is one of the causes of their increased movement and agitation, since it causes a complete movement of the body, the spirit and the constitution. The body inevitably becomes warmer, and the soul increases its movement, seeking pleasure and its fulfilment. The spirit moves also, following the movement of the soul and the body. The primary connection of the spirit with the body is by the heart from which the spirit arises and is sent forth into the parts of the body. The movement of the constitution is in order to send forth that amount of semen which is necessary. In short, intercourse is an inclusive general movement, in which the body and its faculties, its constitution and humours, the spirit and the soul all move. Every movement arouses and thins the humours, and brings about their repulsion and their flow to the weak parts. When the eye is suffering from ophthalmia, it is in its weakest possible state, and the movement of coitus is then most harmful. Hippocrates said in his *Aphorisms*: 'Travel by ship may show that movement agitates the body.' This is true despite the fact that ophthalmia also contains benefits. It requires abstention, evacuation, cleansing of the head and body from their superfluities and decomposed matters, refraining from any anger, worry and grief that may harm the soul and body, and avoiding any violent movement and troublesome work. In a tradition of the ancestors: Do not despise ophthalmia, for it cuts the roots of blindness.

Among the means for its treatment are continual quiet and rest, leaving the eye alone, and not touching it. To disregard these instructions would bring down a flow of matters to the eye. One of our ancestors has said: The friends of Muḥammad are like the eye; and medicine for the eye is to refrain from touching it.

In a *ḥadīth* (*marfūʿ*)—God knows best—we find: 'Treatment for ophthalmia

2 Frenitis: *sirsām*, pleurisy: *birsām*. At an earlier stage there was confusion between the two terms. See discussion in Ullmann, *Medicine*, 28–30.

is to drop cold water into the eye.' This is one of the best remedies for hot ophthalmia, for water is a cold remedy that is used to extinguish the heat of the ophthalmia, when it is hot. Therefore ʿAbd-Allāh b. Masʿūd said to his wife Zaynab, when she suffered from pain in her eye: 'If you were to do as the Messenger of God ﷺ did, it would be best for you and more suitable to bring about a cure. You sprinkle cold water in your eye, then say, "Lord of mankind, expel this evil and cure me, O You Who are the Healer, there is no healing save Yours, a healing which does not leave any illness".'[96]

This treatment, as we have already said frequently, is iṇtended in particular for certain lands and certain types of eye ailments. Do not take as particular and specific of the words of the Prophet ﷺ what is meant to be universal and general, nor the universal and general to be particular and specific, for this would lead to errors and incorrect conclusions.

God knows best.

CHAPTER

20

Paralysis (*khadrān*)[1]

ABU ʿUBAYD in *Gharīb al-ḥadīth,* from *ḥadīth* of Abū ʿUthmān al-Nahdi, said that a group of people passed by a tree and ate from it; then it was as if a wind passed by them and made them numb. The Prophet ﷺ said: 'Cool some water in the water-skins (*shinān*) and pour it over them, during the time between the two calls to prayer.' Abū ʿUbayd continued: 'Cool' (*qarrisū*) means make it cold. For people say 'the cold has become severe' (*qaras*) and it is written with *sīn* not *ṣād*. *Shinān* means the water containers (*asqiya*) and both words are the same as *qirab* and old water-skins *shann* (pl. *shinān*). These types of water-skin are mentioned, rather than water jars, because they are better at cooling water. When the Prophet ﷺ said 'between the two calls to prayer', this indicates between the call for the dawn prayer and the standing for prayer (*iqāma*), but he named the latter also the call to prayer (*adhān*).

Some physicians have said that this treatment recommended by the Prophet ﷺ is one of the best kinds of treatment for this illness, when it occurs in the Ḥijāz, for it is a hot dry country, and the innate heat is weak in the interiors of its inhabitants. So pouring cold water on them at this particular time—the coldest time of the day—would bring together the natural heat, dispersed throughout the body, which carries all its powers. This treatment would strengthen the repulsive faculty, collecting together from the extremities of the body to its interior, which is the site of that illness. Thus it would assist the remainder of the faculties to repel this illness and would repel it, with the permission of God, the Glorious One. Had Hippocrates or Galen or others prescribed this treatment for this illness, physicians would have followed them and been amazed at the perfection of their knowledge.

1 *Khadrān,* a total 'paralysis' or numbness. IQ reports *ḥadīth* with variant terms for water-skins, all indicating the same items, i.e. skins rather than earthenware jars. He draws attention to the time of day and explains that cold water at a cold time will stimulate the body's powers, especially the faculty of repelling external influences (*al-quwwa al-dāfiʿa*).

CHAPTER

21

Rectifying food into which flies have fallen[1]

IN THE two books of the *Ṣaḥīḥ*, from a *ḥadīth* of Abū Hurayra, the Messenger of God ﷺ said: 'If a fly falls into the water container of any one of you, then immerse it; for in one of its wings is illness; in the other a cure.'[97]

In Ibn Māja's *Sunan*, from Abū Saʿīd al-Khudrī, the Messenger of God ﷺ said: 'One of the fly's wings is poison, and the other a cure. When it falls into food, immerse it; for it brings the poison forward, holds back the cure.'[98]

This *ḥadīth* has two main points: legal and medical; the legal aspect is that the *ḥadīth* proves the purity of water and liquid, where flies are found dead. This is the consensus of all scholars, and in no way is it opposed by the ancestors.

So the Prophet ﷺ ordered the fly to be immersed, that is to be immersed completely in the food. Of course it will then die especially if the food is hot. Now if this caused impurity the order of the Prophet ﷺ would have entailed spoiling the food, whereas he in fact ordered its rectification. This judgement is extended to everything without a 'life flow'—such as bees, hornets, spiders, and similar creatures. Thus a rule becomes general when its cause is general, and does not apply when the cause is absent. Since the cause of contamination is blood confined in an animal by its death, the rule does not apply in the case of a creature without any blood flow; it is irrelevant because its cause does not exist.

The jurists who rule that the bones of dead animals contain no impurities cite this latter case in support of their view as this ruling proves the purity of the entire creature (ie. flies etc.) despite all the moisture, superfluities and fluids it contains. Therefore it is even more appropriate to confirm the purity in the case of

1 Flies (*dhubāb*), their poison, and the 'antidote' which they are said to carry. The Prophet's order to immerse a fly in liquid—which would kill the fly within the liquid—did not make the food ritually unclean, since the fly has no 'life flow' (*nafs sā'ila*). A creature without blood cannot therefore cause uncleanness.

bones as they are furthest away from moistures, superfluities and blood. This is a very strong argument which should be favoured.

The first person in Islam who is recorded to have spoken about this, saying: 'that which has no life flow' was Ibrāhīm al-Nakhaʿī, and the jurists have taken this from him. 'Life' here is interpreted as blood. For example the phrase concerning a woman who had *nafasat* means that she loses blood by menstruation, while *nufisat* means that she gives birth.

As for the medical meaning, when Abū ʿUbayd said: 'Immerse it,' it means drown it so that the cure can come out from it, just as the illness has come out. It is said of two men 'they immerse one another' when they push each other under the water.

Flies contain a poisonous faculty, which is shown by the inflammation and itching that occur from their bite, and this is a kind of weapon. When they fall into something which harms them, they use their weapons to protect themselves. The Prophet ﷺ ordered people to oppose this poison by the cure that God, praised be He, had consigned to it within its other wing. One drowns the whole creature in the water and the food, so that the poisonous substance is opposed by the beneficial, and its harm ceases. This is medicine to which the greatest physicians and their leading men could not be guided, and it can only emerge through the light of prophethood. Despite this, the learned, aware, and successful physician accedes to the treatment, and acknowledges that the one who brings it is the most perfect of creation, without exception, and that he is assisted by divine revelation which is beyond human power.

More than one physician has said that, when the place of the sting of the hornet and scorpion is rubbed with flies, this gives clear benefit and relieves it. This is only due to the healing substance which it contains. When flies, after their heads have been cut off, are rubbed on an inflammation that occurs in the eyelash, known as *shaʿra*, the flies cure it.

CHAPTER

22

Pustules (*bathra*), inflammations (*awrām*), and abscesses (*khurājāt*)[1]

IBN AL-SUNNĪ quotes in his book one of the wives of the Prophet ﷺ saying: The Messenger of God ﷺ arrived in my room, and a pustule had broken out on my finger. He asked: 'Do you have any sweet rush?' I replied: 'Yes,' and he said: 'Put that on the place, and then say: "O Lord! You Who reduce what is large, Who enlarge what is small, reduce my affliction".'[99]

Sweet rush (*dharīra*, acorus) is an Indian medicine taken from the stalk of the sweet rush. It is hot and dry, good for inflammation of the stomach and liver and for dropsy, and strengthens the heart by its sweetness.

It is related in the two books of the *Ṣaḥīḥ*, from ʿĀ'isha: I perfumed the Messenger of God ﷺ with my own hand with the sweet rush in the Farewell Pilgrimage, before he put on the two garments for *iḥrām* (state of ritual purity) and whilst he was wearing them.[100]

Pustules are small abscesses that are caused by hot matter rejected by the constitution, so that it seeks a soft place on the body where they can come out; they need what will coct them and expel them. Sweet rush is one of the things which have this effect on them, for it contains a power of coction and dispersal together with a sweetness of scent. But it also contains a power to cool the fieriness that is in that substance. Therefore Ibn Sīnā said: There is naught better for burns by fire than sweet rush with oil of rose and vinegar.

It is reported that ʿAlī said: I went with the Messenger of God ﷺ to visit a man who was suffering from inflammation on his back. They said: 'O Messenger of God, this has pus in it.' He said: 'Incise it.' ʿAlī continued: 'Without delay it was incised, while the Prophet ﷺ was watching.'

It is reported from Abū Hurayra that the Prophet ﷺ ordered a physician to incise the abdomen of a man whose abdomen was afflicted; the Prophet ﷺ

1 Treatment of pustules (*buthra*, pl. *buthūr*) by medication and incantation together. Inflammations (*awrām*) and abscesses (*khurājāt*) which are cured by incision (*baṭṭ*) and lancing (*bazl*).

was asked: 'O Messenger of God, will medicine be of benefit?' He replied: 'He Who sent down illness, sent down healing as He wills.'[2]

Inflammation is matter that locates itself in the organ, from superfluity of an unnatural matter that flows to it. This is found in all kinds of illnesses. The matters from which it arises are the four humours, the watery element and the wind. When inflammation collects together, it is called an abscess. Every hot inflammation will progress into one of three states: to dissolution, to collection of pus, or to change into hardness. If the faculty is strong, it overcomes the matter of the inflammation and dissolves it, which is the best of the circumstances to which the state of inflammation can lead. If less strong, it cocts the matter and changes it to white pus, and it opens a place to make it flow out. If the faculty cannot achieve that, it changes the matter into pus of incomplete coction and is unable to open a place in the organ by which to expel it. So there is a risk of putrefaction in the organ when it remains inside it for a long time. Then, the assistance of a physician is needed to expel, through incision or some other means, the poisonous matter that is harming the organ.[3]

Incision has two advantages: to expel the poisonous matter, and to prevent the collection of other matters to it, which might make it worse.

As for the words of the Prophet ﷺ in the second *ḥadīth*, that he ordered a physician to incise a man's afflicted abdomen, the word for afflicted (*ajwā*) has several meanings, including putrefying liquid that is in the abdomen, whence arises dropsy.

Physicians have differed regarding the use of lancing to expel this matter. One group forbids it because of its danger and the remote possibility of regaining health. Another group permits it, when there is no other treatment. In their opinion that is only for dropsy in the skin. As we have said, there are three kinds of inflammation: (1) membraneous, where the abdomen is swollen with a windy matter. When it is struck a sound is given out like the sound of a drum; (2) fleshy, where the flesh of the whole body increases with phlegmy matter, which diffuses with the blood into the limbs. This is more difficult than the first to treat; (3) cutaneous, where a poisonous matter collects in the lower abdomen, so that with any movement a shaking sound is heard like the sloshing of water in a skin. This condition is the worst kind, according to the majority of physicians, though one group says the worst kind is the fleshy because the damage is widespread.

The various types of treatment for the cutaneous kind includes expulsion of that water by lancing, which is the equivalent to phlebotomy for veins to expel corrupt blood. But it is dangerous, as we have said. If this *ḥadīth* is confirmed then it is a proof of permission to carry out lancing.

God knows best.

2 A man whose abdomen was afflicted (*ajwā baṭnuhu*) ie. with a long-standing complaint. Cf. Chapter 6, n.1.

3 His explanation of the cause of inflammation and abscess seeks to show that incision is merely assisting nature when the faculty (*quwwa*) is unable to expel the corrupt matter. For dropsy (*istisqā'*) see Chapter 6.

CHAPTER

23

Treatment of the sick by reassurance and encouragement

IBN MĀJA relates in his *Sunan,* from a *ḥadīth* of Abū Saʿīd al-Khudrī, that the Messenger of God ﷺ said: 'When you go in to a sick person, reassure him concerning his appointed life-span; for that does not contradict the decree, and it sets the patient's mind at ease.'[101]

This *ḥadīth* contains one of the most noble of all kinds of treatment. This is guidance to whatever will invigorate the soul of the patient, through words which will strengthen his constitution, revive his strength and increase his innate heat. The soul and the innate heat will assist each other to repel or alleviate the illness, which is the aim of the physician.

Giving joy to the patient's soul, and bringing pleasure to his heart and whatever will make him happy will have a wonderful effect in curing and alleviating his illness. For the vital spirits and the faculties grow strong thereby and they assist the constitution in repelling the harmful agent. People have seen the faculties of many of the sick revived at the visit of one whom they love and hold in respect, by seeing such people, by the gracious treatment they are given and their talking with them. That is one of the advantages of visiting the sick. Visiting the sick has four kinds of advantages, one that returns to the patient, one to the person who visits, one to the family of the patient, one to people in general.

It has already been mentioned, concerning the guidance of the Prophet ﷺ, that he used to enquire of the patient what was his trouble and how he felt. He would ask him about what he desired, and would place his hand on his forehead, and sometimes place it at the centre of his chest. He would make supplication for him, and would prescribe for him what would benefit him in his illness.

Sometimes he would perform ritual ablution (*wuḍū'*) and pour some of that water over the sick person.[1] Sometimes he would say to the patient: 'No harm shall come to you, only purification, by the Will of God.' That is the most perfect of treatment, courtesy and consolation.

1 Stressing the psychological side of sickness: the importance of reassuring and encouraging the sick person. The practice of pouring over the patient water to which *baraka* has been imparted—in this case by contact with the Prophet—is seen partly as transference of strength to combat illness.

CHAPTER

24

Treatment by such medicines and foods as patients are accustomed to[1]

(a) *General principles*

THIS IS a very important principle of treatment and is a most useful tenet. If the physician ignores it, he injures the patient just where he thinks that he benefits him. Only an ignorant physician would replace this with such medicaments as he finds in the books of medicine. For the suitability of medicines and foods to the body depends on the body's preparation and acceptance of them. Those meant here are the people of the desert lands and the tillers of the soil and others; they would gain no benefit from draughts of water-lily (*nīlūfar*) or dried rose, nor smilax (*mughlā*), and it would have no effect whatever on their constitutions. Most of the medicines used by those who lead a settled and comfortable life would not be helpful for them. This principle has been proved by experience.

If anyone considers carefully the prophetic treatment we have outlined, he will see it all to be appropriate to the habits and the environment of the patient, and what he has been brought up on. This is one of the important principles of treatment, to which careful attention must be paid. It was pointed out by the most excellent of the physicians. The one known as the physician of the Arabs, or rather the greatest physician, al-Ḥārith ibn Kalada, who was to them what Hippocrates was to his people, said that abstinence is the chief part of medicine, and the stomach is the site of illness; each body must be treated by what it is accustomed to. He is also quoted as saying: abstention is medicine. Abstention

1 Giving accustomed foods and medicines to the sick; this follows on from the previous principle, and is both psychological and medical: familiar items are unlikely to cause anxiety, while the state of the body and its customary environment and habits will influence the efficacy of any treatment. Cf. Chapter 15. IQ again refers to the difference between settled and bedouin life, with their respective diet and customs. Cf. Chapter 1 e, n. 4.

is refraining from food, and means hunger.[2] This is one of the greatest medicines in the cure of all illnesses of repletion, and it is even more excellent in their treatment than evacuants, provided there is no risk from the intensity of repletion, agitation, fierceness and boiling over of the humours.

When he says: 'the stomach is the site of illness', the stomach is a muscular hollow organ, shaped like a gourd, composed of three layers made up of fine, muscular slivers, known as fibres, surrounded by the flesh. The fibres of one layer are lengthwise, of the other breadthwise and of the third diagonal. The mouth of the stomach is more muscular, and its hollow more fleshy, and within it is a rough fibrous surface. It is protected in the centre of the abdomen, inclining somewhat more to the right side. It was created in this form through the subtle wisdom of the wise Creator, praised be He. Yet it is the site of illness. It is the place of the first digestion. Here the food is cocted, and then it flows down to the liver and the intestines. From this process some superfluities are left behind in the stomach, which the digestive faculty is not able to digest completely. This residue may be the result of the excess in the quantity of the food, or its inferior quality, or that it was consumed in the wrong order, or indeed for all these reasons put together. Some of these are things that no human being can in general escape from; therefore, the stomach is the site of illness. This indicates an encouragement to take only a little food, to prevent the soul from following its appetites, and to guard against superfluities.

Habit is like nature for the human being, and for this reason there is a saying: Habit is the second nature.[3] It is an important power in the body, to the point where one and the same substance, in relation to bodies whose habits differ, will have a different relationship to each, even if the bodies are in conformity in other respects. For example, consider three bodies of hot temperament in their youth: one of them is accustomed to taking hot things, the second is accustomed to taking cold things and the third is accustomed to taking moderate things. Now, when the first one takes honey, it will not harm him; when the second one takes it, it will harm him; and the third it will harm only a little. Habit is an important basic pillar of the preservation of health and treatment of illnesses. Therefore, the Prophet's treatment would confirm that everybody keep to his accustomed habits in the use of foods and medicines and other things.

2 Abstinence, *ḥimya*: see Chapter 18. This is properly 'prophylaxis by diet'. The word 'abstention' is here used to translate *azm* which more specifically refers to abstinence from food, rather than precautionary measures of a more general nature.

3 Habit, or custom: *al-ʿāda ṭabʿ thānin*; he calls it also an important basic principle (*rukn ʿaẓīm*). See Chapter 34, n. 4.

(b) *On feeding the patient with the most refined and light food he is accustomed to*[4]

In the two books of the *Ṣaḥīḥ*, from a *ḥadīth* of ʿUrwa, from ʿĀ'isha, it says: Whenever someone from her own people died, the women would gather together for that reason; when all had dispersed except for her family and close friends, she would order an earthenware pot of *talbīna* to be cooked, then a *tharīd* would be made, and the *talbīna* poured over it. Then she would say to the women: Eat of it, for indeed I have heard the Messenger of God ﷺ say: '*Talbīna* is a relaxation for the heart of the sick person, it disperses some of the sorrow.'[102]

In the *Sunan*, also from a *ḥadīth* of ʿĀ'isha: The Messenger of God ﷺ said: 'You must have what you find unpleasant but beneficial: the *talbīna*.'[103] She said: 'Whenever one of the family of the Messenger of God ﷺ was troubled by sickness, the pot never left the fire until he reached one of his two extremes', meaning, until he was cured or died. She related also: When someone said to the Messenger of God ﷺ: 'Such a one is in pain, and he is not eating any food,' he would say: 'You must make *talbīna*; give it to him to drink, like soup.' And he would say: 'By Him Who holds my soul in his hand, it cleanses the belly of any one of you, just as one of you women would wash dirt from her face'.[104]

(c) *Talbīna*

Talbīna is thin soup that has the consistency of yoghurt (*laban*), whence its name is derived. Al-Harawī said: It was named *talbīna* from its resemblance to yoghurt because it is white and thin. This food is beneficial to a sick person because it is thin and cooked, not thick and raw. If you wish to know the merits of *talbīna*, see how good is barley water. Yet this is even better than barley water for the sick. For it is a broth taken from barley flour with its husks. The difference between this and barley water is that the latter is cooked whole while *talbīna* is cooked with ground barley. It is more beneficial, because the special property of the barley is released through grinding.

It has already been noted that habits have an influence on the usefulness of medicines and foods. The habit of a particular people was to make barley water from ground barley, not whole. The former contains more nourishment and is

4 Most refined and light (*alṭaf*), exemplified by *talbīna*, made with barley and water, much of the consistency of milk or yoghurt—hence the name—and *tharīd*, soup with meat. IQ here discusses thin gruelly food, which includes barley water (*ma' al-shaʿīr*). *Talbīna* he considers superior to barley water, which is made with whole barley, since *talbīna* is made of ground (*maṭḥūn*) barley with its husks. See also *talbīna* in Part II. *ḥadīth* on *talbīna*: Bukhārī, *Aṭʿima* 24, VII. 244f., *Ṭibb* 8, VII. 401 f. *Tharīd*: *Aṭʿima* 25, VII. 244–45.

IQ combines humoral and psychological explanations for the effect of *talbīna*. Either its heat disperses the cold of melancholy, or its moisture dispels the dryness of sorrow. These effects in turn influence the heart; or there may be some unhealthy humour which it repels.

stronger in its action, and it has a greater power to cleanse. The physicians in towns used whole barley so that the barley water would be thinner and more refined, and thus not heavy on the patient's constitution. This practice is in accordance with the city folk, whose constitutions are soft, so barley water made from ground barley would be heavy on them.

The point here is that barley water if cooked with whole barley penetrates swiftly, has an obvious cleansing action and provides subtle nourishment. When it is drunk hot, it cleanses better, it is swifter to penetrate, and it is better able to increase the innate heat, and more effectively adheres to the surfaces of the stomach.

His words: 'It has relaxation for the heart of the sick person,' can be read in two ways: *majamma*, and *mujimma*. The former is better known: it means that it brings him happiness, that is, makes him happy and tranquil. The word is from *ijmām* which means rest (*rāḥa*). His words: 'It disperses some of the sorrow'—God knows best—mean that distress and sorrow both make the temperament cold and weaken the innate heat, because they are carried by a spirit which inclines toward the heart where these feelings originate, and as this broth increases the innate heat by increasing its substance, thus it disperses most of the anxiety and sorrow which had come upon it.

It may be said—and this is nearer the truth—that broth removes some of the sorrow because it contains a special property similar to those contained in the foods which cheer. There are some foods that bring delight by their special property. God knows best.

It may be said: The faculties of a sorrowful person are weakened because dryness predominates over his organs, especially over his stomach, because he takes so little food. This broth moistens it, strengthens it and nourishes it, and has much the same effect on the heart of the patient. It often happens, however, that some bilious phlegmy or purulent humour collects in the patient's stomach, and this broth clears the humour from the stomach and dispels it, reduces it and dilutes it, and modifies its quality, breaks its vehemence, and puts the stomach at rest. This is especially so for the person who is accustomed to feed on barley bread. This was a habit of the people of Madīna, at that time. It was their staple food, for wheat was expensive in their region. God knows best.

CHAPTER

25

On poison, magic, and emesis (*qay'*)

(a) *The treatment of the poisoning*[1] *of the Prophet* ﷺ *at Khaybar*[2]

ᶜABD AL-RAZZĀQ reported, from Maᶜmar, from al-Zuhrī, from ᶜAbd al-Raḥmān b. Kaᶜb b. Mālik: A Jewish woman gave the Prophet ﷺ a present of a cooked sheep at Khaybar.[3] He asked: 'What is this?' and she replied: 'A gift.' She was careful not to say that it was from the alms tax, or he would not have eaten any of it. So the Prophet ﷺ ate some of it and so did the Companions. Then he said: 'Hold off!' and asked the woman: 'Have you poisoned this sheep?' She asked: 'Who told you of that?' He replied: 'This bone', indicating a leg that he was holding in his hand. Then she said: 'Yes,' and he asked: 'Why?' She replied: 'I wished that, if you are lying, the people should be rid of you; but if you are a prophet, it will not harm you.' The narrative continues: So the Prophet ﷺ was cupped three times on his upper back, and he ordered his Companions to be cupped, so they were. Yet some of them died.[105]

In another version of the narrative, the Messenger of God ﷺ was cupped on his upper back because of sheep's meat that he had eaten. Abū Hind cupped

1 Poisoning: the accepted remedy is cupping. This is seen as the way to expel poison which has entered the bloodstream, and which, if it reaches the heart in any concentration, causes death. For cupping cf. Chapter 8.

2 Khaybar: an oasis town north of Madīna, inhabited by Jewish tribes. In 7 AH Muḥammad led the Muslim forces against the town, and defeated the Jews. It was during this attack that the attempt on his life took place.

3 In this episode, related in the *ḥadīth*, the magic was of the material kind, not consisting of spells alone, and so had to be physically removed and destroyed. IQ here points out that bewitchment or magic (*siḥr*) does not, anyway in this case, imply imperfection, lack of trust or susceptibility to evil, but is to be assessed like any other hazard or illness. In the next section he explains that magic, in general, has the greatest effect on those who are weak in religion or distracted from God, and thus open to attack. Hence the importance of stressing that the magic put upon the Prophet acted only upon his bodily, and to a certain extent mental, faculties, without damaging his heart and soul; nor could it in any way affect his prophetic status and his veracity. The quotation from Abū ᶜUbayda links *siḥr* more closely with *ṭibb* (see Chapter 26).

him, using a horn and a large knife; he was in a protection pact of allegience with the Banu Bayāḍa, of the Anṣār. This trouble remained for a further three years, until the illness from which he died. He said: 'I still feel pain from that morsel I ate of the sheep, the day of Khaybar, until the severance of my aorta.' Thus the Messenger of God ﷺ died a martyr's death.[106]

Mūsā b. ʿUqba said: Treatment for poison is by means of evacuation, and by medicines that oppose and neutralise the poison's action, whether by their qualities or by their specific properties. If anyone does not have medicine available, he should hasten to carry out a complete evacuation; the most beneficial is cupping, especially in hot countries and at hot seasons. The poisonous force spreads into the blood, and thus is sent into the veins and vessels until it reaches the heart, and then death occurs. The blood is the way by which the poison is brought to the heart and the organs. When the poisoned person hastens to let out the blood, that poisonous quality which has mixed with it also goes out. If it is a complete evacuation, the poison will not harm him: either it will be dispersed or it will be weakened, so that the constitution will overcome, annul and weaken its action.

When the Prophet ﷺ was cupped, this treatment was done in the upper part of his back, which is the closest place to the heart where cupping is possible. And the poisonous water went out together with the blood, but not completely, for its weakening effect remained because God, praised be He, wished to give him the perfection of degrees of excellence (by adding the excellence of martyrdom). When God wished to honour him with martyrdom, the effect of that hidden poison appeared, so that God might carry out a matter already decreed. Then appeared the hidden meaning of the words of the Most High to his enemies among the Jews: *Is it that whenever there comes to you a Messenger with what you do not wish, you are puffed up with pride? Some you called impostors, and some [others] you kill!* (11:87). The phrase: *You called them impostors* was in the past tense, for this had already happened and was confirmed, whereas the phrase *you kill them* was in the future which they expected and awaited. God knows best.

(b) *Treatment for magic*

A group of people have denied this event, saying it could not possibly have happened to the Prophet ﷺ, and they considered it as a sign of weakness and imperfection. Yet the matter is not as they claim, but is like any other illness and pain that befell him since it is an illness and that it happened to him is similar to his being poisoned; thus there is no difference between the two cases.

It is confirmed in the two books of the *Ṣaḥīḥ*, from ʿĀ'isha, who said: The Messenger of God ﷺ was bewitched, so that he was made to imagine that he had had intercourse with his wives yet he had not done so.[107] That is the strongest possible sort of magic.

Said the Qāḍī ʿIyāḍ: Bewitchment is an illness, a condition of sickness which could come upon him, like the various kinds of illnesses that befell him which cannot be denied nor do they impair his status as a prophet. As for his being made to imagine that he had done something when he had not, there is no hint here of anything to impair his veracity, since proofs have been established and a consensus reached regarding his infallibility in this concern. This incident was merely one which might occur unexpectedly concerning his worldly affairs—and these were not what he was sent for, nor were they the reason for which he was given preference; in such matters he was as liable to suffer assaults as the rest of humanity. Therefore it is unlikely that he could be made to imagine affairs of this world which did not exist, and afterwards the real state of affairs would become clear to him.

The point here is to relate his guidance concerning the treatment of this illness. It is narrated in two different versions: the first, which is more effective, is that he removed the cause and made it ineffective, as it is reliably said of him: 'that he asked his Lord, praised be He, about the magic and was shown it. So he removed it from a well, and the spell was contained in a comb and combings of hair, and the spathes of the spadix of a male palm tree. When he had removed this, his trouble left him, as if he had been released from a tethering rope.'[108] This is one of the most effective means of treating one who suffers from magic spells, and this is the equivalent of removing the evil matter and expelling it from the body by evacuation.

The second is evacuation in the place which is affected by the magic. Magic has an effect on the constitution and stirs up its humours, confusing the temperaments. When its effect appears in a certain organ and it is possible to evacuate the evil matter from that organ, it is very beneficial to do so.

Abū ʿUbayd mentioned in his book *Gharīb al-ḥadīth*, with his *isnād* from ʿAbd al-Raḥmān b. Abī Laylā, that the Prophet ﷺ was cupped on his head with a horn, when he was bewitched. Abū ʿUbayd said that the meaning of this term 'bewitched' (*ṭubba*) is enchanted (*suḥira*).

This treatment is somewhat incomprehensible for those whose knowledge is limited; they ask: 'What has cupping to do with magic? What is the connection between this illness and this medication?' Yet, if the one asking this had found this treatment recommended by Hippocrates or Ibn Sīnā or someone else, he would have accepted it with submission and would have said: This treatment is determined by one whose knowledge and excellence we do not doubt.

Know that the core substance of the magic with which the Prophet ﷺ was afflicted settled in his head, in one of his faculties within it, so that he imagined he had done something when he had not. That was one way in which the magician acted upon the constitution and the sanguineous matter, whereby that matter became predominant in the forward cavity of the head, thus changing its temperament from its original constitution.

Magic is compounded from the influences of evil spirits and the reaction to them of the natural powers. This is magic of 'mixtures' and is the most severe kind possible, especially in the place where the magic finally settles.[4] Use of cupping on that place whose actions are injured by magic is one of the most useful of treatments when it is carried out according to the decreed methods. Hippocrates said: The things which need to be evacuated must be evacuated from the places to which they are more inclined and by those things which are appropriate for their evacuation.

A group of people have said: When the Messenger of God ﷺ was afflicted by that illness, and he was made to imagine he had done things which he had not done, he thought that was caused by a sanguineous matter or something else that had inclined towards the side of the brain, and had overcome the front cavity of it, and so had made his temperament depart from the natural state. The use of cupping, at that time, was one of the most powerful medicaments and most beneficial of treatments, and so he was cupped. That was before it was revealed to him that the cause was magic. When he received the revelation from God the Most High, telling him that he had been bewitched, he had recourse to the true treatment, which is to expel and nullify the magic. So he asked God, praised be He, and God showed him where it was, so he removed it. Then he stood up, as if he had been released from a tethering rope. The extent to which this magic affected him was limited only to his body and external limbs, not reaching his mind or heart. Therefore, he did not believe the reality of what he was made to imagine, namely that he had had intercourse with his wives, but rather he knew it was imaginary with no truth in it. Such things can occur in some illnesses. God knows best.

Among the most beneficial of treatments for magic are the divine medicines; rather, they are the medicines beneficial for it by their essence. Magic is from the influences of the evil, lower spirits. Their influence will be repelled by that which opposes and resists them: by invocation of the name of God (*dhikr*), recitation of Qur'ānic verses and supplications which cancel the action and effect of the spirits. The stronger and more sincere these supplications are, the more comprehensive and absolute is the protection they render. This is analogous to the meeting of two armies: each one has its troops and its arms, and whichever overcomes the other conquers it and takes control. Thus, when the heart is filled with God, immersed in remembrance of Him, through a daily portion (*wird*) of devotions, supplications, invocations and taking refuge, and wherein the heart truly matches the tongue—this would be one of the most powerful means to prevent the attack of magic, and among the mightiest treatments for it once it has struck.

Concerning magicians, it is held that their magic has an effect only on hearts which are weak and susceptible and on souls whose appetites are attached to

4 Mixtures: the word is given as *tamrījāt*, but might with addition of a dot to the r be *tamzījāt*, connected with *mizāj* (mixture/temperament or constitution). Here again IQ notes the co-operation of psychical and physical factors.

lower things. Therefore, they mostly have an effect on women, on young men, on ignorant people and on desert folk, and on anyone with a weak share of religion, trust and belief in God, or who has no portion in divine worship and in the prayers and invocations of the Prophet ﷺ. In short, its effects are powerful on weak and susceptible hearts, which are inclined to lower things.

It is said that the person bewitched is the one who assists this. We find his heart is attached to something, turns constantly to it, so it gains mastery over his heart by means of its inclination and attention. The evil spirits only gain control over spirits which they find to be prepared for their control over them, through their inclination towards what is associated with those evil spirits, because of their lack of divine power, and inability to fight them. The evil spirits find these human souls empty, desolate, and unprepared, thus left only with an inclination that draws these evil spirits to manipulate them, gain control over them, and their overwhelming hold is consolidated by magic and other means. God knows best.

(c) *Evacuation by emesis* (qay')

Al-Tirmidhī relates in his *Jāmi*ᶜ, from Maᶜdān b. Abī Ṭalḥa, from Abū al-Dardā': The Prophet ﷺ vomited, and then performed *wuḍū'*. I met Thawbān in the mosque of Damascus, and told him that. He replied: 'True, it was I who poured out the water for his *wuḍū'*.'[109] Al-Tirmidhī commented: and this is the strongest *ḥadīth* concerning this matter.

Emesis is one of the five basic forms of evacuations, these being: purging, emesis, blood-letting, the release of vapours, and sweat. And the *Sunna* deals with all these.

Purging occurs in a *ḥadīth*: the best form of treatment is by a laxative (*mashiy*) and in the *ḥadīth* concerning *Senna*.[5]

Bloodletting has already been mentioned in the *ḥadīth*s on cupping. Evacuation by vapours we shall deal with at the end of this section, God willing.

Evacuation by sweat: this is not generally by any special means but by the constitution's forcing it to the surface of the body, where it finds the pores open and makes its way out through them.

Emesis consists of evacuation from the upper part of the stomach, retention from its lower part and by medication from its upper and lower part. Emesis is of two kinds: one caused when the nature is overcome and stirred up, and one which is brought about by medical means. The first must not be suppressed or prevented except when excessive, and when it gives rise to fear that injury may result. It is checked by things which restrain it. The second is of benefit to the patient who needs it, if care is taken regarding its time and conditions, as already discussed.

5 *Mashiy*, laxative, see Chapter 8, n. 4, and Chapter 11: senna; Chapter 11: cupping; Chapter 8.

Causes of emesis are ten:[6] (1) predominance of the yellow bile, which floats to the surface at the top of the stomach and seeks to rise; (2) predominance of sticky phlegm which has been in motion in the stomach and needs to emerge; (3) weakness of the stomach itself and inability to digest the food which forces it upwards; (4) the digestive juices of the stomach become mixed with some bad humour which flows down to it and thus spoils the digestive process and weakens its action; (5) it may be from an excess of food or drink beyond the amount which the stomach can accommodate, so that it is unable to retain it, but seeks to repel and eject it; (6) it may be that the food and drink are not suitable for the stomach, so that it dislikes them and seeks to repel and eject them; (7) there may occur in the stomach something which stirs up the food by its quality or its nature, so the stomach rejects it; (8) it may be from disgust, which causes the soul to be nauseated and to vomit; (9) it can be from certain psychological accidental causes, such severe worry, anxiety or sorrow. The onset of such causes dominates the constitution and the natural powers, which are thus concerned and distracted from a proper ordering of the body and the rectification, coction and digestion of the food; consequently the stomach then rejects the food. It may be from movement of the humours at the time of the soul's confusion: The soul and the body react one upon the other, and the quality of one affects the quality of the other; (10) by sympathy: when nature copies nature. For someone can see a person vomit and be himself overcome by this without any attempt to provoke it. For nature tends to emulate.

A certain skilful physician told me: 'I had a nephew who was skilled in treating the eyes, and he held sessions as an oculist. When he opened a man's eye and saw ophthalmia there and treated it, he himself developed ophthalmia. That happened to him many times, so he left off holding these sessions. 'I asked him: 'What was the cause of that?' He replied: 'Copying by nature; for it is imitative.' He continued: 'I know another who used to see an abscess in a place on a man's body, which he scratched, and he himself scratched that place. And an abscess came out on him.'

My comment: All this arises when the constitution is affected and the matter is dormant in it and then moves for one of these reasons. These are causes for the movement of the matter, not that in itself it brings about this occurrence.

Since the humours, in hot countries and in hot seasons, become thin and are attracted upwards, in these circumstances vomiting is more useful. And since in cold countries and cold seasons these humours thicken and are hard to attract upwards, their evacuation by purging with laxatives is more useful.

Removal and repulsion of humours can be either by attraction or by evacuation. Attraction is one of the more remote ways, and evacuation one of the nearest. The difference between them is that when a matter is activated, in

6 Causes of emesis include psychological causes. The tenth contains the phrase 'the constitution is a carrier' (*al-ṭabīʿa naqqāla*), ie. one which transmits. IQ's final comment presupposes an actual material cause which is latent and provoked by psychological stimuli.

flowing down or rising up, it has not yet settled, so it needs to be drawn. If it is rising it is drawn from below, and if flowing down it is drawn from above. When it is settled in its place it is evacuated by whichever means is the nearest to it.

When the matter harms the upper organs it is drawn from below, and when it harms the lower organs it is drawn from above; when it is settled it is evacuated through the nearest means to it. Therefore, the Prophet ﷺ was cupped on his upper back sometimes, on his head at other times, and on the back of his heel at yet other times. So the matter of the harmful blood was evacuated from the place nearest to it.

God knows best.

Emesis cleanses and strengthens the stomach, sharpens the sight, removes heaviness of the head, is beneficial for ulcers of the kidneys and bladder, and for chronic diseases such as dropsy, paralysis, and tremor; it also benefits jaundice.

It is necessary for the healthy person to use this treatment on two successive occasions each month, without any interval, so that the second treatment may compensate for whatever the first did not reach and may cleanse the superfluities which flowed down because of it. But to resort to it frequently will harm the stomach and make it receptive to superfluities; also it harms the teeth, the sight and hearing, and sometimes can rupture a vein. It should be avoided by anyone with an inflammation in the throat, weakness in the chest, anyone who has a thin neck or is subject to haemoptysis or anyone who finds this treatment difficult to carry out.

Many people suffer from bad digestion[7]—which means that they are filled with food and then reject it—and these are afflicted by numerous troubles. For instance it hastens the onset of old age, causes serious diseases and makes emesis habitual for them.

Emesis accompanied by constipation, weakness of the intestines, wasting away of thin places, or weakness of the person vomiting, is dangerous. The most recommended seasons for it are summer and spring, not winter and autumn. At the time of vomiting it is necessary to bandage the eyes and bind up the abdomen, and wash the face in cold water when it is finished. Afterwards, one should drink apple juice with a little mastic. Rose water is very beneficial indeed. Emesis evacuates from the upper part of the stomach, and attracts from the lower, whereas purging is the opposite.

Hippocrates said: It is necessary that evacuation in summer from above be more than evacuation by medicine; and in winter it should be from below.

7 'Digestion', lit. 'organisation', *tadbīr*, in this case referring to the digestive system.

CHAPTER

26

The profession and responsibilities of anyone who carries out medical treatment[1]

(a) *Guidance for choosing the best physician*

MĀLIK mentions in his *Muwaṭṭa'*, from Zayd b. Aslam: A man, in the time of the Messenger of God ﷺ, was wounded, and the blood became congested. The man summoned two men from Bānū Anmār, who examined him. He declared then that the Messenger of God ﷺ asked these two: 'Which of you is the more skilled as a physician?' To which they asked: 'Is there then some value in medicine, O Messenger of God?' He replied: 'The One Who sent down illness also sent down medicine.'[110]

This *ḥadīth* shows that it is necessary, concerning every science and craft, to seek the help of the person most skilful in it; the most skilful person will be the one most likely to find the best solution. Thus the person seeking to obtain a legal pronouncement (*fatwā*) has the obligation to seek assistance concerning what has been revealed about it from the most learned of all the learned people,

1 'Anyone who carries out medical treatment', *taṭabbaba*, fifth form of the root *ṭbb*, is explained as meaning to practise medicine, sometimes with the implication of being unlearned. A *mutaṭabbib* is a practitioner, as compared with *ṭabīb*, one with extensive theoretical knowledge. IQ approaches the question in three ways: firstly, concerning the word: the root *ṭbb* itself can have several meanings, connected with rectification (*iṣlāḥ*), skill (*ḥidhq*), custom (*ʿāda*), or magic (*siḥr*) (see Chapter 25 b). Abū ʿUbayd explains the latter use as a case of euphemism merging on prophylactic magic.

Secondly there is the legal aspect, where he goes into unaccustomed detail in discussing variant claims of the different law schools regarding responsibility—in fact a theological question, given the debate concerning God's absolute power in relation to human potentiality and responsibility. Legal punishment (*ḥadd*) and retaliation (*qiṣāṣ*) are possibilities. He considers that anyone untrained who claims medical skill and by his treatment causes harm is totally responsible for the damage caused. An ignorant person is responsible in accordance with the amount of deception involved. A skilled physician may err in actual performance, or in his judgement and such cases do require compensation. If he performs an operation without the required consent, he is responsible. Finally, IQ gives some characteristics of various members of the medical fraternity.

for the most learned is closer to the correct answer than the less learned. Likewise, if anyone is not sure of the true direction of the *qibla*, he will follow the most learned person he can find, for this is the way God created His servants. Thus too, one who travels by land or sea will find tranquillity for his soul and confidence only in the most skilful and best informed of any two guides, and to this one he will betake himself and on him he will rely. In this, the *sharīʿa*, human nature and reason are all agreed.

The saying of the Prophet ﷺ: 'The One Who sent down illness sent down medicine' is a phrase of his that occurs, in very similar forms in many *ḥadīth*. These include the following: narrative of ʿAmr b. Dīnār from Hilāl b. Yasāf, who said: The Messenger of God ﷺ arrived to visit a sick person, and he said: 'Send for a physician.' Someone asked: 'Do you indeed mean that, O Messenger of God?' He replied: 'Yes, for God the Glorious One never sent down illness without sending down medicine for it.'[111] And in the two books of *Ṣaḥīḥ*, from *ḥadīth* of Abū Hurayra (*marfūʿ*): 'God sent down no illness without sending down healing for it.' We have already mentioned this *ḥadīth*, and others.

There have been some differences concerning the precise meaning of sending down of illness and medicine.[2] For one group has said: Sending it down means informing the servants of it, and it is not an actual thing. The Prophet ﷺ informed us of the general purport of 'sending down', for every illness and its medicine, yet most people do not know that. Thus, he said: 'The one who knows this, knows it, the one who does not is ignorant of it.'

Another group have said: Their sending down means their creation and their being placed on the earth, as in the other version of the *ḥadīth*: Indeed God did not place any illness without placing medicine for it. Even if this *ḥadīth* is more precise than the preceding one, the word sending down (*inzāl*) is more specific than creation (*khalq*) or placing (*waḍʿ*); one must not ignore the specific meaning of the expression without good cause.

Another group have said: Their sending down is by the mediation of the angels who are entrusted with direct dealings with humankind, by way of illness and medicine and other things. The angels are entrusted with the affairs of this world and of the human species, from the moment the individual leaves his mother's womb to the moment of his death. So the sending down of illness and medicine is with the angels. This is more accurate than the two preceding explanations.

Another group have said: By far the majority of illnesses and medicines are

2 The variation of terms between variant versions of a *ḥadīth* is not always of great significance; but the use of *anzala*, says IQ, is more specific than, eg., *waḍaʿa*, to put or place. In fact it is the word often used in the Qur'ān of the Qur'ān itself, and implies that it is sent down from above to the world beneath. How then can medicine, or a cure, be 'sent down'? Is the material or the knowledge of it 'sent down'? IQ considers the sending down, or mediation of medicine, is entrusted to the angels, since they have general charge of human affairs. The poetry is quoted to show how one verb can have more than one direct object. See Chapter 1 g.

mediated by the sending down of rain from heaven, whereby are produced foods and nutriment, medicines and illnesses, and all the necessary tools for their perfection. As for all higher minerals, they descend from the mountains, while medicines and rivers and fruits are all included in the wider meaning of the verb *anzala*. Hence there is no need for two verbs, because one verb includes both meanings. This is known from the Arabic language and indeed in the usage of other languages. Thus the poet says:

> I fed her (the steed) with straw and cold water,
> till she left, her eyes shedding tears.
>
> Another said:
>
> And I saw your husband, when he had left,
> wearing a sword and a spear.
>
> Another said:
>
> We pencilled the eyebrows and the eyes.

This is better than the preceding explanation. God knows best.

This is part of the perfect wisdom of the Most Glorious Lord, and His perfect lordship. Indeed, as He tests His servants with illnesses, He assists them against these by such medicines as He makes easy for them to find. As He tests them with sins, He grants them forgiveness through repentance, good deeds that wipe sins out, and tribulations that make expiation for them. As He tries them with wicked spirits, from amongst the satans, He supports them with an army of good spirits, ie. the angels. As He afflicts them with all sorts of desires and appetites, yet He helps them to fulfil these through delicious and delightful things that He decreed, made easy and lawful for them. He does not test them, praised be He, with anything unless He gives them the means whereby to seek help against that thing and to repel it. All that remains is the difference between them, concerning knowledge of that and knowledge of the means of acquiring it and achieving it. From God we seek help.

(b) *Physicians and medical responsibility*

It is related by Abū Dāwūd, al-Nisā'ī and Ibn Māja, from *ḥadīth* of ʿAmr b. Shuʿayb, from his father, from his grandfather: The Messenger of God ﷺ said: 'If anyone carries out medical treatment, yet previously he was not known as a medical man, then he takes the responsibility.'[112]

This *ḥadīth* is concerned with three points, one linguistic, one legal and one medical.

From the linguistic point of view:

1. *ṭibb* in the language of the Arabs has several meanings: rectification, putting right. One says: 'I treated it', when I put it right. Also one says: He had 'practice' *ṭibb* in such things, that is, subtlety and practical skill.

The poet said: 'When the affair of Tamīm altered, I was their physician with a perspicacious view'.

2. Skill (*ḥidhq*) Al-Jawharī said: Every skilled man is a 'physician', according to the Arabs. Abū ʿUbayd said: The basic meaning of the term 'medicine' is skill with various things, and proficiency therein. One calls a man: *ṭabb*, or *ṭabīb*, when he is skilful, even if this does not concern treatment of the sick. Another said: If a man is *ṭabīb*, that means a skilful man; he is called *ṭabīb* because of his skill and cleverness.

Said ʿAlqama: 'If you ask me about women, then I am an expert in the ills of women, a *ṭabīb*; when a man's hair turns white or his wealth decreases, then he has no part in their affection.'

Said ʿAntara: 'If you let down your veil across your face before me, then I am skilled (*ṭabb*) at capturing even the cavalier clad in mail.'

This means: If you veil yourself from me and hide your face, seeking to avoid me; well, I am experienced and skilful at catching the horseman who has dressed in battle armour.

3. Custom. One says: 'That is not my *ṭibb*', meaning my custom.

Said Farwa b. Musayk: 'Indeed our *ṭibb* is not cowardice, but our destiny and the kingdom of others.'

Said Aḥmad b. al-Ḥusayn: 'And pride is not my *ṭibb* among them, except that hateful to me is the ignorant one who pretends to intelligence.'

4. Magic. One says: a man is 'physicked' (*maṭbūb*), meaning bewitched (*masḥūr*). In the *Ṣaḥīḥ* from *ḥadīth* of ʿĀ'isha it says: Now when the Jews bewitched the Messenger of God ﷺ, and the two angels sat at his head and at his feet, one of them asked: 'What is wrong with the man?' and the other replied: 'Bewitched (*maṭbūb*)'. The one asked: 'Who bewitched him?' and the other replied: 'So and so, the Jew.'[113]

Abū ʿUbayd said: They called the person bewitched only because they used the word *ṭibb* as a euphemism for magic; similarly they called one who was stung 'well' (*salīm*), thus seeking a good omen of health. Likewise, they apply the word 'victorious' to the open desert where there is no water; so the word *mafaza* is to draw a good omen of victory over death.

The word *ṭibb* is also used for the actual medicament.

Said Ibn Abī al-Aslat: 'Nay, did not one tell Ḥassān: Was your medicine bewitchment, or madness?'

Consider the words of al-Ḥamāsī: 'If I am bewitched (*maṭbūb*), may I remain so, and if I am sick (*masḥūr*), then let there be no cure to the magic.'

Now by 'bewitched' he meant that one has been put under magic, and by 'sick' one who is ill. Al-Jawharī said: Some call the sick person 'bewitched' (*masḥūr*); and he recited the verse. Its meaning is: If what has befallen me is because of you and love of you, I ask God that it should remain, and I do not wish it to cease, whether it came about through magic or illness.

The root *ṭbb* has three forms of vocalisation: *ṭabb* is one who is learned about matters, and thus the physician (*ṭabīb*) is also called *ṭabb*. *Ṭibb* is the practice of medicine; while *ṭubb* is the name of the place. Ibn al-Sikkīt recited: 'So I said: Have you sent your horseman to assail Ṭubb, the place of water, whose land is good?'

The words of the Prophet ﷺ were: 'Whoever practises medicine (*taṭabbaba*)'; he did not say 'whoever is a physician (*ṭabba*)'. The expression of the fifth form (*tafaʿala*) indicates some constraint in the action, and entering into it with difficulty, and that the one so described is not originally one of its practitioners. Similarly, we find the expressions: to attempt clemency (*taḥallama*), to show courage (*tashajjaʿa*), to adopt patience (*taṣabbara*) and others of this kind. Thus, 'to force oneself' (*takallafa*) is formed upon this pattern. The poet said: 'And Qays of ʿAylān, and whoever sought to be a Qays (*taqayyasa*).

The legal (*sharʿī*) aspect is that this *ḥadīth* establishes the liability of the ignorant practitioner. For if he assumes the knowledge and practice of medicine, without formerly having any acquaintance with it, by his ignorance he risks causing harm to the lives of people; he practises irresponsibly what he does not know and, thus, deceives the sick person. Therefore he must be held responsible. This is the consensus among all scholars.

Al-Khaṭṭābī said: I do not know of any disagreement regarding the fact that when a person carrying out treatment transgresses the limits of his knowledge and expertise and causes harm to the patient he should be held responsible. One who lays claim to knowledge or practice which he does not have is an impostor. When injury is brought about by his action, he is responsible for the blood-money, and he has no right to retaliation (*qawad*); for he has no authority without the sick person's permission. The consequences of the practitioner's felony—according to the opinion of most jurists—falls upon his clan (*ʿāqila*).

My own comment: there are five categories:

1. A skilful physician who practises his craft properly, whose hand causes no harm, yet from his action—permitted by the law, and by the one he was treating—there occurs injury to a limb or loss of life, or the loss of some faculty. Such a man is not held responsible, and this is agreed. This happens to a person who has been given full permission. For example, if someone circumcises a boy at a certain time, who is of the right age for this, and he performs the operation correctly, yet injury occurs to the organ or to the boy himself, he is not held responsible. Similarly, if he peforms an urgent incision on someone, whether the patient be fully conscious or not, at the right time, according to the proper method, yet some injury results, he is not held liable. This principle is applicable in all other cases involving a person with permission, so long as he does not transgress the limits of such a permission. This is similar to the consensus on the applicability of legal punishment, and the majority's agreement on retaliation. This is in contradiction to Abū Ḥanīfa's view, who would hold such a practitioner responsible. This is still the judgement concerning the application of chastisement, or a man's striking his wife, a master his pupil, or an employer

his hired animal; and it is in contradiction to Abū Ḥanīfa and al-Shāfiʿī, who hold the view that such persons are responsible, although al-Shāfiʿī exempted the case of beating an animal.

Now the rules governing in this type of case are reached through both consensus and disagreement. According to consensus, if harm occurs as a result of transgression, liability is established, while if accidentally, it entails no liability. Yet concerning the intermediate categories there is disagreement. For Abū Ḥanīfa required that the person's liability should be absolute while Aḥmad and Mālik denied it; Shāfiʿī drew a distinction between the one compelled to carry out legally prescribed actions who therefore cannot be held responsible, and one who is executing acts that are based on opinion, who was to be held responsible. Abū Ḥanīfa considered that permission is only granted on condition that it is safe. Aḥmad and Mālik considered that the existence of permission revokes liability. Shāfiʿī considered that the one compelled could not be seen as falling short, for this is tantamount to a decree. But for the one who executes actions based on opinion, as in the case of chastisements and punishments that are not textually prescribed, this is a question of independent judgement. If injury occurs thereby then he is to be held responsible, for this can be thought of as aggression.

2. The second example is that of an ignorant practitioner who treats a person and injures him. In this case if the person thus injured knew that he was ignorant, that is to say without knowledge of his profession, yet permitted him to treat him, the practitioner is not held responsible. This kind is not opposed by the obvious sense of the *ḥadīth*. For the context and purport of the words show that he deceived the sick person, and made him think he was a physician, while he was not. If the sick person thinks him to be a physician and permits him to treat him on the basis of his knowledge, the physician is responsible for any injury he commits. Similarly, if he prescribes him some medicine to take, and the patient thinks that he has prescribed it because of his knowledge and skill, yet is injured thereby, he is responsible for that. The *ḥadīth* here is clear and obvious.

3. The third example: A skilful physician, with permission, who performs his craft properly, but his hand makes a mistake, thus causing harm and injury to a healthy limb. For instance, where the hand of the circumciser slips and strikes the organ instead; then this one is responsible, for it is an injury due to a mistake. If the amount of indemnity is equal to or more than a third of the blood money, this is an obligation upon his clan. If there is no clan then should the indemnity be taken from his property or from the public treasury? There are two opinions, both related from Aḥmad. It has been said that if the physician is a *dhimmī* (protected non-Muslim, ie. Jew or Christian) then this should be taken from his property; if he is a Muslim then either of the two possibilities. If there is no public treasury, or if he cannot afford the payment, then should the blood debt lapse, or should it be made an obligation on the estate of the

offender? There are two views here, the most widely accepted being that it should be allowed to lapse.

4. The fourth example: The skilful physician, proficient in his art, who exerts his effort and prescribes a medicine for the patient, but he arrives at the wrong judgement and kills the patient. There are two opinions regarding such a case: (1) that the blood money for the patient should come from the public treasury; (2) that it should come from the tribe of the physician. These have been specified by the Imām Aḥmad concerning the mistake made by an imām or a judge.

5. The fifth example: A skilful physician who performs his work properly, but who cuts a cyst on a man, a child or a deranged person, without permission of the patient or of the guardian and causes injury; or one who circumcises a young boy without the permission of his guardian and causes injury. Some of the leading authorities in our school of thought have said: he is responsible, for the injury resulted from an action for which permission had not been given. But if he had permission from the adult, or the guardian of the child or the deranged person, he is not held responsible.

It is also possible that he is exempt from responsiblity in an absolute sense, because he was seeking to do good, and there is no fault held against those who are doing good. Had he committed any transgression, the permission of the guardian has no effect in letting the responsibility lapse; as he did not, then he is in no way responsible.

You may say: he is an aggressor when he does not have permission but not when he does. Then I would reply: aggression, or its absence, only refers to his own action, and no effect is brought about by permission or the lack of it, in this case. But here there are divergent views.

The physician—in this *ḥadīth*—includes all those carrying out treatment either through general prescriptions or the practice of a specialized method of healers. If he uses a *koḥl* stick he is an oculist; if a scalpel and ointments, he is a surgeon; if a knife, a circumciser; an incising instrument, a phlebotomist; cupping glasses and sharp knife, a cupper. He is known by his bonesetting equipment and his bandages if a bonesetter; by his irons and fire if a cauteriser; by his waterskin-bag if one who administers clysters.

It is the same whether the medical treatment is for dumb animals or for humans, the name of 'physician' is given in general parlance for all of these, as has already been mentioned. The introduction of categories of specialists for various kinds of physicians is only a recent practice, similar to the particular terms given to a riding animal (*dābba*), according to the purpose that it is predominantly used for.

(c) *Characteristics of the skilful physician*

The skilful physician is the one who in his treatment carefully takes into account the following twenty matters:

1. Diagnosis of the illness, identifying its category.

2. Consideration of its cause: where did it strike at first, and what is the effective cause?

3. The strength of the patient; his physical resistance; his weak points; and if such resistance can withstand and overcome the illness. If so, he lets his body deal with the illness, and does not stir it up.

4. The natural temperament of the body.

5. The changes to the normal temperament.

6. The age of the patient.

7. His habits.

8. The season of the year, and what is appropriate to it.

9. The patient's homeland and environment.

10. The state of the atmosphere (polluted or otherwise) at the time of the illness.

11. Consideration of the medicine which is the opposite to that illness.

12. Considering the strength and degree of that medicine, and the balance between these factors and the strength of the patient.

13. The whole aim of the physician should not be restricted only to removing that illness, but to remove it in such a way that there is no danger that something worse might result. When its removal is not free from the risk that another worse illness might occur, he leaves it as it is, and it is necessary to deal very gently with it. This condition is like the illness of the 'mouths' of the veins, for when this is treated by cutting and restricting them there is the risk of something more serious occurring.

14. He should proceed by using simple treatments, and build up progressively, so he should not proceed from treatment by food to treatment by medicine except when he is compelled to do so, or proceed to compound medication except when the simple medicine is not effective. It is the physician's good fortune that he may treat with foods instead of medicines, and with simple medicines instead of compound.

15. He should look into the ailment: is there a known treatment for it? If not, then he preserves the inviolability of his craft and his own professional integrity, and he must not be impelled by greed to carry out any treatment which will be of no apparent use. If it is possible to treat it, then he considers whether or not it can be removed. When he knows that it is not possible to remove, then he considers whether or not it can be eased or confined. If it cannot be confined, and he sees that the only possibility is to stabilise it and prevent it advancing, then he seeks that by his treatment, and he assists the faculty and weakens the substance of the illness.

16. He should not meddle with any humour before its coction, by means of evacuation, but should seek to bring about its coction, and when this is completed, then hasten to its evacuation.

17. He should have knowledge of the illness and the medicines of hearts and

spirits, for that is a great basis for physical treatment. That the body and its constitution are affected by the soul and the heart is an obvious matter. And when the physician is acquainted with the sicknesses and treatment of the heart and spirit, then he is the perfect physician, but the one who has no such knowledge, even if he is skilful in the treatment of the constitution, and the states of the physical body, is only half a physician. Any physician who does not treat the patient by inspection of his heart and what is good for it, strengthening of his spirits and active faculties by righteousness, doing good, beneficence, and turning towards God and the eternal abode is no physician, but an inadeqate practitioner. Among the greatest means of treatment for illness are charity, beneficence, remembrance of God, supplications, humility and humble prayer to God, and repentance. These matters are very effective in warding off illness and bringing about healing, far more so than natural medicines. But this is in accordance with the readiness and preparation of the soul, and its belief in such things and their benefit.

18. Gentleness towards the patient and dealing kindly with him, like the gracious treatment of a young child.

19. That he should use both natural and divine types of treatment, and treatment by positive imagination and uplifting of the spirit (*takhyīl*). Indeed the skilful physicians can carry out marvels through positive thinking, such as medicine cannot attain. The skilful physician seeks every means of help to fight disease.

20. The twentieth—the foundation of the physician's business—is that his treatment and planning should be based upon six principles: preservation of the present state of health; restoration of health which is lost, to the best of his ability; removal, or confining, of the illness, so far as he can; tolerating the lesser of two evil factors for the removal of the greater; abandoning the lesser of two benefits, in order to acquire the greater. Around these six principles does treatment revolve. Any physician who is not bound by these guiding principles is no real physician.

God knows best.

CHAPTER

27

On the progression of illness and contagious disease

(a) *Stages and conditions of illness*

AN ILLNESS has four stages : its onset, its increase, its decline, its end;[1] so the physician has the specific duty of watching carefully over each of the stages of the illness, with the knowledge of what is suitable and appropriate for them, and during each stage he employs what ought to be used then. If he sees, during the onset of the illness, that the constitution needs something to move and to evacuate the superfluities, because of their state of coction, then he makes haste to do this. If he misses his chance to make the constitution move during the onset of the illness because some hindrance prevents that, or because the faculty is weak and unable to bear evacuation, or because the season is cold, or because some negligence has occurred, then extreme caution is necessary not to do this at the time when the illness increases. If he does so, the constitution becomes confused because it is distracted by the medicine and it is quite unable to regulate and oppose the illness. This could be likened to coming to a horseman who was busied with the overthrow of his enemy and causing him to be distracted from that by something else. What is necessary in this stage is to make sure the constitution is assisted to preserve the strength as much as possible.

When the illness nears its end, stops, and becomes quietened, one can begin its evacuation and the eradication of its causes. When it begins to decline this is more fitting. A similar example to this would be that of an enemy, who when his powers are at an end and his ammunition used up, can easily be captured; when he turns and begins to flee, he can be captured more easily still. The violence and disturbance of the illness are only at the beginning and

1 Conditions, stages, or states (*aḥwāl*) through which most illnesses will progress. These are the onset (*ibtidā'*), increase (*ṣuʿūd*), decline (*inḥiṭāṭ*), ending (*intihā'*). Treatment must always be in accordance with the state prevailing at the time, and should never exceed what is appropriate (e.g. regulation of diet to be employed before medicaments—cf. Chapter 1 e). That the nature must not be distracted, cf. Chapter 15, Chapter 18, n. 5, Chapter 24.

during its evacuation, and when its power is extensive. In this way the illness and the medicine are equal.

It is part of the physician's skill that, when he is able to undertake the easier kind of measures, he does not turn to the more difficult, and he progresses gradually from the weaker to the stronger, unless he fears the patient's strength may collapse at that time. Then, it is necessary to begin with the stronger and in the course of treatment not to persist in one single state. For the constitution would become accustomed to it, and its reaction would be limited. One would not dare to use strong medicines during the strong seasons. It has already been stated that when treatment is possible by means of diet, then treatment is not given by medicines. When the illness is not apparent to him—is it hot, or cold?—then he must not take any further steps until this has become clear to him, and he does not carry out any experiment with anything where he fears the outcome. But there is nothing wrong with experimenting with something which cannot have a harmful effect.

When various illnesses occur at the same time, the physician starts on that one which has one of three characteristics:

1. That the cure of the other will be dependent on its cure, such as inflammation and ulceration, for he begins with treating the inflammation;

2. That one of the two is the cause of the other, such as obstruction and putrid fever; then he begins with removing the cause;

3. That one of the two is more serious than the other, such as the acute and the chronic; then he begins with the acute, though he must not neglect the other.

When both illness and symptom are combined, he begins with the illness, unless the symptom is more fierce, as is the case with colic; so he first alleviates the pain, then treats the obstruction. If he can replace evacuation with treatment by hunger, fasting, or sleep, then he does not carry out evacuation. The preservation of every state of health is sought by what is similar or its like, and if the aim is to transfer it to what is more excellent, it is transferred by the opposite.

(b) *Precautions against contagious disease*[2]

It is confirmed in the *Ṣaḥīḥ* of Muslim, from a *ḥadīth* of Jābir b. ʿAbd-Allāh: in the deputation of Thaqīf there was a man suffering from leprosy. So the Prophet ﷺ sent to him saying: 'Return, for we have given the oath of allegiance (*bayʿa*) to you.'[114] And Bukhārī relates in his *Ṣaḥīḥ*, as commentary, from *ḥadīth* of Abū Hurayra concerning the Prophet ﷺ, that he said: 'Flee from the one with leprosy, as you flee from the lion.'[115]

It is related in the *Sunan* of Ibn Māja, from *ḥadīth* of Ibn ʿAbbās, that the

2 Illnesses which are contagious by their nature (*al-adwāʾ al-muʿdiyya bi-ṭabʿihā*).

Prophet ﷺ said: 'Do not let your glance rest long on those afflicted with leprosy.[116]

It is quoted in the two books of the *Ṣaḥīḥ*, from a *ḥadīth* of Abū Hurayra, who said: The Messenger of God ﷺ said: 'A sick person must not be in contact with one in good health.'[117] It is reported, from the Prophet ﷺ: 'Talk to the person with leprosy, but leave between you the length of one or two spears.'[118]

Leprosy[3] is a serious disease that arises from the spreading of the black bile throughout the entire body, so that the temperament as well as appearance and the shape of the organs is corrupted. Sometimes in the last stages the organs are corrupted to the point where they are eaten away and fall off. It is called 'the lion's disease'. In this name, the physicians note three points:

1. Because of the amount that the lion tears away;
2. Because this illness makes the sufferer's face very grim, and gives it the appearance of a lion;
3. Because his illness causes him to carry out such ravages on whoever approaches or comes near, as a lion does.

This disease—in the physicians' opinion—is one of the contagious and hereditary diseases. The one who approaches the sufferer from leprosy or consumption falls sick through his breath.

Now such was the compassion of the Prophet ﷺ for the community and his concern to advise them, that he forbade them any circumstances which would expose them to the arrival of harm and corruption to their bodies and their hearts.

Undoubtedly there may be in the body some latent preparedness and readiness to succumb to this disease, and the nature may be quite susceptible, disposed to accept disease from the bodies of those it has contact with. For indeed it is able to transmit disease in this way. Now the constitution's fear and imagination concerning that can be among the most potent causes for that disease to attack it. Indeed imagination has a powerful influence upon faculties and constitutions. Also the breath of the sick person may reach the healthy one and cause him to fall sick. This can be clearly seen in the case of some illnesses. Breath is one of the means of contagion. Despite this, the body has to be prepared for and susceptible to the illness. The Prophet ﷺ had married a woman, but when he wanted to consummate the marriage, he found on her hips some leucoma and said: 'Stay with your own people.'

Now a group of people have thought that these *ḥadīth* are opposed to others which make them void and contradictory. These include al-Tirmidhī's narrative, from a *ḥadīth* of ʿAbd-Allāh b. ʿUmar, that the Messenger of God ﷺ took the hand of a man suffering from leprosy, and he put it with his own into the large food bowl, saying: 'Eat in the Name of God, trusting in God, and

3 Leprosy, *judhām*. IQ speaks of an objective contagion, and also a psychological 'preparedness' to succumb to a disease. The imagination, *wahm*, can influence the body in this way and cause illness, much as faith can assist in its cure.

relying upon Him.[119] Ibn Māja related this, from *ḥadīth* of Jābir b. ʿAbd-Allāh. It is confirmed in the *Ṣaḥīḥ*, from Abū Hurayra, from the Prophet ﷺ, that he said: 'There is no contagion, and there is no evil portent.'[120]

We declare that there is no contradiction—by the praise of God—between these sound *ḥadīth*. If any occurs, then it maybe that one of the two *ḥadīth* is not of the Prophet's own speech. Rather it is an error of one of the narrators, for even a reliable narrator can make a mistake. Alternatively one of the two *ḥadīth* could be abrogating the other. A third possibility is that if the two *ḥadīth* impart superficial contradiction or opposition as understood by the hearer, but not in the actual words of the Prophet ﷺ, then inevitably the explanation of that contradiction lies in one of these three ways.

Two sound clear *ḥadīth*, opposed in every way, where one does not abrogate the other, could never be found. God forbid that such should occur in the speech of one truthful and trusted, the one from whose mouth naught but truth can ever come. But the defect is from inadequate knowledge of what is transmitted and the distinction between what part of it is sound and what is defective, or from incapacity in the understanding of the Prophet's ﷺ intent and attributing to his words a meaning which he did not intend; or from both reasons together. From this has occurred a great deal of disagreement and harm. Success comes from God.

In his book *The Variance of* Ḥadīth, Ibn Qutayba related a narrative concerning the enemies of the science of *ḥadīth* and its scholars. They have said: There are two mutually opposing *ḥadīth* which you have narrated from the Prophet. Firstly, that he said: 'There is no contagion, and no evil portent;' and someone said to him: 'Scab occurs on the snout of a camel, and the whole herd becomes scabby from that one.' He asked: 'And what caused the trouble of the first one?' Then you have narrated: 'Let the one who has a physical disease not come into contact with the healthy one,' and 'Flee from the leprous person as you flee from the lion.' Also a leprous man came to him to give his allegiance to Islam, so he sent to him accepting his allegiance, and gave him permission to go back without seeing him personally. He said: Ill omen is in a woman, a house and a riding animal. They have said: All of this is contradictory; part of it does not resemble the other. Abū Muḥammad said: But we declare that there is no variance at all in this, but for every meaning of it there is a time and a place. When the context is given, the variance ceases.

Now contagion is of two kinds:

1. Contagion of leprosy, for the leprous person's breath intensifies until he gives the disease to anyone who spends a long time sitting near him or talking with him. Similarly, if a woman sleeps with a leper, and is with him beneath the same covering, he transmits the harm to her, and she may become leprous. Likewise, his offspring when older may have this tendency. The same is true of one suffering from consumption or hectic fever or scab. Physicians order that one should not sit with the consumptive nor the leper. They are not imme-

diately considering the concept of contagion, but their prime concern here is to prevent the exchange of breath as it may cause sickness to anyone who inhales it for a long while. Physicians are the people least likely to believe in good or evil portents. Similarly, scab (*nuqba*) occurs to the camel—this is moist scab (*jarab*)—and when the animal mixes with the herd or rubs against them or shelters in their stopping places, the liquid which streams from it or falls in drops will transfer to them the same illness. This is the concept which the Prophet ﷺ had in mind: 'A sick person must not be in contact with the one in good health.' He did not wish the one blighted to mix with the healthy, so that the like of his trouble should not afflict the healthy one through drops of moisture and scab.

2. The other kind of contagion is the plague (*ṭāʿūn*); this befalls a town, and then everyone leaves out of fear of contagion. Now the Prophet ﷺ had said: 'If it occurs in a town while you are there, do not leave the place; but when plague is in some other town, do not enter there.' By his words 'Do not leave the town where it occured' he means it is as if you think that flight from God's decree will rescue you from God. And by his words: 'When it is in a town, do not enter there' he means that remaining in the place where there is no plague will calm the hearts, and will promote confidence and safety.

In the same way, if a woman or a house is known for bringing misfortune, in the event that something unpleasant befalls the husband or some calamity occurs for the inhabitants, then one would say: It gave me contagion by its misfortune. It is the kind of 'contagion' of which the Messenger of God ﷺ said: 'There is no contagion.'

Another group said: Rather, the command to avoid the leper and to flee from him is a matter of recommendation, choice, and guidance. As for eating with him, his action was to show clearly that this is permitted and it is not forbidden.

Another group said: But the speech in both these cases is particularly intended, not general. For the Prophet ﷺ addressed every individual according to what was appropriate for his condition. If the person is strong in his faith and his trust in God, then the strength of his trust would repel the power of contagion, just as the strength of the constitution repels the power of the illness and makes it of no avail. Another person has no such strength, so he counselled him to be careful and to take precautions. The Prophet ﷺ himself practised both options: so that the Community might draw an example from both, and the member of his Community who is strong might adopt the way of trust and confidence in God, while the one among them who is weak might take the way of precaution and care. They are both valid paths—one for the firm believer, the other for the one whose faith is weak. Thus each of the two groups should find proof and example in the practice of the Messenger ﷺ according to their state and what is appropriate for them. This is similar to when he performed cautery, yet praised the one who did not do so, and connected his omission of it with trust and with rejecting augury. There are many similar instances. This is a very gracious and good way; if anyone follows it rightly, and is given real spiritual understanding thereby, this will remove much contradiction which he may suspect in the sound *Sunna*.

Yet another group have concluded that the command to flee from the leper and to avoid him concerned a physical matter, which is the transmission of the disease from him to a healthy person by means of touch, contact, and breath. This occurs if such contact and touch are repeated, whereas eating with him, over a short period of time, for a specific purpose, holds no harm; nor can contagion be acquired from one occasion and a brief moment. The prohibition was to prevent harm, and to protect health. Yet he associated with such a one but for need and interest. So there is no opposition between the two commands.

Another group have said: It is possible that this leper with whom he ate had only a slight infection of leprosy, the like of which is not contagious. Not all lepers are the same, nor can contagion be acquired from all of them. But among them is the one with whom contact is neither harmful nor contagious, and he is the one who is only slightly afflicted. In him the leprosy halts and remains in the same state, and it does not spread to the rest of the body. It is more appropriate and likely that it will not spread to anyone else.

Another group have said: In the pre-Islamic times (*Jāhiliyya*) people believed that the contagious diseases spread by their own nature and without reference to God, praised be He. So the Prophet invalidated their belief in that, and he ate with a leper to make clear to them that God, praised be He, is the One who causes illness and healing. He forbade people to come close to the leper, so that it might be clear to them that this is one of the causes which God has made to bring about certain definite results. In his prohibition there is confirmation of the causes, and in his action is clarification that they are not autonomous in any way, but the Lord, praised be He, if He wishes can remove their powers, so that they have no influence at all, or vice versa.

Another group have said: But these *ḥadīth* contain the abrogating (*nāsikh*) and the abrogated (*mansūkh*) so one should examine their history, and once one knows which is the later, this will be the one which cancels out the other. If not, we should accept both of them as valid.

Another group have said: But some of them are memorized, some are not memorized. They have discussed the *ḥadīth* on 'No contagion', and have declared: Abū Hurayra related it in the first place, but subsequently he was in doubt and left it aside; they tried to get him to repeat it, saying: we have heard you relate this. But he refused to do so.

Abū Salma said: I do not know whether Abū Hurayra forgot it or whether one of the two *ḥadīth* abrogated the other. As for the *ḥadīth* of Jābir, that the Prophet ﷺ took the hand of a leper and put it with his own into the large food bowl, this is a *ḥadīth* unconfirmed and unsound. Al-Tirmidhī said of it no more than that it was strange, but he did not call it sound nor fair. Shuʿba and others have said: Be wary of these strange *ḥadīth*. Al-Tirmidhī said: This is related also as an action of ʿUmar, and that is better confirmed.

Such is the case of these two *ḥadīth* which are opposed by the *ḥadīth* of prohibition; one of them Abū Hurayra refrained from relating and denied, and the second is not soundly attributed to the Messenger of God ﷺ. God knows best.

We have given a full discussion of this question in *Kitāb al-Miftāḥ* (the Book of the Key), at greater length.[4] And God gives success.

4 *Kitāb al-miftāḥ*, probably *miftāḥ al-saʿāda*, one of the works attributed to IQ in the preface to the Cairo edition. The title is given in full as *Miftāḥ dār al-saʿāda wa-manshūr ʿalawiyāt al-ʿilm wa-l-irāda* (Key of the abode of happiness and proclamation of the loftiness of knowledge and will), GALL II. 128.

CHAPTER

28

Prevention of treatment with forbidden substances[1]

ABŪ DĀWŪD related in his *Sunan*, from *ḥadīth* of Abū al-Dardā': The Messenger of God ﷺ said: 'Indeed God sent down both illness and medicine, and for every illness He gave a remedy. So carry out medical treatment, but do not use therein anything unlawful.'[121]

Bukhārī mentioned in his *Ṣaḥīḥ*, from Ibn Masʿūd: 'God did not place your healing in anything which has been made unlawful for you'.[122] And in the *Sunan*, from Abū Hurayra, who said: The Messenger of God ﷺ forbade medication with impure medicines (*khabīth*).[123]

In the *Ṣaḥīḥ* of Muslim, from Ṭāriq b. Suwayd al-Jaʿfī, we read that he asked the Prophet ﷺ about wine. The Prophet ﷺ forbade it, or disapproved of Ṭāriq's making it.[2] So he said: 'I only make it for medicinal purposes', to which the Prophet ﷺ replied: 'It is no medicine, but it is an illness.'[124]

In the *Sunan*, it is related that he was asked about the use of wine in medicine, and replied: 'It is an illness, and is not a medicine.'[125] This tradition is related by Abū Dāwūd and Tirmidhī.

In the *Ṣaḥīḥ* of Muslim, from Ṭāriq b. Suwayd al-Ḥaḍramī, it says: I asked: 'O Messenger of God, in our land there are grapes which we press, so may we drink from them?' He replied: 'No.' I persisted, saying: 'But we use this product seeking to cure the sick.' He replied: 'That is not healing, but sickness.'[126]

In the *Sunan* of al-Nisā'ī: A physician mentioned a frog as an ingredient of a medicine, in the presence of the Messenger of God ﷺ, and he forbade him to kill it.[127]

The Prophet ﷺ is quoted as saying: 'If anyone uses wine as a medicine, may God not heal him.'[128]

1 On the fact that medical treatment must always conform to the religious law.

2 One of the forbidden things most likely to be recommended was wine, whether prescribed for internal or external use. IQ insists that under no circumstances may it be used medicinally. Wine is forbidden in the Qur'ān, II : 219 and V : 93, the term being *khamr*.

Treatment with forbidden things is repulsive both to the intelligence and to the religious law. The legal aspect can be seen in these and other *ḥadīth*. As for the intelligence, the point is that God, praised be He, made these matters forbidden because of their impurity; He did not make unlawful to this Community anything which is good by way of punishment for them, as He did in the case of Children of Israel, in His words: *For the iniquity of the Jews, We made unlawful for them, certain good foods which had been lawful for them* (IV : 160). However, for this Community whatever was forbidden, was forbidden only because of its intrinsic evil. God's prohibition of it is to protect them and to safeguard them from drinking it. It is not appropriate that through it healing from sicknesses and illnesses should be sought. Even if it has some effect in removing them, yet it results in a sickness which is far greater, in the heart, by the force of impurity which it contains. Thus the one who uses it as medicine, in seeking to remove sickness of the body, brings about sickness of the heart.

Also, its being made unlawful requires that it should be avoided and that one should keep a safe distance from it, in every way. Its use as a medicine could be an inducement to desire it and become acquainted with it. This is against the intention of the Lawgiver.

It is a disease, just as the Messenger has ordained, thus it is not permitted to take it as medicine. It imparts to the constitution and spirit the characteristic of impurity, for the bodily constitution has a manifest reaction to the quality of medicine. When its quality is impure, then the medicine imparts to the constitution the impurity: so how should it be, when it is impure in its very essence! Therefore God, praised be He, banned for His servants all impure foods, drink and clothing, lest the soul might acquire the appearance and characteristic of impurity.

Furthermore, in permission to use it as medicine, and especially if people are inclined to like it, there is the possibility of a pretext for taking it for appetite and pleasure. This is particularly so if they know that it is beneficial for them and a cure for their sicknesses. This is what they most desire. The Lawgiver, therefore, prevented any pretext for its consumption in any possible form. Undoubtedly there will always be contradictions and conflicts found when considering the legal principle of blocking of the means (*sadd al-dharā'iʿ*) as to allowing or prohibiting the use of alcohol in medicine. In this forbidden medicine there are impure things, which far exceed any healing power which might be expected from it. So one should talk about this greatest of evils, in which God never placed any healing for us at all. Indeed, it is exceedingly harmful to the brain, which is the seat of intelligence according to the physicians and many of the experts in the revealed law and theologians.

Hippocrates declared in the course of his teaching on *Acute Diseases*: wine has a damaging effect on the head, for it rises swiftly thereto, and with its ascent there arise also the humours which go to the upper parts of the body. For this reason it harms the intellect (*dhihn*).

Al-Majūsī, the author of the *Kāmil*,[3] said: 'The property of alcoholic drinks (*sharāb*) is that it harms the brain and nerves.'

Other forbidden medicines come in two categories:

1. That by which the soul is repulsed and which the constitution is not mobilised to assist in order to repel the illness, such as medicines found in poisons and viper's flesh, and other unclean substances. Once such medicines are administered, they remain as a burden on the body, causing fatigue to the constitution, and become harmful not medicinal.

2. That by which the soul is not repulsed, for instance *sharāb* being used by pregnant women, where its harm exceeds its benefit. Now reason would entail that it still be prohibited. Therefore reason and natural disposition are in agreement with the revealed law.

There is a subtle meaning in the fact that forbidden things cannot be used for healing. Healing is achieved by medicine when the soul readily accepts it and believes in its usefulness, and in the blessing of healing which God has put into it. What is beneficial is that which is blessed and the most beneficial is that with the greatest blessing. And blessed among the people is he from whom benefit comes wherever he may be.

It is well known that the belief of the Muslim in the unlawfulness of this matter, ie. of wine, is something which prevents him from having confidence in its blessing and utility, having a good opinion of it, and hinders his human nature from readily accepting it. But the greater the servant's faith (*īmān*), the more he disapproves and the less he will trust it, and his nature will consider it the worst thing possible. If he takes it, in this condition, it will be a cause of disease to him, not a medicine, unless he ceases to consider it as impure and evil; his bad opinion of it changes and his dislike of it turns to liking. But this would be contradictory to faith. So the believer cannot take it without its being a cause of sickness. God knows best.

3 ie. *Kāmil al-ṣināʿa al-ṭibbiyya*, Perfection in (or complete book of) the art of medicine, by ʿAlī b. al-ʿAbbās al-Majūsī, d. 994 A D. GAL I. 273, S.I. 423.

CHAPTER

29

Treatment for lice (*qaml*)[1]

IT IS related in the two books of the *Ṣaḥīḥ*, from Kaᶜb b. ᶜUjra: There was something wrong with my scalp. I was taken to the Messenger of God ﷺ. Now the lice were moving onto my face, and he said: 'I did not know your trouble had reached as far as I can see now.' So he ordered him to shave his head, and to divide a *farq* (a measure of weight equalling 12 *mudd*, ie. 6,516 grammes), or give a sheep (as alms), or fast for three days.[129]

Lice (*qaml*) are generated on the head and body from two causes, one external to the body and other internal. The external cause is dirt and stains combined on the body surface. The internal is an evil putrid humour, which the constitution forces between the skin and the flesh, so it grows putrid with the sanguineous moistures in the skin layer. When the moistures have gone out through the pores, lice are produced. Mostly this occurs after ailments and sicknesses, because of unclean matters. The reason for its more frequent occurrence in the heads of children is simply the abundance of their moistures and the fact that they are generally involved in activities that generate lice. Therefore the Prophet ﷺ ordered 'that the heads of the young boys of the Banū Jaᶜfar should be shaved.'[130] One of the greatest of treatments for lice is shaving the head, so that the pores open up: the evil vapours make their way out, and the substance of the humour grows weak. The head must be anointed after that, with medicines which kill lice and prevent their generation.

Shaving the head is done for any one of three purposes: firstly as a religious act of piety and drawing near to God; secondly as religious innovation and associating with God; and thirdly for need and medical reasons. Firstly: shaving the head for one of the two pious duties, the greater or lesser Pilgrimage (*hajj* or ᶜ*umra*). Secondly: shaving of the head for the sake of any other than God, praised be He, as the disciples do for the sake of their shaykhs, so that one of them says: I have shaved my head for such a one, or you have shaved your head

1 Lice, *qaml*. *ḥadīth* concerning ailment on the head: Bukhārī, *Ṭibb* 16, VII. 406. Shaving of the head is seen here not primarily as a health measure but as a vow and then in acknowledgement of overlordship: where this is given to other than God, IQ argues, the action amounts to worship of that other, and thus unbelief.

for such a one. This is as if one said: I have prostrated myself to such a one. Shaving of the head signifies humility, submission, and lowliness; therefore it comes as the completion of the Pilgrimage. In al-Shāfiʿī's opinion it is even one of its necessary pillars, without which the pilgrimage is not correctly concluded. It signifies the placing of one's forehead in the hands of his Lord in obeisance to His might and in humility before His glory, and it is among the profoundest types of servanthood. Therefore, the Arabs, when they wished to humiliate a prisoner of war of theirs and then release him, used to shave his head and set him free. Then came the shaykhs of misguidance and those who compete for lordship—whose status as shaykhs is based on association with God and innovation—and wished that their disciples should pay homage to them; so they demanded of their disciples to shave their heads for them, just as they demanded that they should kneel before them. They named it by another name, saying: this signifies placing the head between the hands of the shaykh. But, by the Eternal One! prostration to God is placing the head between His hands, praised be He. Also, they demanded of those disciples to make a vow to them, turn to them in repentance and swear by their names. This means that the disciples are taking them as lords and gods other than God. The Most High has said: *It is not for any man, that he should be given the Book and Wisdom and the prophetic office, and then should say to people: Be worshippers of me rather than God, but he would say: Be true worshippers of the Lord, for you have taught the Book and you have studied it. Nor would he command you to take the Angels and the Prophets as lords. What! would he command you to unbelief after you have become submitted to God?* (III: 79–80).

The most noble kind of servanthood is the servanthood during ritual worship (*ṣalāt*). But it has been divided up by the shaykhs, those who pretend to be scholars and tyrants, and the shaykhs have taken from it the most noble element, which is the prostration (*sujūd*). Those who pretend to be scholars have taken from it the bowing (*rukūʿ*), so that when one of them meets another he bows just as the worshipper does to his Lord. The tyrants have taken over the standing upright (*qiyām*), so that free men and slaves alike stand beside them in servitude to them, while they are seated.

Now the Messenger of God ﷺ forbade these three things specifically. To carry them out is a clear contravention. He forbade prostration to any but God, and said: 'No one must prostrate to any other!' He rebuked Muʿādh when he knelt to him, saying 'Desist'. The unlawfulness of this is an established fact of religion. For anyone to permit it, to other than God, is disobedience to God and His Messenger ﷺ. It is one of the profoundest forms of servanthood. When the polytheist permits this prostration to other than God, he is permitting servanthood to other than God. It is a sound tradition that the Prophet ﷺ was asked: 'When a man meets his brother, may he bow to him?' and he replied 'No'. They asked: 'May he hold him and embrace him?' He replied 'No'. They asked: 'May he shake his hand?' and he replied 'Yes'.[131]

Furthermore: to bow, when greeting one another, is a type of prostration. Here we have the words of the Most High: *Enter the gate prostrating* (II: 58), that is, bending low. Otherwise, prostration and entering would not be possible on one's forehead.

There is a sound tradition concerning his prohibition of others standing while he sat, in the way in which non-Arabs pay honour to one another. He even forbade that during prayer; when he prayed seated, he ordered them also to pray seated, even though they were healthy with no excuse of illness. This was so that they should not be standing beside him while he was sitting, even though their standing was to honour God. How then would it be, to stand upright in giving honour and worship to anyone other than God, praised be He!

The point is that ignorant, misguided souls had devalued the servanthood to God, praised be He, and associated in this homage those created beings whom they honour. So they prostrate themselves to other than God, and bow to this other, stand before him as they stand in prayer, and swear by another, and make vows to another, shave their heads in honour of another, perform sacrifice and the circumambulation (of the Kaʿba) to another, magnify him with love and fear, hope and obedience, as they magnify the Creator, or to an even greater degree. This created being that they worship they put on an equal level with the Lord of the Worlds. These men oppose the preaching of the messengers and make another equal to their Lord. These are the ones who, when they are in the fire of hell along with their gods, arguing with them, will say: *By God, we were indeed in clear error, when we held you as equal with the Lord of the Worlds* (XXVI: 97–8). They are the ones of whom it is said: *And among men there are those who take others as equals besides God; they love them as they should love God. But those who believe have much firmer love for God* (II: 165). All this is polytheism, and God does not forgive the association of any creature with Him.

This is a section albeit outside his guidance on shaving of the head, yet we saw it necessary to include, and perhaps it is more important than what was intended on this subject. God knows best.

CHAPTER

30

Prophetic guidance concerning treatment with spiritual medicines[1]

(a) *Treatment of the Evil Eye*

MUSLIM relates in his *Ṣaḥīḥ*, from Ibn ʿAbbās, the Prophet ﷺ said: 'The Eye is true, and could anything precede the divine decree, it would be the Eye.'[132] In the same source, from Anas, we find that the Prophet ﷺ authorised incantation to be recited for fever, the Eye, and itching (*namla*).[133] In the two books of the *Ṣaḥīḥ* from Abū Hurayra it is related that the Prophet ﷺ said: 'The Eye is true.'[134] And from the *Sunan* of Abū Dāwūd, on the authority of ʿĀ'isha: 'The one with the Eye was commanded to carry out *wuḍū'*, then the one afflicted used that water for washing the whole body (*ghusl*).'[135] In the two books of the *Ṣaḥīḥ*, from ʿĀ'isha, it says: 'The Prophet ﷺ ordered me (or, the Prophet gave orders) that we should recite incantations to guard against the Eye.'[136]

Al-Tirmidhī gives a *ḥadīth* from Sufyān b. ʿUyayna, from ʿAmr b. Dīnār, from ʿUrwa b. ʿĀmir, from ʿUbayd b. Rafāʿa al-Zurqī relating that Asmā' bint ʿUmays asked: 'O Messenger of God, the Banū Jaʿfar have been afflicted with the Eye, so shall we recite incantations on their behalf?' and he replied: 'Yes; for could anything precede the decree, it would be the Eye.'[137] Al-Tirmidhī said: This is a good (*ḥasan*) and sound (*ṣaḥīḥ*) *ḥadīth*.

Mālik related, from Ibn Shihāb, from Abū Umāma b. Sahl b. Ḥunayf: ʿĀmir b. Rabīʿa saw Sahl b. Ḥunayf washing himself, and said: 'I have not seen such skin before today, not even the skin of a young secluded virgin.' Sahl fell to the ground, and the Messenger of God ﷺ came to ʿĀmir and was angry with him, saying: 'Why should one of you kill his brother? You should have said a

1 Concerning divine (divinely inspired) spiritual medicines, *al-adwiya al-rūḥāniyya al-ilāhiyya*. Treatment for the (Evil) eye, *ʿayn*, which could cause illness, damage and death to humankind or animals. The Eye is a belief long prevalent in the Arab and the Middle Eastern world in general, with a variety of measures to ward it off.

blessing. Then cleanse yourself on his behalf.' So, for him, ʿĀmir washed his hands and face, his elbows and knees, the extremities of his feet, and the interior of his loincloth in a bowl, then poured that water over him. By this he regained strength, and he was able to move with the people.[138]

Mālik related also, from Muḥammad b. Abī Umāma b. Sahl, from his father, this *ḥadīth*, in which he said: 'The Eye is true,'[2] and one should perform *wuḍū* for it,[139] and so he did this for him.

ʿAbd al-Razzāq related, from Maʿmar from Ibn Ṭāwūs from his father (*marfūʿ*): 'The Eye is real, for could anything precede the decree, it would be the Eye. If one of you is asked [by one who is afflicted with the Eye] to perform the washing of the whole body (*ghusl*), then let him do so.' The continuous chain of this *ḥadīth* is sound.

Al-Tirmidhī said: The man with the Eye is ordered to take a bowl, to put his palm into his mouth and rinse it, then spit out into the bowl; to wash his face in the bowl, then introduce his left hand, to pour water over his right knee in the bowl, then introduce his right hand and pour water over his left knee, then wash the inner part of his loincloth, but not put the bowl on the ground; then he pours water over the head of the man afflicted with the Eye from behind, in one pouring.

The Eye is of two sorts: the Eye of humankind, and the Eye of the Jinn. It is said truly, on the authority of Umm Salama, that in her house the Prophet ﷺ one day saw a servant girl with *saʿfa* on her face, and said: 'Recite incantations[3] for her, for the "Glance" is on her.'[140] Al-Ḥusayn b. Masʿūd al-Farrā said: 'His word *saʿfa* means glance,'[4] that is from the Jinn. It is said: She is suffering from an Eye which has afflicted from the glance of the Jinn, whose piercing is more deadly than the points of spears. There is a saying from Jābir (*marfūʿ*): 'The Eye can bring a man to his grave, and a camel to the cooking pot.'[141] From Abū Saʿīd: 'The Prophet ﷺ used to seek refuge from the Jinn and from the Eye of humankind.'[142]

One group of people, of those who have but a small share of transmitted knowledge and intelligence, have denied this matter of the Eye, saying this is merely imagination, with no truth in it. These are among the most ignorant of people, in knowledge and intelligence, and have the thickest veil over their eyes, the heaviest of natures, and are furthest of all from the knowledge of spirits and souls and their qualities, deeds, and effects.

The intelligent people of all nations—with their differences of community and of belief—neither reject nor ignore the question of the Eye, even though they differ concerning its cause and the impact of the Eye. One group says: the

2 The Eye is true (a reality), *al-ʿayn ḥaqq*.

3 We were to recite incantations: IQ argues at length for the logicality of belief in the power of the Eye, though he insists the effect is finally due not to the eye of a person but to the spirit or spirits working through it.

4 The text gives *saʿfa*, but the *ḥadīth* has *sufʿa*, a black or brown mark or excoriation. Bukhārī, *Ṭibb* 35, VII. 426.

one with the Eye, when his spirit has taken on an evil quality, emits from his eye a poisonous power which reaches his victim, causing injury. They have said: This cannot be denied, just as one does not deny the emission of a poisonous substance from the viper, once it reaches the human being and kills him. This is a well known fact concerning a certain type of viper: when their glance falls upon a man he dies. Thus it is with the possessor of the Eye.

Another group say: It is not impossible that from the eye of some people there can go forth subtle, invisible substances, which reach the one afflicted and permeate the pores of his body, and thus he is injured.

Yet another group say: God has made it the custom that He creates such harm as He wishes, when the possessor of the Eye meets the one he afflicts, without any power or cause or influence which he can himself originate.

This is the way of those who deny the presence of causes, powers and influences in the world. These have isolated themselves, denying cause, effect, and interaction, and thus opposed all people of wisdom. There is no doubt that the Almighty has created in both bodies and spirits a variety of powers and natures, and has placed in many of them influential characteristics and qualities.

It is not possible for the intelligent man to deny the effect of spirits upon bodies, for this is a fact both seen and felt. You see how a face can become very red, when someone looks at the person whom he is ashamed to face or of whom he is embarrassed, and a face can become very yellow and pale when someone looks at one he fears. It has been known for a person to become ill from a glance, and his faculties weaken. All this comes about through the effect of spirits. Because they are so closely connected with the Eye, this action is attributed to it, although it is not the active agent, but the effect is through the spirit. Spirits vary in their nature and powers, their qualities and characteristics. The spirit of the envier inflicts very obvious damage on the one envied. For this reason God, praised be He, instructed His Prophet to take refuge with Him from the evil of the envier.[5]

The influence of the envious person in injuring the one envied is a fact denied only by one who is not aware of the real meaning of human nature. This influence is the basis of the affliction by the Eye. For the evil, envious soul takes on an evil quality, and confronts the one envied and affects him through that special quality. The nearest parallel is the viper: for its poison is latent and potential; when it confronts its enemy, a hostile power is emitted from it, which is then transformed into an evil, injurious quality. Among these creatures, there are those whose evil quality is so strong and fierce that it can bring about a miscarriage, while others can destroy the sight. Thus the Prophet ﷺ said, regarding stump-tailed serpents and those with white stripes: Indeed they seize hold of the sight, and cause miscarriage.[143] Others can have an effect upon

5 To take refuge . . . ie. in the two last *sūras* (113 and 114) of the Qur'ān, each beginning with 'Say: I take refuge with God from . . .'

human beings merely through the sight of them, without any contact with them, because the evil of that spirit is so strong and its evil quality so effective because of the intensity of the evil qualities in such a soul and its harmful effect.

The effect is not conditional on physical contact, as is thought by some who have little learning or knowledge of nature and the revealed law (*sharīʿa*). But the effect is sometimes by contact or contiguity, sometimes sight, or by the spirit directing its energy towards the one it affects; sometimes through prayers and incantations and seeking refuge; sometimes by hallucination and imagination.

The influence of the one with the Eye is not directly related to sight, for he may be blind; then something can be described to him and his spirit affects it even if he does not see it. Many such persons with the Eye can have this effect through description, without seeing their victim. The Most High said to His Prophet: *And the unbelievers would almost trip you up with their eyes, when they hear the message* (LXVIII: 51). And He said: *Say: I seek refuge with the Lord of the Dawn, from the evil of created things, from the evil of darkness as it descends, from the evil of those who blow upon knots, from the evil of the envious one as he envies* (CXIII: 1–5).

Every one with the Eye envies, but not every envious person has the Eye. Envying is more general than possession of the Eye, so to seek refuge from the envious is really to seek refuge from the Eye. These are arrows which leave the soul of the envier and the one with the Eye, aiming for the one envied and afflicted; sometimes they strike him, sometimes they miss him. If they come upon him unaware and unprotected, they will certainly affect him. If they come upon him alert and fully armed, the arrows cannot penetrate. They will not affect him, and sometimes the arrows are even deflected upon their owner. This is the equivalent to the casting of some physical weapon. This kind concerns souls and spirits, while the other concerns bodies and physical forms.

The origin is from the person with the Eye being mightily pleased at something; then he follows it up with the evil quality of his soul. Then he seeks help for his poison to penetrate with a glance at the one affected.

A man can even afflict himself, and he may cast the Eye without wishing to, merely through his nature. And this is the worst possible of the human variety.

Our companions, and other Jurists, have said that if anyone is recognised as having that power, the Imām should confine him, and pay his expenses for the rest of his life. This is quite definitely the right thing to be done.

Abū Dāwūd has related in his *Sunan*, from Sahl b. Ḥunayf: We passed by a stream, and I went in and washed in it; when I came out I was suffering from fever. This was told to the Messenger ﷺ and he said: 'Command Abū Thābit to seek God's protection for him.' So I said: 'O my master, and is incantation suitable?' He replied: 'Incantation is only for the Eye, for bites (*ḥuma*), or for poisonous stings (*ladgha*).[144] *Nafs* means the Eye. The expression goes: Such a one has been afflicted by *nafs*, which means, the Eye. And the *nāfis* is the

ʿĀ'in, the one who casts the Eye. 'Poisonous stings' means the stinging of a scorpion and similar creatures.[6]

Included among seeking of protection and incantations are repeated recitation of the two *Suras* of seeking refuge and of the *Fātiḥa* and the Throne Verse. Also, there are the Prophet's formulae of seeking protection, such as: 'I seek refuge with God's perfect words from the evil of what He has created,' and 'I seek refuge with God's perfect words from every satan and every reptile and from every Eye which is deranged,' and 'I seek refuge with God's perfect words, which cannot be surpassed by the pious or the impious, from the evil of that which He has created, fashioned and formed, and from the evil of what descends from the sky, and the evil of what rises into it, and from the evil of that which He has created in the earth, and the evil of that which comes forth from it, from the evil of temptation of the night and of the day, and for the visitors by night and day, except the one who brings tidings of good; O most Merciful!'

And: 'I seek refuge with God's perfect words from His anger and His punishment, from the evil of His servants, from the temptations of the satans, and from their presence;' 'O our Lord! I seek refuge with Your most noble countenance and Your perfect words, from the evil of the one whom You seize by the forelock; O our Lord! You uncover sins and offences. O our Lord! Your army is not defeated, Your promise does not fail, praise and glory be to You!' And: 'I seek refuge with the countenance of God, the Mighty One than Whom nothing is mightier, and with His perfect words which are not surpassed by the pious nor the impious, and by the Beautiful Names of God—those I know and those I do not know—from the evil of what He has created, fashioned and formed, and from the evil of everything which is evil, whose evil I cannot bear, and from the evil of everything which is evil which You seize by the forelock; indeed my Lord is upon a straight path.'

And: 'O our Lord! You are indeed my Lord, there is no god but You; unto You have I entrusted myself, for You are the Lord of the mighty throne. Whatever God wishes comes to pass, whatever He does not wish does not come to pass. There is no power nor strength save with God; I know that God is powerful over all things, and that God has encompassed all things with His knowledge, and has reckoned and counted all things. O our Lord! Indeed I take refuge with You, from the evil of my soul, the evil of Satan and his polytheism, from the evil of every creeping thing which You seize by the forelock. Indeed my Lord is on a straight path!'

And if he wished, he said: 'I have taken my protection with God; there is no god but God, my God and the God of all things; I take shelter with my Lord, the Lord of all things. I have entrusted myself to the Living One Who never dies. I have warded off evil by the words: 'There is no power and no strength except with God. God is sufficient and an excellent protection. The Lord is sufficient

6 *Nafs*, literally 'soul', here interpreted in usage as the Eye, representing the soul of the person casting the harm. Incantation, *ruqya*. Bites, *ḥuma* (from serpents etc.).

for His servants, the Creator is sufficient for His creation, the Provider is sufficient for the one nourished. Sufficient is God; He is sufficient alone, sufficient is the One in Whose hand is the kingship over all things. He protects and cannot be oppressed. God is sufficient, and enough. God hears the one who calls. Nothing can reach beyond Him. God is sufficient! There is no god but He, to Him have I entrusted myself, and He is the Lord of the mighty throne.'

Whoever tests these supplications and means of seeking protection knows to what extent they are beneficial, and how great is the need for them. They prevent the influence of the one with the Eye from reaching its victim and repel it once it has reached him, in accordance with the strength of faith of the one who utters these formulae, the power and the preparedness of his soul, and the strength of his commitment to God and the firmness of his heart. For they are arms for the fight, and arms are effective in accordance with the one who will use them.

If the possessor of the Eye fears the harm and the drastic effect it may cause to the one struck, then let him repel its evil by saying: 'O our Lord! Bless him!' as the Prophet ﷺ said to ʿĀmir b. Rabīʿa, when he cast the Eye on Sahl b. Ḥunayf: 'Have you not spoken a blessing?' That is, you said: O our Lord, bless him!

One of the ways to avert the effect of the Eye is to say: 'Whatever God wills: there is no strength but with God!' Hisham b. ʿUrwa related from his father that whenever he saw something which delighted him, or entered one of his walled gardens, he said: 'Whatever God wills; there is no strength but with God!'

Another way is with the incantation which Jibrīl, peace be on him, spoke for the Prophet ﷺ. This is related by Muslim in his *Ṣaḥīḥ*: 'In the Name of God I recite this spell over you, from every ill which can harm you, from the evil of every possessor of the eye or envious eye God heals you. In the Name of God I recite this spell to protect you.'[145]

A group of the early Muslims have considered that for this sufferer the Qur'ānic verses should be written, and then he should drink them (i.e. the water in which they have been soaked). Mujāhid said: There is no harm in writing the Qur'ān, washing it in water, and giving it to the sick person to drink. The same is reported from Abū Qilāba. It is mentioned, on the authority of Ibn ʿAbbās: for a woman who was having a difficult childbirth, he ordered two verses of the Qur'ān to be written, soaked in water and given to her to drink. Ayyūb said: I saw Abū Qilāba write some verses from the Qur'ān, then wash this in water and give it to a man who was in pain.

(b) *Washing to cure the Evil Eye*

The possessor of the Eye should be ordered to wash his groin and armpits, his hands and feet, and the inner part of his loincloth. (This last term, *izār*, has two interpretations: firstly, his private parts, secondly, the extremity of his loincloth which is contiguous to his body on the right side). Then water is poured over the head of the one afflicted by the Eye, suddenly from behind. This practice is a treatment which is not offered by physicians, nor can anyone benefit by it who denies it or despises or doubts it, or carries it out as an experiment without believing it to be effective.

If there are in the natural order special features of whose causes the physicians are totally unaware—which in fact, in their opinion, are outside any analogy of the natural order but have to do with these special features—what is it that the unbelieving and ignorant among them deny of the special features appertaining to the religious law (*sharīʿa*)? Yet this treatment with ablution contains that which sound intellect approves of and confirms as appropriate. Know then, that *tiryāq* (antidote) for the poison of a serpent is from its flesh; and that the treatment for the influence of an angry spirit lies in appeasing its anger and extinguishing its fire, by placing your hand on it, stroking and calming it. That is like the case of a man who has a blazing torch which he wants to hurl at you. So you pour water over it, while it is still in his hand, to extinguish it. It is for this reason that he ordered the one with the Eye to say: 'O our Lord, bless him!' so as to repel that evil quality through prayer, which means benevolence towards the one afflicted. Indeed medication works through its opposite. Because this evil quality appears in the thin places of the body and it seeks to penetrate the body and it finds nothing thinner than armpits and groins and the interior of the loincloth (as an allusion to the private parts), then when these are washed with water its influence and action are neutralised. Also, these places are especially attractive to satanic spirits. The point of this is that washing with water extinguishes that fiery substance and eliminates that poison. This has another aspect: that the effect of ablution reaches the heart from the places which are the thinnest and most swiftly penetrated; so that the fiery and poisonous elements are both extinguished with water, and the person afflicted with the Eye is cured. This is similar to the case of poisonous creatures which are killed after they have bitten, and thus the effect of the bite upon the victim is alleviated and he obtains respite. Their souls extend their harmful power after they have bitten and make it reach their victim: but when they are killed, the pain is relieved. This has various aspects, although one of its causes is the pleasure of the victim and the alleviation his soul finds in killing his enemy. Thus his nature is able to master and repel the pain. In short: the ablution of the one with the Eye disperses that quality which had gone forth from him, but his ablution is only effective when his soul is in conformity with that quality.

The question may be raised: Now the appropriateness of the ablution is made clear, so what is the suitablity of pouring water over the one afflicted? The reply is: It is exceedingly suitable. For that water extinquishes that fiery quality and counteracts that evil quality from the agent. Just as in this way the fire existing in the agent was extinguished, so it was extinguished and kept away from the person affected, after his association with the one who affected him with the Eye. The water with which iron has been quenched enters into many natural medicines mentioned by physicians. As for that whereby the fiery substance of the possessor of the Eye is extinguished, it is not inconceivable that it should enter into medicine which is appropriate for this illness.

In short, relationship between the medicine and treatment of those who follow natural principles, and the prophetic treatment, is like the medicine of itinerant practitioners in relation to 'natural' physicians, or even less. For the difference between the latter and the prophets is far greater than the difference between them and the itinerants, much more so than anyone can realise. Now it has become apparent to you that a bond of friendship exists between wisdom and the religious law, and that there is no contradiction between them. God leads whom He wills towards what is right, and to the one who continues knocking at the door of success which comes from Him, He opens every door. His is the bounty which precedes and the authoritative proof.

Among the methods for treatment of the Eye, and taking precautions against it, is concealing all attributes in a person at risk from the Eye by that which will avert it. As al-Baghawī mentioned, in the book of Commentary on the *Sunna*: ʿUthmān saw a good-looking child and said: 'Grease his dimple, so that the Eye may not fall on him!' The Commentary explains the meaning of 'grease his dimple' as 'blacken it'; and the dimple is the hollow on the chin of the young child.

Al-Khaṭṭābī, in his *Gharīb al-ḥadīth*, from ʿUthmān: He saw a child afflicted by the Eye, and said: 'Grease his dimple.' And Abū ʿAmr said: I asked Aḥmad b. Yaḥya about this, and he replied: By the 'dimple' he meant the hollow on his chin, and to 'grease' means to blacken. So he meant: 'Blacken the place on his chin, so as to repel the Eye.' Of this type is a *ḥadīth* from ʿĀ'isha: that the Messenger of God ﷺ preached one day, wearing on his head a greasy turban, that is, a black one. This was given as an example of the word. Again, we have here the words of the poet:

> How great is the need of the perfect
> for a fault which will protect him from the Eye!

Among incantations which avert the Eye is one mentioned from Abū ʿAbd-Allāh al-Tayyāḥī. On one of his journeys, for pilgrimage or a raid he was on a lively she-camel. In the company there was one man with the Eye, who could hardly ever glance at anything without damaging it. Abū ʿAbd-Allāh was told: 'Protect your she-camel from the evil of so and so who has the Eye.' He replied: 'He has no way of getting at my she-camel.' But the one with the Eye was told of these words, so he waited until Abū ʿAbd-Allāh was absent, and he came to his tethering place and looked at the she-camel, which became disturbed and fell down. Abū ʿAbd-Allāh returned and was told: 'That one with the Eye has cast his eye upon her, and she is as you see her.' So he said: 'Point him out to me,' and he was shown him, and then stood over him and said: 'In the Name of God, a construction that confines, a dry stone, a blazing fire; I have returned the eye of the evil-eyed one upon himself, and upon those dearest to him. *So return the sight; do you see any flaw; then return the sight twice; your sight will come back to you dull and discomforted, in a state worn-out'* (LXVII:3–4). The pupils of the eyes of the evil-eyed one fell out, while the camel got up again none the worse.

CHAPTER

31

Incantation[1]

(a) *Incantation for general treatment*

ABŪ DĀWŪD relates in his *Sunan,* among *ḥadīth* of Abū Darda': I heard the Messenger of God ﷺ saying: 'If anyone of you complains of anything, or if a brother of his is suffering, let him say: Our Lord God, you who are in heaven; Holy is Your Name, and Your command is in heaven and on earth; just as Your mercy is in heaven, so place Your mercy on earth, and forgive us our offences and sins. You are the Lord of the pure ones. Send down mercy from Your presence, and healing from Your healing, upon this pain, and it will be healed with God's permission.'[146]

In the *Ṣaḥīḥ* of Muslim, from Abū Saʿīd al-Khudrī, we read that Jibrīl came to the Prophet ﷺ, and said: 'O Muḥammad, are you in pain?' He replied: 'Yes.' So Jibrīl said: 'In the Name of God I recite this spell over you to free you from every ill that harms you, and from the evil of every *nafs* or envious Eye, God heals you. In the Name of God I recite this spell over you.'[147]

It may be asked: What do you say about the *ḥadīth* which Abū Dāwūd related: 'There is no incantation except for the Eye or bites (*ḥuma*).'[148] ('Bites' refers to all kinds of poisonous creatures). The reply is: The Prophet ﷺ did not intend thereby to deny the possibility of incantation in other cases, but the meaning is that there is no incantation more fitting and benificial than that for the Eye and bites. This is shown by the sequence of the *ḥadīth*. For Sahl b. Ḥunayf asked him, when he was struck by the Eye: 'Is there any good in incantation?' and he replied: 'There is no incantation except for *nafs* or bites.' This is indicated by both the general and particular *ḥadīth* on incantation. Moreover, Abū Dāwūd related, from the *ḥadīth* of Anas: The Messenger of God ﷺ said: 'There is no incantation except for the Eye, or bites, or blood which will not be staunched.[149] In the *Ṣaḥīḥ* of

1 Concerning incantation, *ruqyā,* following on from the previous section, but more specifically for healing. *Ladgh* : sting (of snake etc.); *ḥuma* : bite.

Muslim also, from him: 'The Messenger of God ﷺ permitted incantation for the Eye and bites and *namla*.'[150]

(b) *Incantation for stings with the Opening Chapter of the Qur'ān* [Fātiḥa]

Both the books of the *Ṣaḥīḥ* contain this *ḥadīth* of Abū Saʿīd al-Khudrī: A group of the Companions of the Prophet ﷺ set out on a journey and stopped at a certain tribe of the Bedouin. They asked for hospitality, but the Bedouin refused to receive them as guests. The chief of that tribe was stung, and his people tried all kinds of remedies but nothing was of any use. One of them said: 'If you were to approach the group which asked hospitality, maybe one of them would know of a remedy.' So they went to them and asked: 'Travellers, our chief has been stung, and we have tried everything but nothing is of use. Do you have anything for it?' One of them replied: 'Yes, by God, I can recite incantations. But we asked hospitality of you, and you did not welcome us. I shall not recite a spell until you offer a reward.' So they settled with them for a portion of their flock. Then the man at once spat upon the person who was stung and recited the chapter: 'Praise be to God, Lord of the Worlds . . .' It was as if the man had been unfettered, he began to walk about and had nothing the matter with him. The tribe paid the reward they had agreed with the group, and one of these said: 'Share it out.' The one who had recited the spell said: 'Do not do this until we go back to the Messenger of God ﷺ, and tell him what took place, and we can see what he commands us.' So they went to the Messenger of God ﷺ and told him the whole story. He asked: 'And what led you to think that it was an incantation? You have done right; divide it up, and give me a share with you.'[151] Ibn Māja related in his *Sunan*, from the *ḥadīth* of ʿAlī: The Messenger of God ﷺ said: 'The best medicine is the Qur'ān.'[152]

It is well known that certain words have particular value and well-tried benefits, and the opinion concerning the speech of the 'Lord of the Worlds' is that its excellence over all other speech is like the superiority of God over His creation; that it is the complete healing, and effective protection, and guiding light, and universal mercy, such that were it made to descend upon a mountain this would shatter from its might and glory. The Most High has said: *And We cause to descend of the Qur'ān what is a healing and a mercy to the believers* (XVII: 82).[2] The word 'of' here is used in clarification, not partitively, this being the more correct of the two opinions. As with His words: *God has promised those of them who believe and do good works forgiveness and a mighty reward.*(XLVIII: 29).

All of them are of those who believe and do good works. The opinion regarding the *Fātiḥa* is that nothing similar to it has been revealed in the Qur'ān

2 IQ explains 'of', *min*, as being for specification and clarification of that which had descended: *li-bayān al-jins*. If it were considered as 'partitive', *lil-tabʿīḍ*, that could grammatically indicate that only part of the Qur'ān, that part which was a healing and mercy, had descended.

nor in the Torah nor in the Gospel nor the Psalms, for it comprises all the meanings of the Books of God, which include the origin and the entirety of the Names of the Lord. These are: God, the Lord, the Merciful and the Compassionate; and confirmation of the Return, and the two types of the declaration of the oneness of God (*tawḥīd*): *tawḥīd* of Lordship and *tawḥīd* of Divinity; and mention of need of the Lord, praised be He, in the seeking of help and of guidance, and His unique role in that. It mentions too what is absolutely the most excellent, most beneficial and most obligatory prayer, and that which the servants are most in need of: guidance to His straight path, which includes the perfection of His knowledge, His unity and His worship, through carrying out what He has ordered and avoiding what He has forbidden and persevering therein until death. It also mentions the types of created being, and their divisions into those who have received His favour through knowledge of the Truth, and acting thereby, loving Him and choosing Him above all else; those who have incurred His anger, through deviating from the Truth after being aware of it; and those who go astray through lack of knowledge of Him. Such are the divisions of created being.

Moreover it comprises confirmation of the Decree and the revealed law, the Names and attributes, the Return, Prophethood, purification of souls, and restoration of hearts. It states God's justice and benevolence, and rejects all people of innovation and falsehood.

Similarly we have discussed this matter in our larger commentary, on the *Fātiḥa*. In truth, a *Sūra* of such value should be used in healing from illnesses and should be recited to cure one who has been stung.

In summary—all that the *Fātiḥa* comprises, sincerity of servanthood, praise of God, commitment of all one's affairs to Him, seeking help from Him, complete confidence in Him, and asking Him for all blessings, and guidance which brings down blessings, and repels evil—are all among the mightiest of healing and sufficient medicines.

It has been said that the focal point of the incantation is 'Thee alone do we worship, and Thee alone do we ask for help.' There is no doubt that these two phrases are among the strongest portions of this medicine since they contain the totality of commitment and confidence, seeking of refuge and help, expression of need and request, and integration of the highest intentions, namely worship of the Lord alone, and the most noble of means, namely: seeking His help in order to be able to worship Him. Such cannot be found in other similar verses.

It once happened to me in Mecca that I became ill, and could find neither physician nor medicine, so I treated myself with the *Fātiḥa*, by taking a draught of water of Zamzam, reciting the *Fātiḥa* over it several times, and then drinking it, and I obtained a complete cure. Thereafter I came to rely on it in the case of many kinds of pain and received supreme benefit.

The effect of incantation of the *Fātiḥa* and other verses in treating the sting of poisonous creatures, contains a splendid secret. For poisonous creatures cause an effect through the qualities of their evil souls, as has been explained, and their weapons are their poison with which they sting. They do not sting until they are angered, and once they are angry the poisons are stirred up within them to be cast by their special means.

God, praised be He, has made for every illness a remedy, and for everything an opposite. The soul of the person reciting the incantation works upon the soul of the one so treated, and between their souls there takes place an action and a reaction, as there does between an illness and a medicine. So the soul and power of the person recited over becomes stronger through the incantation over that illness, and he repels it by God's permission. As the influence of medicine on illness in the natural order is dependent upon action and reaction, so is the case when using spiritual treatments and in those combining natural and spiritual means. In spittle and in blowing there is an assistance through the moisture and the air, together with the direct breath for the incantation and *dhikr* and supplication. The incantation comes out from the heart and the mouth of the person casting the spell, and when it includes something from within himself—such as saliva, air and breath—this is more influential and stronger in its action and effectiveness. The pairing between them brings about some influential quality like the quality which arises when medicaments are compounded.

To conclude, the soul of the person making an incantation opposes those evil souls and increases by the quality of his breath, and seeks assistance by the incantation and the blowing to remove that influence. The stronger the quality of the soul of the reciter, the more complete is the spell. His recourse to blowing is like the recourse those evil souls have to their biting. Blowing has yet another secret: it is a source of assistance for both good and evil spirits. Therefore, the sorcerers practise it, just as do people of faith. The Most High has said: *From the evil of those who blow upon knots* (CXIII:4). That is because the soul is in conformity with the quality of anger and hostility, and it sends forth its breaths as its arrows. It reinforces these with spittle and breath, which are accompanied by a saliva that has an effective quality. The sorcerers have very clear recourse to blowing, even though they do not reach to the body of the one bewitched. However, one blows on the knot, ties it, and recites the spell. This takes its toll upon the one bewitched through the mediation of lower evil spirits, which however can be opposed by the pure, good spirit, through the quality of repulsion and by reciting incantations and by recourse to blowing. Whichever of the two is strong has the victory. Opposition of spirits to one another, and their hostility and the means employed, are like the opposition, hostility, and means used by physical bodies. Indeed, the origin, regarding opposition and hostility, is with the spirits, while physical bodies are their tools and their armies. But the person who is predominantly concerned with the senses is not aware of the influence of the spirits nor their actions and reactions because of the dominance which sensory things have over him, and his distance from the world of spirits and their judgements and actions.

In short, when the spirit is strong, and is in harmony with the meanings of the *Fātiḥa*, and seeks assistance from blowing and spitting, it opposes that influence which occurs from the evil spirits and removes it.

And God knows best.

(c) *Incantation for scorpion sting; itching; and serpent bite*

Ibn Abī Shayba related in his *Musnad*, from the *ḥadīth* of ʿAbd-Allāh b. Masʿūd: While the Messenger of God ﷺ was praying, he prostrated and a scorpion stung him on his finger. The Messenger of God ﷺ turned away, saying: 'May God curse the scorpion! It does not leave alone a prophet nor anyone else.' The narrative continues: He called for a vessel containing water and salt, and began to soak the place of the sting in water and salt and to recite: 'Say! He is God, One. . .' and the *Muʿawwidhatayn* (the two *sūras* of Taking Refuge), until the pain subsided.[153] In this *ḥadīth* we find treatment which is composed of two elements, natural and divine.

Sūrat al-Ikhlāṣ[3] has a special property of its own: it has the perfect profession of God's Unity, both intellectually and as an article of faith, and it confirms the Oneness of God, thus utterly and inevitably denying any association with Him. The confirmation of Everlastingness itself necessarily confirms that all perfection is His, as well as the fact that all created beings betake themselves to Him in their needs: that is, creation, from the highest to the lowest, seeks Him and directs itself towards Him. It denies the begetter and the begotten, and any equal, and this includes denial of origin of any derivation, of any similitude or likeness. All this is specific to this *sūra*, and therefore it is said that it equals a third of the whole Qur'ān. His Name the 'Eternal' (*ṣamad*) confirms all perfection; the denial of any equal declares none is like unto Him. 'The One' denies any partner to the possessor of all Majesty. These three fundamental principles are the essence of the declaration of God's Oneness.

The *Muʿawwidhatayn* contain the seeking of refuge from everything hateful, both in general and in detail.[4] Seeking refuge from the evil of that which He has created comprises all evil from which refuge is sought, whether it be physical or spiritual. Seeking refuge from the evil of the twilight (*ghāsiq*), which is in the night, and its sign— the moon hidden—includes seeking refuge from anything which is diffused during it. Now the evil spirits are prevented by the light of the day from going around; but when the night grows dark over them and the moon is absent, they spread about and cause havoc. Seeking refuge from those who blow upon knots comprises protection from the evil and

3 *Sūrat al-Ikhlāṣ*, S. 112. 'Everlastingness', *ṣamadiyya*, from the term used to describe God: *qul, huwa Allah aḥad, Allāh al-ṣamad*, translated in various ways, including 'Eternal', 'Everlasting', 'the Eternal Absolute'. It has almost a sense of solidity, 'lastingness'.

4 *Muʿawwidhatayn*, see Chapter 30, n. 5.

magic of sorcerers. Seeking refuge from the evil of the envious one includes protection from evil souls which cause harm by their envy and their glance.

The second of the two *sūras* comprises seeking refuge from the evil of the satans of mankind and jinn.

So the two *sūras* have included the seeking of protection from every evil, and together they carry immense impact on safety and protection against evils before they occur. Therefore the Prophet ﷺ commended to ʿUqba b. ʿĀmir to recite them at the end of each prayer—al-Tirmidhī mentions this in his *Jāmiʿ*.

There is here a great secret for warding off evil between one time of worship and the next. He said: 'No one can find a means like this for protecting themselves.'

It has been said that the Prophet ﷺ was put under a spell with eleven knots, and that Jibrīl descended to him with these two *sūras*. It came about that every time he recited a verse from them, one knot became loosened, until all the knots were undone and it was as if he was loosed from fetters.

As for the natural treatment for this: salt is beneficial for many poisons, especially for a scorpion's sting. Ibn Sīnā said: 'It is made into a poultice, with linseed, for the sting of a scorpion.' Others also have spoken of it. Salt contains a power of drawing and loosening, such as can draw out and release poisons. When the bite contains a fiery power which needs to be cooled, drawn and extracted, one combines water which cools the fire of the bite with salt which contains power to draw forth and extract. This is the most complete kind of treatment, and the easiest and simplest; and it contains a clear statement that the treatment of this complaint is by cooling, drawing, and extracting. And God knows best.

Muslim has related in his *Ṣaḥīḥ*, from Abū Hurayra: A man came to the Prophet ﷺ and said: 'O Messenger of God, how I have suffered from a scorpion which stung me yesterday!' He replied: 'Had you but said, in the evening: I take refuge with the perfect words of God, from the evil of that which He has created, it would not have harmed you.'[154]

Know then, that divine medicines relieve a disease after it has settled, and they can prevent its occurrence. If it does occur, it is harmless even though it would normally cause injury. Natural medicines can be of use only after the disease has settled. So these practices of taking refuge and remembrance of God can either prevent the occurrence of these causes, or work to ward off the full force of their effect. This will be in accordance with the perfection, the strength or weakness of the one seeking refuge. So incantation and seeking refuge are for two purposes: to preserve health and to remove sickness.

Now the first type is like that which we find in the two books of *Ṣaḥīḥ*, from the *ḥadīth* of ʿĀ'isha: The Messenger of God ﷺ, when he went to his bed, would blow on his palms reciting: 'Say, He is God, One...' and the *Muʿawwidhatayn*. He would wipe his hands over his face and whatever parts of his body his hands could reach.[155] Another example is in the *ḥadīth* of the Refuge-seeking of Abū al-Dardā' (*marfū*ᶜ): 'O my God, You are my Lord, there is no god but You, in You I have trusted; You are the Lord of the mighty Throne,' and has already been narrated.

There is, too, the following: 'If anyone recites these words, at the start of his day, no affliction will befall him before the evening; and if anyone recites them at the end of his day, no affliction will befall him before the morning.'

Likewise, in the two books of *Ṣaḥīḥ*: 'If anyone recites the two verses from the end of the *sūra* of the Cow, at night they will be sufficient for him.[5][156]

Likewise, in the *Ṣaḥīḥ* of Muslim, from the Prophet ﷺ: If anyone stops at a dwelling, and says: 'I seek refuge with the perfect words of God from the evil of what He has created,' nothing can harm him until he departs from that place where he is staying.[157]

In the *Sunan* of Abū Dāwūd it says: the Messenger of God ﷺ when on a journey used to say at night: 'O earth, God is my Lord and your Lord, I seek refuge with God from your evil and the evil of whatever is contained in you, and the evil of whatever creeps upon you. I seek refuge with God from any lion and any black beast, from the serpent and the scorpion, from the dweller in the town, from any who begets and whatever is begotten.'[158]

We have already mentioned the second type of incantations for removal of illness such as the recitation of the *Fātiḥa*; and the incantation for scorpions and the rest will follow.

We have already reported among the *ḥadīth* of Anas, in the *Ṣaḥīḥ* of Muslim 'that the Prophet ﷺ allowed incantation for bites, the Eye and *namla*'.[6][159]

And in Abū Dāwūd's *Sunan*, from al-Shaffā' bint ᶜAbd-Allāh: The Messenger of God ﷺ entered the house, while I was with Ḥafṣa and said: 'Will you not teach this woman incantation for *namla*, as you taught her to write?'[160]

Namla denotes ulcers which break out on both sides of the body, and it is a well-known malady. It is call *namla* (ants) because the sufferer feels, in the places affected, as if ants were crawling on him and biting him. It is of three types.

Ibn Qutayba and others have said: the Magians used to claim that if the son of a man, from his own sister, touched the *namla*, then the sufferer would be cured. Here we have the words of the poet:

> There is no shame among us except the degradation of a noble tribe, and we do not touch *namla*.

Al-Khallāl related that al-Shaffā' bint ᶜAbd-Allāh used to practise incantation for *namla*, in the pre-Islamic period, and when she emigrated to join the Prophet ﷺ—for she had made her allegiance to him in Mecca—she said: 'O

5 End of the *Sūrat al-Baqara*, S. 2:258–56. These contain the words: 'On no soul doth Allāh place a burden greater than it can bear. It gets every good that it earns and it suffers every ill that it earns.'

6 That incantation is permitted for *namla*, ulcers and wounds: see Chapter 30 a.

Messenger of God, I used to practise incantation for skin irritation before Islam, and I wish to present it to you.' So she demonstrated it to him, saying: 'In the name of God, smoothness, until it returns from their mouths; let it not harm anyone. O our Lord! Remove the affliction, Lord of the people.' She recited this incantation over a stick seven times, found a clean place, and rubbed it on a stone, with sharp wine vinegar, and smeared it on the afflicted skin.

This *ḥadīth* indicates that it is permitted to teach women to read and write.

We have already reported his saying: There is to be no incantation except for the Eye or serpent bite (*ḥuma*).

It is related in the *Sunan* of Ibn Māja, from *ḥadīth* of ʿĀ'isha: 'The Messenger of God ﷺ permitted incantations for serpents and scorpions.'[161] There is a narrative from Ibn Shihāb al-Zuhrī: One of the Companions of the Prophet ﷺ was stung by a serpent, and the Prophet ﷺ said: 'Is anyone here able to recite incantations?' They replied: 'O Messenger of God, the family of Ḥazm used to recite incantations for serpents, but when you forbade incantation, they abandoned this.' He said: 'Summon ʿUmāra b. Ḥazm.' So they summoned him, and he demonstrated his incantations to the Prophet ﷺ, who said: 'There is no harm in them', and gave him permission, so he recited them over the sick man.[162]

(d) *Incantations for ulcers, wounds, and pain*

It is reported in the two books of the *Ṣaḥīḥ*, from ʿĀ'isha: 'When anyone complained of pain or suffered from ulceration or wounds, he would put his finger like this (and Sufyān put his index finger on the ground, then raised it) saying: 'In the Name of God, the soil of our land, with our saliva, that our patient may be cured, by the permission of our Lord.'7[163]

This is of the order of treatment which is easy, simple, useful and composite: it is a gentle treatment to be used for ulcers and fresh wounds, especially when there is no other medication on hand, for it is available everywhere. It is a known fact that the nature of pure earth is cold and dry, dessicative to the moistures of ulcers and wounds,which are prevented by the constitution from developing well and rapidly healing; this is especially so in hot countries and for people with hot temperaments. Ulcers and wounds are as a general rule followed by a corrupt hot temperament, so the heat of the region combines with the temperament and the wound itself. The nature of pure earth is cold and dry, stronger than the coldness of all the cold simple drugs, so the coldness of the earth opposes the heat of the illness, especially when the earth has been washed and dried. These ulcers and wounds are followed by an increase of harmful moistures and by pus, which the earth is able to dry up through the strength of its dryness and dessicative power, and it is able to remove the harmful moisture which prevents their healing. Together with this, it brings about the balance of

7 Earth of various sorts was an ancient treatment for external use. On ulcers: Bukhārī, *Ṭibb* 38, VII.429.

the affected limb. When the temperament of the limb is moderate, its healing powers grow strong, and repel the pain with God's permission.

The meaning of the *ḥadīth* is that he takes his own saliva upon his index finger, then places it on the soil, taking up a little on the finger, and with it wipes the wound, while saying these words which contain the blessing of the mention of God's Name and commitment of the matter to Him and confident trust in Him. Thus the two treatments are joined together, and the effect becomes manifold.

Do his words: 'the soil of our earth' mean all kinds of earth, or the earth of Madīna in particular? There are two opinions here. There is no doubt that some kinds of soil possess special properties whereby they can be beneficial to numerous diseases, and can heal serious sicknesses.

Galen said: In Alexandria I saw many suffering from complaints of the spleen or from dropsy, and they would use Egyptian clay, smearing this on their legs, thighs, forearms, backs and ribs, and they obtained a manifest benefit therefrom. And in this way, this embrocation is used for putrid inflammations, or the soft and flabby. Indeed I know some people whose bodies are quite soft from the amount of blood which is evacuated from below, and they gain great benefit from this clay. Other people I know used it to cure chronic pains which had been long-established and firmly fixed in the limbs, and found in it a total cure.

The author al-Masīḥī said: The power of clay from Chios—which is the island of mastic—is a power which cleanses and washes, and it causes flesh to grow on ulcers, sealing them.[8]

If this is the power of these earths, then what should one expect of the best and most blessed soil on the face of the earth, especially as it was mixed with the saliva of the Messenger of God ﷺ, and where the incantation has been joined to the Name of his Lord and the matter entrusted to Him? We have already stated that the powers and effect of the spell are in accordance with the one reciting it and the reaction of the one being so treated. This is a matter which cannot be denied by any intelligent and worthy Muslim physician; but if one of these descriptions does not apply, then let him say what he wishes.

Muslim relates in his *Ṣaḥīḥ*, from ʿUthmān b. Abī al-ʿĀṣ, that he complained to the Messenger of God ﷺ of a pain which he had noticed in his body since he became a Muslim. The Prophet ﷺ said: 'Place your hand on that part of your body where the pain is, and say: In the Name of God, three times, and say seven times: I take refuge with the might and power of God, from the evil of what I find and what I guard against.'[164]

This treatment—the invocation of the Name of God, entrustment to Him, seeking protection by His might and power from the evil of the pain—contains that which will expel it. The repetition is to make it more successful and

8 The text gives the island of Kinus or Knus, probably indicating Chios. Ibn al-Bayṭār, II. 110, speaks of the 'island of gum' as being Ḥiyūs (Khiyūs, Chios).

complete, just as the repetition of medication is to expel the evil substance. In the number seven there is a special property not found in other numbers.

It is related in the two books of the *Ṣaḥīḥ*: When the Prophet ﷺ visited one of his family (who was ill), he would stroke him with his right hand, saying: 'O my God, Lord of mankind, remove all evil, and heal—for You are the healer, there is no healing but Yours—with a healing which does not let any sickness remain.'[165]

In this incantation there is seeking of intercession to God through the perfection of His Lordship and the perfection of His mercy manifest in healing. He alone is the healer, and there is no healing but His. It comprises all means of intercession to Him, through declaring His unity, His beneficence, and His Lordship.

CHAPTER

32

Treatment of calamity

(a) *Burning and grief of calamity*

THE MOST HIGH said: *Give glad tidings to those who patiently persevere, those who say, when afflicted with calamity:*[1] *To God we belong, and to Him is our return. They are those on whom descend blessings from God, and mercy, and they are the rightly guided* (II:155–57).

In the *Musnad*, it is reported that the Prophet ﷺ said: 'If anyone is afflicted by disaster, and he recites: "Indeed, to God we belong, and to Him we return. O God! Reward me for my calamity, and give me hereafter what is better"; then assuredly God will reward him in his distress, and recompense him with what is better than that.'[166]

These words are among the most effective treatments for the person afflicted, and the most beneficial in his worldly life and the Hereafter. They comprise two great principles: when the servant truly and rightly knows them, he will receive consolation from his affliction.

1. That the servant, his family, and his wealth are in reality the property of God, the Most Glorious; that He has placed all this with him as a loan, and when He takes it from him it is like the one who lends, taking back his own goods from the borrower. Also, he is enclosed within two types of want, one precedes and the other succeeds. The servant's ownership is thus temporary as it is borrowed for a short space of time. Again, he is not the one who brought this into existence out of nothingness, making it really his possession; nor is he the one who preserves it from disasters once it does exist; nor does he cause its existence to continue. Throughout he has neither influence nor real ownership.

He is acting in this whole matter with the extent of freedom granted to a servant who is under commands and prohibitions, not in the way of one who really possesses property. Therefore he is not permitted any rights of disposal

1 Calamity, *muṣība*, or misfortune. Misfortune and grief are seen as ills which need healing especially by patient endurance, *ṣabr*, and by reflection; most of all by confidence in, and reliance upon, God the Creator and Giver of all good.

over his possession, except as is in accordance with the command of the real owner.

2. That the servant's destiny and his return are to God his true master, and he must inevitably leave this world behind and come to his Lord on his own—as He created him in the first place—without family, wealth, or tribe, with only his good and bad deeds. If such be the servant's beginning, the permission he has been granted, and his end, then how can he rejoice at what exists, or be in despair at what is lost! Hence the servant's reflection on his beginning and his end is the greatest sort of treatment for this sickness.

Part of his treatment is that he should know with certainty that what has afflicted him was not to miss him, and what missed him was not to bring disaster on him. The Most High said: *No misfortune can happen on earth or in your souls but is recorded in a decree before We bring it into existence; that is truly easy for God; in order that you may not despair over that which passes you by, nor exult over that which is bestowed on you; for God does not love the one who is proud and boasts* (LVII: 22–3).

Part of his treatment is that he should consider his affliction and realize that his Lord has preserved for him something similar or even better, and has stored up for him—if he is patient and compliant—what is far greater than the passing things of that calamity, many times multiplied, and that if He wished He could make them greater still.

Another part of his treatment is that he should quench the fire of his misfortune with the coolness of consolation of those who suffer disasters, and that he should know that in every valley there are sons of good fortune. Let him look to the right: does he see aught but trials? Then turn to the left: does he see aught but loss? And he should know that even if he were to search throughout the world he would find among all people only those under trial, whether by loss of a beloved one, or the coming of something undesired, and that good fortunes of this world are but as dreams, or as passing shadows. If they make one laugh a little, they make one weep much, and if they cause happiness for a day, they are a cause of misery for an age. If they grant enjoyment for a short while, they prevent it for a long while; if they ever fill a house with good, they also fill it with tears, and joys cannot make one happy for a day unless trials hide them for another day.

Ibn Masʿūd said: To every joy is a distress, and no house can be filled with joy, unless it is filled with sorrow.

Ibn Sīrīn said: There is never any laughing that is not followed by weeping.

Hind bint al-Nuʿmān said:[2] I have looked upon us, when we were among the

2 Hind bint al-Nuʿmān: Nuʿmān b. al-Mundhir was the last ruler of the Lakhmid house of Ḥīra, a small kingdom to the east of the Arab land and subject to the Great King of Persia. Nuʿmān ruled for some twenty years around the turn of the sixth/seventh century AD, was finally imprisoned by the King of Persia and died in prison. His family's fate, with legends added, was taken as an example of disaster suddenly striking the wealthy and powerful, and hence as a warning to others. EI[1] 3, 953.

noblest and wealthiest of people; then the sun had no sooner set than I saw us as the least of people. It is incumbent upon God that He should not fill a house with good, unless He fills it with tears. A man asked her to recount her story, and she said: One morning, when we arose, there was not one of the Arabs who did not ask our favour; then one evening, not one of the Arabs but felt pity for us.

One day her sister, Ḥurqa bint al-Nuʿmān, was weeping—and this was during their time of power and glory—and was asked: 'What makes you weep? Perhaps someone has harmed you?' She replied: 'No, but I have seen opulence in my family, and seldom is a house filled with pleasures, unless it is filled with grief.'

Isḥaq b. Ṭalḥa said: I went to see her one day, and asked her: 'How do you consider the tears of kings?' She replied: 'What we enjoy today is far better than what we had yesterday. In our books we find that if ever the people of a house live in a pleasant state, they will end after that in tears. Time never brought forth for any people a day they loved, without it concealing for them a day which they would dislike.' Then she recited:

'While we led the people, the command was ours;
then behold we were among them subjects, subordinate;
So away with a world whose blessings do not last;
it turns aside at times with us, and departs'.

Part of the treatment for such disasters is that one should know that anxiety cannot turn them away, but will multiply them; and in truth it only increases the sickness.

Furthermore, as to their treatment one should know that losing the reward of patience and submission—which is the blessings and mercy and guidance that God warranted for patience and resignation—is truly greater than the disaster.

For such treatment a man should know that anxiety causes his enemy to gloat, and causes ill to his friend, angers his Lord, and rejoices his Satan, lessens his reward and weakens his soul. But when he is patient and resigned to God, he drives his Satan away rejected and pleases his Lord, makes his friend happy and his enemy unhappy, and relieves the burden of his brethren and comforts them before they comfort him. This is the greatest stability and perfection: not striking of the cheeks or beating of the chest, or prayer of grief and destruction, or bitterness at what is decreed.

Part of this treatment is that one should know that the pleasure and joy that follow patience and anticipation of reward from God are many times greater than he would have acquired if what was destroyed remained in his possession. Fully sufficient for him is the house of praise which is built for him in Paradise as reward for his praise of his Lord and his anticipation. And let him consider which of the two disasters would be the greater: loss in the present life or the disaster of losing the house of praise in the Paradise of Eternity.

In al-Tirmidhī (*marfūʿ*) we read: 'People would wish, on the Day of Resurrection, even that their skins might be cut with sharp instruments in this life, for the sake of such reward as they see prepared for those who have suffered trials.'[167]

One of the ancestors said: Were it not for the calamities of this life, we would come to the Resurrection bankrupt.

This treatment includes giving rest to his heart with the solace of hope in the recompense to come from God. For there is a substitute for everything except God, for He has no substitute. As has been said:

'For everything you may lose, there is compensation, but should you lose God, there is no compensation for Him.'

Another part of this treatment is that one should know that his portion of misfortune is what it brings for him; so if he is content then he will attain God's pleasure, and if he is resentful he will obtain God's displeasure. Your portion thereof is what it induced for you. So choose either the best of lots or the worst. So if it brings about in him displeasure and disbelief, he will be inscribed in the register of those due to perish. If it brings about in him anxiety and neglect, in leaving aside some duty or in committing what is forbidden, he will be inscribed in the register of the neglectful. If it causes complaint and lack of patience, he will be inscribed in the register of the deceived. If it causes opposition to God, and depreciation of His wisdom, he has knocked at the door of heresy, or entered it. If it causes patience and steadfastness towards God, he is inscribed in the register of the patient; if it causes contentment, he is inscribed in the register of the approved. If it causes praise and thankfulness he is inscribed in the register of the grateful, and will be included under the banner of praise among those who are continually giving praise. If it causes love and longing to meet his Lord, then he is inscribed in the register of lovers and sincere ones.

In the *Musnad* of Imām Aḥmad, and al-Tirmidhī, from *ḥadīth* of Maḥmūd b. Labīd (*marfūʿ*): 'When God loves a people He tests them, and whosoever is contented will attain God's pleasure, and whosoever is resentful will obtain God's wrath.' Aḥmad adds to this: 'Whosoever is anxious, will incur regret.'[168]

Furthermore, a person should know that even if he is exceedingly anxious, at the end he will have to be patient under duress. He will be neither praised nor rewarded.

A wise man has said: On the first day of his misfortune, an intelligent person does what the foolish waits many days to do. Whoever is not patient in the manner of the noble will have the consolation of dumb animals.

It is related in the *Ṣaḥīḥ* (*marfūʿ*): Patience comes at the first shock of calamity.[169] Al-Ashʿath b. Qays said: If you are patient in faith and anticipation well and good; otherwise you will be consoled as are dumb animals.

Part of the treatment is that a man should know that the most beneficial of medicines for him is to be in conformity with his Lord and God, in what He loves and desires for him; and that the special property and secret of love is conformity with the beloved. Whoever claims to love a beloved, but resents what he likes and likes what he resents, demonstrates that he is lying, and makes himself hateful to the loved one.

Abū al-Dardā' said: 'When God decrees anything, He wishes that one should be content therewith.' And ʿUmrān b. al-Ḥuṣayn used to say, in his illness: 'What is best loved to me, is the best loved to Him;' Abū al-ʿĀliya said the same.

This medicine and treatment can only be used with the lovers of God; not everyone can use it as treatment.

Another element in the treatment is that one should weigh up between the two types of pleasure and enjoyment, which is the greater and the more lasting: pleasure of undergoing affliction, or pleasure of enjoying God's reward. If a person clearly perceives the difference and prefers what is superior, let him praise God for the success He gave. If he prefers what is lower, in every way, then let him know that the disaster in his intelligence, his heart and his religion is greater than the disaster that afflicted him in his worldly affairs.

A further part of the treatment is that one should know that the One who so tests him is the Wisest of all Wise, the most Merciful of all Merciful ones, and that He, praised be He, has not sent the trial upon him to destroy him, nor to punish him thereby, nor sweep him away. But he simply scrutinised him, to examine his patience, his contentment, and his faith; so as to hear his humble entreaty and supplication, and to see him prostrate at His door, seeking shelter under His protection, broken-hearted in His presence, raising a tale of woe to Him.

Shaykh ʿAbd al-Qādir said: 'O my son, disaster has not come in order to destroy you, but it has come only to examine your patience and your faith. O my son, the decree is like a lion, and the lion does not eat a dead body.'

The meaning is that misfortune is like the bellows, working on the servant who thereby produces his cast metal, to see whether he brings forth red gold or brings forth all the dross. It has been said:

> We cast it, and we reckoned it as silver,
> and the bellows showed up dross of iron.

If these bellows do not bring him benefit in this world, then he will have to face the greater bellows. When the servant knows the suffering of the bellows and foundry, and that he cannot escape one or other of the two bellows; then let him know the volume of God's grace towards him in subjecting him to the bellows of the present life.

Again, part of the treatment is that one should know that were it not for this world's tests and disasters, the servant would be afflicted by such ills of pride and self-glory, and regal haughtiness and hardness of heart, as would be the cause of his destruction in this world and the hereafter. So it is the mercy of the Most Merciful that he should treat him at times by certain kinds of medicines of disasters, which protect him from these other ills and preserve the soundness of his servanthood and expel from him the corrupt, destructive evil matters. So glory be to the One who shows mercy through testing, and tests with His blessings! As has been said:

> God gives blessings through His trials, although they are great;
> and God tests some people with favours.'

Were it not that He, praised be He, treats His servants with the medicines of tests and trials, they would transgress and commit injustice. And God, praised be He, when He wishes good for a servant, gives him medicines to drink, of trials and tests, according to the capacity of his condition, whereby He expels his deadly diseases. This continues until He has disciplined him, cleansed and purified him, and He then qualifies him for the noblest degrees of this world—this is servanthood to Him—and the highest reward in the next world, which is to see and be near to his Lord.

Another part of the treatment is that one should know that the bitterness of this life is in itself the sweetness of the next. God, praised be He, transforms them thus; and sweetness of this life is in itself bitterness of the next. To cross over from a temporary bitterness to a lasting sweetness is better for one than the reverse.

If this is hidden from you, then look at the words of the truthful one, the one believed: Paradise is encompassed by unpleasant things, and the fire is surrounded by pleasures.

In this whole matter, the intellects of created people are very diverse, and their true natures are apparent. Most of them prefer the temporary sweetness to the lasting sweetness which never ends, and do not bear the bitterness of an hour for the sake of the sweetness of eternity, nor the wretchedness of an hour for the sake of the glory of eternity, nor the suffering of an hour for the health of eternity. What is present is manifest, while that which is awaited is hidden; faith is weak, the power of desire is predominant. Thence comes about the preference for what is present and passing and the rejection of what is still to come.

This is the condition of the glance which falls upon the external appearance of matters, their beginnings and early stages. As for the piercing glance which penetrates the veils of this present life, and crosses over it to reach the results and goals, this is of quite another quality.

So summon your soul to what God has prepared for His friends and those obedient to Him, in the way of lasting joy, eternal happiness and the greater victory; and consider what He has prepared for the people of vanity and waste, in the way of disgrace and punishment, and everlasting sorrow. Then choose which of the two divisions is more fitting for you. *Everyone acts according to his own disposition* (XVII:84). Everyone aspires to what is suitable for him and more appropriate. Do not underestimate this treatment because of its length, as the desperate need of it—on the part of physician and patient—calls for this extended presentation. God gives success.

(b) *Treatment for anxiety, worry, sorrow, and grief*[3]

It is reported in the two books of the *Ṣaḥīḥ*, from *ḥadīth* of Ibn ʿAbbās, that the Messenger of God ﷺ, in time of anxiety, used to say: 'There is no god but God, the Mighty, the Clement; there is no god but God, the Lord of the mighty throne; there is no god but God, Lord of the seven heavens and Lord of the earth, Lord of the noble throne.'[170]

It is related in al-Tirmidhī's *Jāmiʿ*, from Anas, that the Messenger of God ﷺ, when some serious matter troubled him, would say: 'O Everliving, O Eversubsistent! Through Your mercy I seek help.'[171] In the same source, from Abū Hurayra, it says that when something troubled him the Prophet ﷺ raised his eyes to heaven and said: 'Praise be to God the Mighty'. When he was making earnest supplication, he would say: 'O Everliving, O Eversubsistent'.[172]

In the *Sunan* of Abū Dāwūd, from Abū Bakr al-Ṣiddīq, we read that the Messenger of God ﷺ said: 'The supplications of the anxious are: O my God! In Your mercy I hope, so do not leave me to myself for a single instant, and make all things well for me. There is no god but You.'[173] Here also Asmā' bint ʿUmays said: The Messenger of God ﷺ said to me: 'Shall I not teach you words which you may recite at a time of anxiety: God is my Lord, I do not associate anything with Him.'[174] One narrative quotes that this is to be repeated seven times.

In the *Musnad* of Imām Aḥmad, from Ibn Masʿūd from the Prophet ﷺ, we read: If ever a servant is afflicted with worry or grief and he recites: 'O my God, I am Your servant, the son of Your servant and of Your maidservant, my forelock is in Your hand; Your judgement is carried out with me, Your decree regarding me is just. I ask you by every Name which is Yours, whereby You have named Yourself or which You have revealed in Your book or taught to any one of Your creation, or have exclusively kept in the knowledge of the unseen with You—that You would make the mighty Qur'ān the pasture of my heart, the light of my breast, the cleanser of my grief and dispeller of my worry'—then indeed God disperses his grief and worry and gives in its place joy.'[175]

In al-Tirmidhī, from Saʿd b. Abī Waqqās it says: the Messenger of God ﷺ said: 'Consider the supplication of Dhū'l-Nūn (Jonah), when he called on the Lord from within the fish's belly: *There is no god but You, praise to You, indeed I am among the wrongdoers* (XXI:87)—now if ever any Muslim calls upon his Lord with this prayer in any matter, then he will certainly be

3 In which IQ sets out to explain why and how the spiritual remedies described are effective in trouble, disaster and grief. These are in fact the true 'Medicine of the Prophet'; *tawḥīd* 'opens the door' to true happiness, for it puts the believer in touch with the source of all life.

answered.'[176] And in another narrative: Indeed I know a word which, if ever a troubled person calls on the Lord with it, God will rescue him; and that is the supplication of my brother Jonah.

It is related in the *Sunan* of Abū Dāwūd, from Abū Saʿīd al-Khudrī: The Messenger of God ﷺ entered the mosque one day, and there he saw a man of the Anṣār, called Abū Umāma. He asked: 'O Abū Umāma, wherefore do I see you in the mosque outside the hours of worship?' He replied: 'Worries which have attacked me, and debts, O Messenger of God.' He said: 'Shall I not teach you a word which, when you recite it, God the Most Glorious will disperse your worry, and discharge your debt?' 'Yes, O Messenger of God'. He then recited: 'Say, in the morning and the evening: "O my God, I take refuge with You from worry and grief, I take refuge with You from incapacity and laziness, and I take refuge with You from cowardice and miserliness; and I take refuge with You from overwhelming debt and the power of men".' The man said: 'So I did that, and God the Most Glorious dispersed my worry and discharged my debt for me.'[177]

In the *Sunan* of Abū Dāwūd, from Ibn ʿAbbās we read: The Messenger of God ﷺ said: 'If anyone continues to seek forgiveness, God will give him for every worry joy, and for every trouble a way out, and will grant him his livelihood whence he does not expect it.'[178]

In the *Musnad*: the Prophet ﷺ, 'when some serious matter troubled him, would seek protection in the prayer',[179] for the Most High has said: '*Seek God's help with patient perseverance and with prayer*' (11:45).

In the *Sunan* is reported: 'You must strive, for striving is one of the gates of Paradise, and thereby God repels from souls their worry and concern.'

It is reported from Ibn ʿAbbās, from the Prophet ﷺ: If anyone has many worries and concerns, then let him say often: 'There is no power and no strength save with God'. It is confirmed in the two books of the *Ṣaḥīḥ*: 'It is one of the treasures of Paradise'[180] and in al-Tirmidhī: 'It is one of the gates of Paradise'.

These remedies comprise fifteen types of medicine; and if these are not strong enough to disperse the disease of worry, sorrow and grief, then this is a disease which has taken firm hold and whose causes have become deep-seated, and it needs complete expulsion: (1) acknowledging the unity of Lordship; (2) the Divine unity; (3) intellectual and credal acknowledgement of unity; (4) declaration that the Lord Most High is free from any unjust treatment of His servant and would never punish him without due cause on the part of the servant to deserve this; (5) admission by the servant that he is the wrongdoer; (6) seeking access to the Lord Most High through what is most dear to Him, that is through His Names and Attributes—and among those which best encompass the meanings of the Names and Attributes, are 'The Everliving, the Eversubsistent'; (7) seeking help from Him alone; (8) affirmation of the servant's hope in Him; (9) affirmation of confident trust in Him, and entrustment of all to Him, admitting to Him that his forelock is in His hand, that He can dispose of him as He wishes, and that His judgement is carried out in him, His decree regarding him is just; (10) that his heart should pasture in the gardens of the Qur'ān, that he should make it for his heart like the spring pasture for animals, and that he should find in it guidance in the darknesses of doubts and desires, consolation for all that passes away and comfort from every disaster; that he should seek healing thereby from ills of the heart; that it may clear his grief and heal his worry and concern; (11) seeking forgiveness; (12) repentance; (13) striving; (14) prayer; (15) disclaiming all power and strength, and leaving them in the hand of the One to whom they belong by right.

(c) *Influence of medicine on these worries and diseases, through seeking access to God*

The Almighty created the human being, his organs and parts, and for each one of these organs He appointed a state of perfection, at the loss of which he feels pain. For the chief organ, the heart, God appointed a perfect state, at a loss of which it is visited by its illnesses and pains, consisting of worries, sorrows, and grief.

When the eye loses that power of sight for which it was created, and the ear loses that power of hearing for which it was created, and the tongue that power of speech for which it was created, then these organs lose their perfection.

Now the heart was created for the knowledge and love of its Creator, to acknowledge His Oneness, to delight in Him and rejoice in His love; for contentment with Him, for complete trust in Him, for love and hatred in Him, friendship and enmity for Him, and to continue in remembrance of Him. And the Creator should be more dear to the creature than all else, desired above all, and more splendid in his heart than anything else. There is no blessedness, no happiness nor pleasure—nay more, no life—except in this way. This for him takes the place of nourishment, health, and life. If the heart loses these blessings, then worries, anxieties, and griefs come hastening upon it from every side, and insecurity stands over it.

Among the heart's worst ills are association (*shirk*), sins and negligence, and disdain for what He likes and what pleases Him, abandoning of complete trust in Him, not relying enough on Him and being dependent on other than Him, resentment at His decree and doubt concerning His promise and threat.

When you reflect on the diseases of the heart, you will find that they are caused by these and similar matters, and no others.

So the ultimate medicine is often contained in these prescriptions of the Prophet ﷺ which will oppose such ills. For a disease is brought to an end by its opposite, and health is preserved by its similar. The health of the heart is preserved by these treatments of the Prophet ﷺ and its illnesses are treated by their opposites.

Tawḥīd (the profession of God's Oneness) opens for the servant the door of goodness, joy, pleasure, happiness, and rejoicing. Repentance is the expulsion of corrupt mixtures and substances which are the cause of his illnesses, and it is a protection for him from confusion, for it shuts securely the door of evils. Through *Tawḥīd*, the door of happiness and wellbeing is opened, while through repentance and seeking forgiveness the door of evils is locked.

Some earlier authorities on medicine have said: If anyone seeks health of the body, let him be sparing in food and drink; and if anyone seeks health of the heart, let him abandon his wrong action. Thābit b. Qurra has said: Repose of the body lies in eating little food, repose of the spirit in avoiding wrong action, and repose of the tongue in minimizing speech.

Wrong action is like poison to the heart. If it does not quite destroy it, it inevitably weakens it; when its power is thus weakened, it cannot withstand diseases. The physician of hearts, ʿAbd-Allāh b. al-Mubārak, has said: I saw how sins bring death to hearts. Addiction to them is but disgrace. Renouncing sins is life for hearts. Defying yourself is your best path.'

Desire is the greatest of its illnesses, and opposing this is the strongest of its remedies. The self (*nafs*) in its original state, is created ignorant and sinful, and because of its ignorance it thinks that its healing lies in following its desire and appetites; yet therein lies only its destruction and ruin. Because of its sinfulness, it will not accept advice from a wise physician, but considers its illness as if it were a remedy and relies upon it, while it considers the remedy as though it were the illness and avoids it. Thus—from both its preference for the disease and its avoiding of the remedy—there are generated various kinds of sicknesses and illnesses which baffle the physicians, and with these healing is impossible.

The greatest disaster is that the ego should blame that upon destiny, and exonerate itself, and blame its Lord silently, while the sense of grievance would grow stronger so that the tongue would express only blame.

When the sick person reaches this state, there is no hope for a cure, unless mercy from his Lord should pursue and reach him, and He should renew his life and grant him to follow a praiseworthy path. For this reason, the *ḥadīth* of Ibn ʿAbbās, on the prayer of distress, included the profession of oneness of divinity and lordship; he ascribed to the Lord, praised be He, might and clemency. These two attributes are necessary consequences of the perfection of omnipotence, mercy, beneficence, and forgiveness. Further, he described Him as possessing absolute lordship over the upper and lower worlds, and the Throne which is the highest level and the most magnificent of all created things. Complete Lordship is of necessity unique, and it requires that worship, love, fear, hope, veneration, and obedience are due to Him alone. His absolute might requires that all perfection is acknowledged as belonging to Him, and that He lacks nothing and can be compared to none. His clemency requires the perfection of His mercy and beneficence towards His creation.

When the heart knows and realises all this it is obliged to love and glorify Him and confess His unity. Thus it attains such delight, pleasure, and joy as will repel from it the pain of anxiety, worry and sorrow. When the sick man receives that which brings him joy and happiness, and strengthens his soul, you will see how his nature will grow strong to repel the physical disease. That the heart should acquire this healing is even more suitable and fitting.

When you compare the narrowness of distress and the breadth of these characteristics—which the prayer of distress has included—you will see it is exceedingly appropriate to release one from this restriction, and that the heart can come forth from it into the abundance of joy and happiness. These matters can only be believed by one on whom their light has shone and whose heart has direct experience of their truth.

The influence of his words: 'O Everliving, O Eversubsistent, I seek help from your mercy' has astonishing relevance for repelling this illness. For the attribute of Life contains all the attributes of perfection which necessarily accompany it; and the attribute of Self-Subsistence contains all the attributes of actions. Therefore the mightiest of God's Names is the name the Living, the Subsistent by which when He is called He replies; when He is asked He gives. Full perfect life is contrary to all sicknesses and pains. Thus when the life of the People of Paradise is fulfilled, they cannot be touched by any worry, grief, sorrow, nor any distress. But any deficiency of life harms actions, and contradicts the quality of Self-Subsistence. Perfection of Self-Subsistance entails perfection of life. The Living One, absolute and complete, cannot in any way fall short in the attribute of perfection, and the Eversubsistent cannot be incapable of any possible action whatever. So supplication by the attribute of Life and Everlasting Subsistence is influential for eliminating whatever opposes life and harms activity.

An equivalent to this is the Prophet's ﷺ supplication of his Lord—by His Lordship to Jibrīl and Mīkā'īl and Isrāfīl—that He should guide him to the truth concerning doubtful matters, by His permission. For the life of the heart comes through guidance, and God, praised be He, has given these three angels charge over life. Gabriel is entrusted with the Revelation which is life for hearts, and Michael with rain which is life for human bodies and animals, and Isrāfīl with the blowing of the trumpet, which will cause the resurrection of the world and the return of spirits to their bodies. So supplication to Him, praised be He, by acknowledging his Lordship of these great spirits who watch over all life, carries great weight in obtaining one's request.

In short the name of the Living, the Eversubsistent has special power to answer supplications and relieve anxieties.

In the *Sunan*, and in the *Ṣaḥīḥ* of Abū Ḥātim (*marfūᶜ*): The mightiest Name of God is in these two verses: *Your God is One God, there is no god but He, the Merciful the Compassionate* (II:163) and the opening of Āl ᶜImrān: *Alif Lām Mīm. God: there is no god but He, the Living, the Self-Subsisting, Eternal.'* (III: 1–2)[181] According to al-Tirmidhī, this is a sound *ḥadīth*.

In the *Sunan*, and the *Ṣaḥīḥ* of Ibn Ḥibbān also from the *ḥadīth* of Anas: A man supplicated, saying: 'O God! I call upon You, by the fact that Yours is the praise, there is no god but You, the Bounteous who gives; Creator of the heavens and earth, O Thou who possess majesty and honour, O Living, O Everlasting! 'And the Prophet ﷺ said: 'He has called upon God by His mightiest Name, that one by which when He is called upon He answers, when He is asked He gives.'[182]

Therefore when the Prophet ﷺ was supplicating especially fervently, he would say: 'O Living, O Self-subsisting!' His words: 'O God! I wish for your mercy, so do not leave me to myself for an instant, and make all things well for me, there is no god but You,' contain confirmation of hope in the One in whose hands is all good, and reliance on Him alone, and the entrusting of all to Him, and humble supplication to Him; that He would take responsibility to put right all his affairs, and would not leave him to himself; and earnestly pleading through declaration of His oneness; all of which is of such a nature as to have great influence in warding off this illness. Thus too, his words: 'God is my Lord, I associate nothing whatever with Him.'

Now the *ḥadīth* of Ibn Masᶜūd: 'O God! I am Your servant, the son of Your servant' has such divine knowledge, and secrets of true servanthood, as no book could adequately cover. For it acknowledges that he is a servant, as were his forbears, and that God's hands have control of his forelock and over him, to dispose of him as He wishes, and that without Him the servant possesses nothing for himself, good nor ill, death nor life, nor resurrection. For one who is controlled by someone else has nothing of his own affair, but he is subservient, in his grasp, in humility beneath the authority of his power.

His words, 'Your judgement is carried out in me, Your decree regarding me is just', contain two important principles, which are central to *Tawḥīd*: firstly, acknowledgement of the Decree, and that the judgements of the Lord Most High are effective in His servant and carried out, for he can not separate himself from them, nor plot to reject them; secondly, that God, praised be He, is just in these judgements, never oppressing His servant, and He never goes beyond the bounds of justice and beneficence.

Oppression is caused by need, or ignorance, or foolishness on the part of the oppresser, and this could not possibly issue from the One who is knowledgeable of all things, who has no need of anything, but all are in need of Him and He is the most Just of all judges. Not an atom of His creation is outside His wisdom and praise, nor outside His power and His will. His wisdom is effective wherever His will and power take effect.

Therefore God's Prophet, Hud ﷺ, said when his people were threatening him about their gods: *I call God to witness, and do you bear witness, that I am free from the sin of ascribing to Him other (gods) as partners! So plot against me, all of you, and give me no respite. I have put my trust in God, my Lord and yours. There is no moving creature but He takes hold of its forelock. Indeed my*

Lord is on a straight path (XI: 54–6). That means that: with the Most High's taking control of His creatures and disposing of them as He wishes, He is on a straight path. He disposes of them exclusively in a just and wise manner, in beneficence and mercy. His words: *There is no moving creature but He takes hold of its forelock;* and his words: 'Your decree regarding me is just' conform to His words: *Indeed my Lord is on a straight path.*

Next, the Prophet ﷺ pleaded by His Names with which He named Himself, those which the servants know, and those which they do not know, and those which He has exclusively kept with Him in the knowledge of the Unseen, i.e. those which He has not told to any angel close to Him nor to any prophet. So this prayer is the most pleasing to God, and the shortest way for the granting of a request.

Then he asked Him to make the Qur'ān for his heart, like the spring pasture on which the animals graze; and thus the Qur'ān is the pasture for hearts; and that He might make it a healing for his worry and his sorrow, so that it takes the place of a remedy to eliminate illness, and restores the body to its health and equilibrium. And that He might make it, for his grief, like a cleanser which clears stains and rust and all such things. So it is more appropriate with his treatment, when the patient uses it with sincerity, that it should remove his illness from him, and bring him finally to complete healing, health and well-being. God brings success.

Now the supplication of Dhū'l-Nūn contains such perfect acknowledgement of the unity (*tawḥīd*) and incomparability (*tanzīh*) of the Lord Most High, and the servant's confession of his own wrongdoing and sin, as to be among the greatest of medicines for anxiety, worry, and sorrow, and the greatest of means of intercession with God, praised be He, in the fulfilment of need. For the acknowledgement of God's unity and incomparability together comprise the confirmation that all perfection belongs to Him, and the distancing and negation of any defect, blame or comparability from Him; while confession of wrongdoing indicates the servant's faith in the religious law (*sharīʿa*), and reward and punishment, which entails his humility and his return to God, and to ask pardon for his lapse admitting his servanthood and utter dependence on his Lord. There are four things through which one pleads: by affirming God's oneness; by affirming His incomparability; by servanthood; and by humble confession.

As for the *ḥadīth* of Abū Umāma: 'O God, I take refuge with you from worry and grief,' the seeking refuge comprises eight aspects, which fall into matching pairs: worry and grief, incapacity and laziness, cowardice and miserliness, and oppression of debt and subduing of man.

When that which is disliked and harmful reaches the heart, then if it is caused by a past event, it produces grief; if caused by a future event, it produces worry. When the servant pays no attention to his interests and fails to achieve them, this may be either from lack of ability, which is incapacity, or from lack of will, which is laziness. If he withholds what is good and beneficial from himself and from his own people, this is either restriction of the benefits that come through his body, which is cowardice, or through his wealth, which is miserliness. When people overwhelm him it may be through a just cause, which is the oppression of debt, or unjustly, which is subduing by men. So the *ḥadīth* has included seeking refuge from all evil.

The benefits of seeking forgiveness, in the repelling of worry and sorrow and distress, is common knowledge among the people of different religions and the learned men of every nation. That is to say that evil deeds and corruption bring about worry and sorrow, fear and grief, distress and sickness of the heart. It is even true that those who commit such deeds when they have fulfilled their desires, and their souls grow to detest it, continue the practice, only to repel the distress, worry and sorrow they find in their breasts.

As that master of the profligates has said: 'One glass I drank for pleasure, another I took as a remedy'.

But if this is the influence of sins and offences on hearts, then there is no remedy save repentance and seeking forgiveness.

As for prayer, it has an exceedingly important place in giving joy and strength to the heart, so that it expands, rejoices and has pleasure. For it contains the capacity to let the heart and the spirit come near to God and approach Him, to take delight in remembering Him, to rejoice in having intimate dialogue with Him, to stand in His presence, to use the whole body and its powers and faculties in His worship, to let every limb share therein, and stay free from any attachment to created beings or involvement, or converse with them, to allow the powers of his heart and limbs to be attracted to His Lord and Creator, and rest from his enemy at the time of prayer. All this can be among the greatest of remedies and causes of joy, and of the foods which are suitable only for sound hearts. But unhealthy hearts are like unhealthy bodies, in that excellent foods are not appropriate for them.

Prayer is among the greatest helps to obtain benefits and ward off evils, in this world and the next; for it forbids offences, and repels illnesses of hearts, casts out illness from the body; it enlightens the heart, brightens the face, gives energy to the limbs and soul, and brings sustenance, repels oppression, helps the one oppressed, restrains the humours of the appetites, preserves grace, wards off misfortune, causes mercy to descend, lifts away sadness, and is beneficial for many of the pains of the belly.

Ibn Māja related in his *Sunan* a *ḥadīth* of Mujāhid from Abū Hurayra: The Messenger of God ﷺ saw me while I was lying down, complaining of a pain in my belly. He asked me: 'O Abū Hurayra, do you suffer from pain (*ishkam dard*)?' I replied: 'Yes O Messenger of God'. He said: 'Rise up and pray, for the prayer contains healing.'[183]

And this *ḥadīth* is also related (*mawqūf*) on the authority of Abū Hurayra, and that it was he who said that to Mujāhid; and this is more likely. The meaning of the phrase (quoted in Persian, from the Prophet), is 'Does your belly pain you?'

If the heart of the unbelieving physician does not expand to accept the description of this treatment, then one should speak about the art of medicine, and he should be told: Prayer is exercise for both the soul and the body, since it contains a variety of movements and positions: standing upright (*intiṣāb*), bowing (*rukūʿ*), prostration (*sujūd*), sitting back on the thighs (*tawarruk*), and moving from one position to another (*intiqalāt*); whereby most of the joints move, and most of the internal organs are moved around, such as the stomach and intestines, and the other organs of breathing and alimentation. And it is a known fact that these movements contain power to strengthen, and to dissolve matters, especially through the power of the soul, and its delight in the prayer; so the constitution is strengthened, and the pain is removed.

But the illness of unbelief (*zandaqa*) and turning away from the prophets' teaching and substituting for it heresy is an illness which has no remedy except *fire blazing fiercely; none shall reach it but the most wretched who give lie to Truth and turn their backs* (XCII:14–6).

As for the influence of earnest striving to ward off worry and sorrow, this is something well-known in the sphere of the emotions. For when the soul abandons its pursuit of vanities and search for dominance and mastery, its sadness and anxiety grow strong, and its worry and fear. When it fights these, for the sake of God the Most High, God turns that sadness and anxiety into joy, energy and strength. Just as the Most High has said: *Fight them; God will punish them at your hands and put them to shame, and give you victory over them and heal the breasts of a believing people, and disperse the indignation of their hearts* (IX:14–5). Nothing is swifter than striving (*jihād*) in dispersing the grief, worry, anxiety, and sorrow of the heart; and God is the One we ask for help.

As for the effect of the saying: 'There is no power nor strength save in God', in repelling this illness: this comes from its perfection of trusting and disclaiming the possibility of power or strength belonging to any other than He, and submitting everything absolutely to Him, and avoiding any kind of conflict in this regard, and applying this to every change from one state to another in the upper and the lower world, and the power over that change; and acknowledging that all such power belongs to God alone. And nothing whatever can oppose this word.

In one of the traditions we read that no angel descends from heaven nor rises to it, except by this phrase 'there is no power nor strength save in God'. It has a wonderful effect in casting out Satan.

God is the One we ask for help.

(d) *Treatment for terror and insomnia*[4]

Al-Tirmidhī relates in his *Jāmiᶜ* from Burayda: Khālid complained to the Prophet ﷺ, saying: 'O Messenger of God, I cannot sleep at night, from insomnia.' The Prophet ﷺ replied: 'When you go to your bed, say: O my God! Lord of the seven heavens and all beneath their sway, Lord of the earths and what they carry, Lord of the satans and whatever they lead astray, be close to me to keep me from the evil of Your creation, all of them whatsoever, lest any one of them should abuse me or oppress me; Your protection is mighty, Your praise glorious, there is no god but You.'[184] In the same source, from ᶜAmr b. Shuᶜayb, from his father, from his grandfather: The Messenger of God ﷺ used to teach them this formula, as a protection from terror: 'I take refuge with the perfect words of God from His anger, His punishment, the evil of His servants and from the temptations of the satans; I take refuge with You my Lord that they come not.' He said: ᶜAbd-Allāh b. ᶜUmar used to teach these words to any of his sons who were able to learn them, and for the one who would not, he would write these words and tie the writing round his neck.'[185]

It is well-known that this formula of taking refuge is appropriate for the treatment of this illness.

(e) *Treatment for burning*

It is related from ᶜAmr b. Shuᶜayb from his father, from his grandfather, saying: The Prophet ﷺ said: 'If you see a burning, then pronounce the *takbīr* (God is Most Great), for the *takbīr* extinguishes it.'[186]

Since burning is caused by fire—for this is the substance from which the devil was created—and it contains such widespread corruption as is related to the devil through his own substance and action, it is a help to the devil, giving him influence, for fire by its nature seeks to rise and to corrupt. These two matters, that is, rising up in the earth, and corruption, are the devil's guidance to which he calls, and thereby he causes the sons of Adam to perish. Fire and the devil both seek to rise in the earth and to cause corruption.

The magnification of the Lord, the Glorious, through *takbīr* subdues the devil and his works.

Therefore the *takbīr* has influence in extinguishing burning. Indeed nothing can withstand the magnification of God, and when the Muslim glorifies his Lord, his praises have an effect of putting out the fieriness of the fire and suppressing the devil whose substance it is, and this exinguishes the burning. We ourselves, and others, have tested this and have found this to be so. God knows best.

4 Terror, *jazaᶜ*; insomnia, *araq*.

CHAPTER

33

The Prophet's guidance on the preservation of health[1]

HEALTH, stability and the body's state of equilibrium are regulated through moisture which opposes the heat; the moisture is the body's substance, and the heat brings it to maturity, expelling its superfluities, thus correcting and refining it. Otherwise it would harm the body, which could no longer subsist. Thus too the moisture is the food of the heat, and were it not for the moisture, it would burn up, dry and destroy the body. Each of the two qualities upholds the other, and the body is upheld by them both. Each one is a material for the other. Heat is a material for moisture, preserving it, preventing it from corruption and change; and moisture is a material for heat, feeding and supporting it. When one of them exceeds the other, the body becomes indisposed accordingly. For heat always dissolves moisture, and the body needs that which is necessary for its survival, namely food and drink, to replace what the heat dissolves.

When food increases beyond the extent of dissolution, the heat is too weak to dissolve its superfluities, and these turn into harmful substances. They cause havoc in the body and corrupt it, and bring about various types of illness, according to the various types of harmful substances and the susceptibility of organs and body.

All of this is deduced from God's words: *eat and drink and do not be excessive* (VII:31). He thus guided His servants to consume such food and drink as will support the body, replacing what has been dissolved and to such quantity and quality as is beneficial to the body. Whatever goes beyond that is excess. Each extreme is deleterious to health and conducive to illness: either lack of food and drink or an excess thereof.

The whole of the preservation of health lies in these two divine utterances.

1 Preservation of health, *ḥifẓ al-ṣiḥḥa*, first of the two main aims of medicine. Equilibrium, or the 'mean', *iʿtidāl*, stability, *baqāʾ*; just proportion, *ʿadl*. The humoral theory applies here: two of the four qualities, heat and moisture, need to be kept in balance, and a lack of balance causes illness.

There is no doubt that the body is continually in a state of being dissolved and being replaced. Whenever there is much dissolution, the heat grows weak because its own substance passes away; much dissolution destroys the moisture, which is the substance of the heat, and when the heat is weakened the digestion grows weak and continues in that state till the moisture is destroyed and the heat extinguished entirely. In this way, the servant completes the allotted time which God had decreed for him to reach.

The utmost goal of the human being's treatment of himself and others is to safeguard the body until it reaches this state. It is not that he seeks the lasting continuance of the heat and moisture, which themselves ensure continuance of youth, health and strength, for this indeed is something which does not accrue to any man during this life.

For the highest aim of the physician is simply to guard the moisture against putrefaction and other factors which would corrupt it, and guard the heat from factors which would weaken it, and to keep them in right proportion, whereby the human body is upheld in balance, just as heavens, earth, and all of creation are upheld in balance through the just proportion.

Whoever reflects upon the guidance of the Prophet ﷺ finds it the most excellent guidance whereby health can be preserved. Its preservation is dependent on good organisation of food and drink, clothing and dwelling place, climate, sleep and waking, movement and rest, marriage, purging and retention (of substances of the body). When these are managed according to suitable preparations appropriate to the body, environment, age, and habit, it is more likely to preserve health and well-being, throughout life, up to the end of the appointed time.

Since health is one of the most precious favours God has given to His servants, the most generous of His gifts, and most plentiful of His bounties—nay more, absolute health is the most precious of all favours, without exception—it is fitting for whoever is granted a portion of this good fortune to cherish, preserve, and to guard it against harm.

Bukhārī has related in his *Ṣaḥīḥ*, from *ḥadīth* of Ibn ʿAbbās: The Messenger of God ﷺ said: 'Two favours about which many people are not aware: health and being devoid of anxiety.'[187]

In al-Tirmidhī, and elsewhere, from *ḥadīth* of ʿAbd-Allāh b. Muḥṣin al-Anṣārī: The Messenger of God ﷺ said: 'Whoever awakes with good health of body, safe in his mind, possessing the food for that day, it is as if the world is granted to him.'[188] Also, in al-Tirmidhī, from *ḥadīth* of Abū Hurayra, on the authority of the Prophet ﷺ, who said: 'The first question the servant will be asked about on the Day of Resurrection concerning blessings received will be "Did We not make your body healthy for you? and give you cold water to drink?"'[189] Thence we have the Qur'ānic interpretation reported from the ancestors regarding the words of the Most High: *Then you shall be questioned that day about blessings* (CII : 8) that it refers to health.

In the *Musnad* of Imām Aḥmad, the Prophet ﷺ said to al-ʿAbbās: 'O ʿAbbās, uncle of the Messenger of God, ask of God health in this world and the next.'[190] Here too, from Abū Bakr al-Ṣiddīq: I heard the Messenger of God ﷺ say: 'Ask God for certainty and well-being; for after certainty, no one is given any gift better than health.'[191] Thus he combined health of religion and of worldly matters. The true well-being of the servant, in the two abodes, is completed only by certainty and by health. Certainty wards off from him the punishments of the next life, and health wards off the sicknesses of this world, from both his heart and body.

In the *Sunan* of al-Nisāʾī from *ḥadīth* of Abū Hurayra (*marfūʿ*): 'Ask God for pardon, health and well-being, for after certainty no one is given any greater gift than well-being.' These three things encompass the removal of the past evils by pardon, present ones by health, and future ones by well-being. They assure permanence and continuance in good health.

In al-Tirmidhī (*marfūʿ*) it says: 'God is not asked for any gift dearer to Him than health.'[192]

ʿAbd al-Raḥmān b. Abī Laylā said, from Abū'l-Dardāʾ: I said: 'O Messenger of God, that I may be healthy and grateful is dearer to me than that I should suffer trials and be patient.' The Messenger of God ﷺ replied: 'The Messenger of God, likewise, wishes for health.'

It is reported from Ibn ʿAbbās that an Arab bedouin came to the Messenger of God ﷺ and said to him: 'What shall I ask of God, after the five prayers?' He replied: 'Ask God for good health'. This was repeated, and the third time he added: 'Ask God for health in this world and the next'.

Seeing that this is the importance of health and well-being, we shall mention of the guidance of the Prophet ﷺ such points concerning the management of these matters as will make evident, to whoever considers it, that it is absolutely the most perfect guidance whereby one can preserve health of the body and heart, and the life of this world and the next. And of God we seek help, our trust is committed to Him, and there is no power nor strength save with God.

CHAPTER

34
Food and drink

(a) *Types of food*

CONCERNING food and drink, it was not the custom of the Prophet ﷺ to restrict a man to any one kind of food, excluding others. For that is very harmful to the constitution, and could be very difficult for him to accept at times. If anyone restricts himself to one kind of food and takes nothing else then he grows weak or dies; and if he takes something else the constitution might reject it and is harmed thereby. So to restrict the food always to one type, even if it be the most excellent, is dangerous and harmful.

On the contrary, the Prophet ﷺ used to eat what was customary for the people of his country to eat: meat, fruit, bread, dates and such other items as we have mentioned in his guidance concerning foods, to which the reader may refer.

When one of the two foods has a quality which needs to be altered and modified, then he did this by taking its opposite, wherever possible, as he modified the heat of fresh dates by water-melon. If that was not to be found, he would take it, when he felt a need for it, and his appetite desired it, in moderation and without excess; thus it is no longer harmful to the constitution. But when his soul felt an aversion to some food he did not eat it, and did not force himself to take it unwillingly. This is an important principle in the preservation of health. For when a person eats what he dislikes and has no appetite for, it does him more harm than benefit.

Anas said: The Messenger of God ﷺ never denounced any food. If he liked it he ate it, otherwise he left it and did not eat any.[193] Now when he was offered a roasted lizard, he did not eat it. He was asked :'Is it forbidden (*ḥarām*)?' and replied: 'No, but it is not found in our land, and I for myself dislike it.'[194] So he followed custom and his own appetite: when something was not usually eaten in his land, and he himself had no liking for it, he refrained from eating it, but did not prevent anyone else who wished to eat it and who was accustomed to it from doing so.

He liked meat, and especially the foreleg and the front part of the sheep. For this reason, it was this part which was poisoned. In the two books of the *Ṣaḥīḥ* it is said: 'The Messenger of God was brought some meat, and the foreleg was offered to him, for he enjoyed that.'[195]

Abū ʿUbayd and others reported, from Ḍubāʿa bint al-Zubayr, that she had slaughtered a sheep in her house, and the Messenger of God ﷺ sent to her asking: 'Will you feed us from your sheep?' She told the man who came to ask: 'Only the neck is left, and I should be ashamed to send this to the Messenger of God ﷺ.' The man returned and reported this, and he said: 'Go back to her, and tell her: Send it to me, for it is the front part of the sheep, the nearest to what is good and the furthest from harm.'[196]

There is no doubt that the lightest of mutton is the flesh of the neck, the foreleg and the upper foreleg. This is lightest on the stomach, and is fastest to be digested. In all this, there is attention to food which contains three qualities: (1) the abundance of its benefit and effect on the faculties; (2) its lightness on the stomach, and absence of heaviness; (3) the swiftness of its digestion. This is the most excellent food. Nourishment with a little of this is more beneficial than with a larger quantity of some other food.

The Messenger of God ﷺ liked sweetmeats and honey. These three—meat, honey and sweetmeats—are among the most excellent of foods and the most beneficial to the body, the liver and the organs. Nourishment from these brings great benefit in preserving health and strength, and no one can be harmed by it unless he has some illness and affliction.

He used to eat bread with seasoning (*idām*): sometimes he would season it with meat and would say: 'This is the chief food of the people of this world and the next.'[197] This is related by Ibn Māja and others. Sometimes he would eat it with water-melon; sometimes with dates. He put a date on a morsel of bread, saying: 'This is the proper seasoning for that.' This is an example that indicates the importance of balancing different types of food in order to obtain a proper diet. For barley bread is cold and dry, while dates are hot and moist (this is according to the more reliable of the two sources). To season barley bread with dates is the best arrangement, especially for those who are accustomed to them, like the people of Madīna.

Sometimes, too, he would use vinegar, and he said: 'Vinegar is good as a seasoning'. This was in appreciation of it, according to the exigencies of the current situation, not indicating preference for it over other things, as the ignorant may think. The circumstances of the *ḥadīth* are that he went in to his family one day, and they offered him bread. He asked: 'Have you anything to flavour it with?' They replied: 'We have only vinegar.' Then he said: 'Vinegar is good as a seasoning.'[198] The point here is that eating bread with seasoning is one of the ways of preserving health, rather than restricting oneself to either. Seasoning or flavouring (*idām*) is so called because it modifies the bread and makes it appropriate for preserving health. The meaning of the Arabic word for 'seasoning', *idām*', is further explained when we consider the words of the Prophet ﷺ permitting the one proposing to see his prospective bride, saying 'It is more likely that they will be better suited [if they see each other]', meaning it is likely to bring harmony and suitability as the partners would be acquainted in advance and thus proceed with the marriage with knowledge, and there would be no regret.[1][199]

The Prophet ﷺ used to eat the fruit of the land when it was in season, and did not refrain from it. This too is among the greatest means of preserving health; for God, praised be He, in His wisdom created in every land such varieties of fruit and crops as to give nourishment and benefit to the local inhabitants. When consumed at its season it brings health and maintains well-being, and makes unnecessary the use of many medicines. Among those who avoid eating the produce of their own land, for fear of illness, few escape much suffering from bodily illness and these are deprived of health and vigour.

The moistures fruit contains will be cooked by the heat of the season and of the earth, and by the heat of the stomach, which repels any harm it may have. This is provided one does not eat it to excess, nor overload the constitution with more than it can bear, nor corrupt by it other food which is still undigested, nor corrupt the fruit by drinking water or eating food immediately afterwards. For colic is often the result of such eating habits. Whoever eats the right amount of fruit in season, in the proper manner, finds it a most beneficial medicine.

(b) *Eating manners*

It is reliably reported that the Prophet ﷺ said: 'I do not eat when reclining'.[200] And he said: 'I sit simply as a servant and eat as a servant eats'.[201] Ibn Māja relates in his *Sunan*: He forbade any man to eat lying forward on his face.[202]

'Reclining' has been explained as sitting cross-legged; as 'reclining upon something' that is, leaning on it; and also as reclining on one's side. Of these three sorts of 'reclining', one is harmful during eating, and that is reclining on one's side. This hinders the natural course of food from its usual position, and obstructs it from swiftly reaching the stomach, and oppresses the stomach, so that it is not completely open to receive food. Moreover, it leans to one side rather than being upright, and thus food does not easily reach it.

The other two kinds are the ways in which tyrants sit, which is contradictory to true servanthood. Therefore he said: 'I eat as a servant eats', and he would eat while sitting in a position where the buttocks are placed upon the heels.

1 The *ḥadīth*, of which part only is here quoted, concerns the Prophet's advice to a Companion intending marriage. 'Have you seen her?' 'No.' 'Then see her. For it is more fitting that there should be compatibility (love and agreement) between you both (*an yu'dam baynakumā*).' The verb can be taken in two senses: to season, mix and thus make pleasant the food; to mix with, become familiar with people.

It is said of him that he would sit down to eat, leaning onto his knees, and put the sole of his left foot over the back of his right foot. This was out of humility to his Lord the Exalted, being courteous in His presence and showing respect for the food and the companion at table. This position is the best, most appropriate position for eating: for the organs are all in their natural place, as God, praised be He, created them, together with it being the most courteous position. The best position for the human being to take food is when his limbs are in their natural place; this is only possible when man is properly set in his natural posture. The worst way to sit at food is reclining on one's side, for the reason already explained: the gullet and the organs of swallowing are restricted in this position, and the stomach is no longer in its natural place, for it is pushed to the side of the belly by the ground and to the back by the diaphragm dividing the organs of food from those of breathing.

If the sense of 'reclining' is leaning on pillows and cushions placed beneath the one seated, then the meaning is: When I eat, I do not sit reclining on cushions and pillows, as do tyrants and those who intend to eat much, but I eat barely sufficient, as the servant eats.

He used to eat with his three fingers, which is the best way to eat. Eating with one finger or with two does not allow the one eating to derive pleasure, nor does it give him any benefit, and it is a long while before he has enough; nor do the organs of taste or the stomach gain any pleasure by such small morsels. Eating thus becomes mechanical and functional, rather than out of pleasure; just as when a man takes a large portion (of grain), only a grain or two, at a time, then he finds neither pleasure nor satisfaction in doing so. To eat with five fingers and the whole hand causes the food to crowd the organs and the stomach—and it may even happen that the swallowing organs are blocked and death ensues—so the organs are forced to pass it through, and the stomach to bear it. This gives neither pleasure nor relish. The most excellent way of eating is that adopted by the Prophet ﷺ and those who follow him, with three fingers.

Anyone who thinks carefully about his food and what the Prophet ﷺ used to eat will find that he never combined milk and fish, nor milk and acid foods, nor hot foods, nor two cold, nor two viscous, nor two costives, nor two laxative, nor two solid, nor two loose, nor two which cannot be mixed into one; nor did he combine two which were different, like a costive and a laxative, one swift and one slow to digest; nor roast and boiled, nor fresh and dried, nor milk and eggs, nor meat and milk. He never ate any food while it was very hot, nor anything cooked and left overnight to be warmed up on the next day. Nor did he eat putrid and salty foods, like pickles or foods preserved in vinegar or salted. All of these kinds are harmful and cause a loss of health and deviation of the equilibrium in various ways.

He used to rectify the harm of some foods by using others, whenever possible. He would modify the heat of one with the cold of another, the dryness of one with the moisture of another, as he did cucumber and fresh dates, and as he used to eat dried dates with clarified butter, and used to drink the infusion of dried dates, thereby lightening and refining the juices of strong foods.

He used to call for an evening meal, were it only a handful of dates, and would say: 'To abandon the evening meal is a cause of ageing'.[203] This is mentioned by al-Tirmidhī in his *Jāmiʿ* and Ibn Māja in his *Sunan*.

Abū Nuʿaym reported that the Prophet ﷺ used to forbid sleep straight after food, mentioning that this hardens the heart. Therefore, physicians recommend to those who wish to preserve their health that one should walk some little way after the evening meal, be it only a hundred yards, and not sleep immediately following it, for this is very harmful; Muslim physicians say that one can pray after it. The food may thus be settled in the lower part of the stomach, making its digestion easier and more efficient.

It was not part of his guidance that one should take drink immediately after food, for that corrupts it, especially when the water is hot or cold, which is very bad.

The poet said:

> Drink not water after hot or cold food, nor while having a bath.
> If you truly abide by that, fear no stomach disorder as long as you live'.

He disliked drinking water after exercise and fatigue, and after intercourse, and both after and before food, also after eating fruit—although drinking after some kinds is less harmful than drinking after others—and after the bath, and on waking up from sleep. All of this is contrary to the preservation of health. One takes no notice here of habits, for they are only second nature.

(c) *Guidance on drink*

As for his guidance concerning drink, this is among the most perfect guidance for guarding health. He used to drink honey mixed with cold water. This contains value for the preservation of health that only the most excellent of physicians could know. For if it is drunk and swallowed on an empty stomach it will dissolve the phlegm, wash the stomach's surface, cleanse its viscosity, expel superfluities from it, heat it moderately, and repel its obstructions: it will do the same for the liver, the kidneys and the bladder. It is more useful to the stomach than any other sweet substance which enters it. It may have some bad side effect for the sufferer of yellow bile, because of its strength and the strength of the bile, for it may sometimes stir it up. Any harm it may cause to such a person is removed by vinegar, and then it regains its very beneficial effect for him. The drinking of honey is more beneficial than many other drinks, which are in large part compounded from sugar, especially for whoever is not accustomed to these drinks and whose constitution is not familiar with them. When he drinks them they do not suit him as honey does, nor do they come anywhere near this. The decisive factor here is custom: it contradicts some principles and confirms others.

When a drink combines the two qualities of sweet and cold, it is one of the most beneficial things for the body and one of the greatest means of the preservation of health; the spirits, the faculties, the liver and the heart have a great longing for it, and are nourished by it. When it combines the two qualities, nourishment is acquired, and the penetration and distribution of the food to the organs is fully achieved.

Cold water is moist: it calms heat and preserves in the body its original moistures; it replaces what is dissolved, and dilutes the essence of food, enabling it to penetrate the veins.

Concerning the question of whether water nourishes the body, physicians are divided into two opinions.

One group affirms that the body is nourished by water; this is based upon the evidence of growth, increase and strength generated, especially when urgently needed. They argue: Among animals and plants there is a shared similarity in numerous ways as to growth, nourishment and moderation. Plants have a relative appropriate faculty of sensation and movement while their nutriment comes from water. Therefore there is no denying that animals could possibly also draw nourishment from water as part of their overall nourishment. They continue: We do not deny that energy and a major portion of nutriment is found in food; we only deny that there should be no nourishment whatever in water. Moreover, food gives nourishment only by the watery quality it contains, and which would not be possible otherwise.

They say: Because water is the substance of life for animals and plants, there is no doubt that nourishment is greater the closer the source of nourishment is to the substance of life (ie. water), let alone being that very substance. God Most High has said: *We made from water every living thing* (XXI: 30). So how can one deny that nourishment is gained by that which is in the absolute sense the substance of life?

Finally they say: We have observed that when the thirsty man is given cold water to drink, he regains his powers, his energy and his movement, and he is able to go without food, and benefits from just a small amount of it. We have observed that the thirsty man does not benefit from a large quantity of food, nor does it give him strength and nourishment. We do not deny that water conveys food to the parts of the body, and to all the organs, and that alimentation is incomplete without it. We would only argue against the one who would divest it of every power of nourishment whatever, and we consider that to say this is almost a denial of existential realities.

Another group deny that nourishment is obtained by water. These argue on several grounds: that the one who takes water will find it insufficient, and that it does not take the place of food; that it does not increase the growth of the organs, and does not leave any replacement for what the heat has dissolved; and similar points which are not denied by the supporters of the theory of nourishment by water. They consider its nourishment in accordance with its essence, its subtlety and fineness, and the nourishment of each element is measured in accordance to these. It has been observed that the moist, cold, soft, sweet air nourishes in accordance with these qualities. Sweet scents provide a kind of nutriment. The nourishing power of water is much more evident.

In short, when water is cold and is mixed with something that sweetens it—like honey, raisins, dates or sugar—it is one of the most useful items to enter the body and preserve it in a state of health. Therefore the favourite drink of the Prophet ﷺ was the cold and sweet. Warm water inflates and works the opposite to these things.

Since water which has waited overnight is more beneficial than that which is drunk at the time it is drawn, the Prophet ﷺ, after going to visit Abū Haytham b. al-Tayhān, asked: 'Is there any water which has been kept overnight in its skin?' He brought him some, and he drank from it. Bukhārī relates this, with the words: 'If you have any water which has been kept overnight in its skin, well and good; otherwise, we shall sip some.'[204]

Water left overnight is comparable to leavened dough, and that which is drunk immediately is like the unleavened. Moreover, the dusty and earthy parts are separated out when it is left overnight; it has been said that the Prophet ﷺ would select water for its sweetness and would choose that which had been left overnight. ʿĀ'isha said: 'The Messenger of God ﷺ would be given fresh water to drink from the irrigation well.'[205]

Water that is kept in various water-skins (*qirab* and *shinān*) is sweeter to taste than that which is kept in a vessel of earthenware, stone or other such materials; especially good quality water-skins of hide (*adam*). Therefore, the Prophet ﷺ would request water which had been kept overnight in its skin, rather than any other container. Water placed in skins and vessels of hide has a subtle property, because these contain opened pores through which the water can percolate. Therefore, water which is in earthenware that allows it to percolate is more tasty and colder than that in containers which do not allow percolation. Blessings and peace of God be upon the most perfect of creation, the one of the noblest soul, of most excellent guidance in everything. He has shown his community those things which are most excellent and beneficial for them, concerning hearts and bodies, in this world and the next.

ʿĀ'isha said: 'The favourite drink of the Messenger of God ﷺ was the sweet and the cold.'[206] It may be that this means pure water, like water of springs and sweet wells, for they used to select sweet water for him. It may be that this means water mixed with honey, or that in which dates or raisins were infused. It can be said—and this is the most obvious explanation—that it means all of them.

His words in the sound *ḥadīth*: 'If you have any water which has been kept overnight in a skin; otherwise we shall sip some' indicates the permission to sip water, which means to drink with the mouth from a basin, water trough or something similar. This—God knows best—may refer to the case of a spring, in which necessity called for a sipping by mouth; or he may have said this to make clear that it is permitted. For there are some people who dislike it, and physicians almost forbid it, saying it harms the stomach. It is related in a *ḥadīth*—I have no details of how sound it is—from Ibn ʿUmar: the Prophet ﷺ forbade us to drink lying on our bellies, that is, to lap, and he forbade us to scoop up with one hand. He said: 'No one of you is to lap up as a dog does, nor drink at night from a container until he examines it, unless it be covered over.'[207]

Bukhārī's *ḥadīth* is sounder than this. Yet if the former one is also sound, then there is no contradiction between them. Maybe drinking with the hand was not possible at the time, and so he said: 'Otherwise we shall sip'. Drinking with the mouth is harmful only when the drinker is leaning over onto his face and belly, like one drinking from a river or a pool. But when he drinks with his mouth in an upright position, from a raised basin or similar, there is no difference whether he drinks with his hand or his mouth.

It was part of his guidance to drink sitting, this being his custom. It is reliably reported that he forbade drinking while standing. Similarly that he ordered anyone who drank standing to vomit. Similarly, that he did drink standing.

One group have said that this last abrogates the prohibition. Another group have said: rather, it is clear that the prohibition is not because it is unlawful, but for counsel and to indicate the possibility of leaving aside the most appropriate way of drinking, ie. while seated.

Still another group have said: There is basically no contradiction between the two, for he drank standing only when necessary. Now he came to Zamzam, and they were all seeking water from the well, so he asked for water and they handed him the bucket; he drank while standing. This was a case of necessity.

To drink standing up causes many troubles; for it does not really quench one's thirst; the water does not settle down in the stomach until the liver distributes it to the organs. It descends swiftly and sharply to the stomach, so there is fear lest the water might cool its heat and disturb it, and that it might penetrate swiftly to the lower parts of the body without graduation. All this harms the drinker; but if he does this rarely, or in case of necessity, it does not harm him.

Nor do customs oppose this view; for customs are 'second natures', which come under other provisions, and they are similar to unrelated matters that are not to be used for analogy, according to the Jurists.

In the *Ṣaḥīḥ* of Muslim, from *ḥadīth* of Anas b. Mālik, it says: 'The Messenger of God ﷺ used to pause to breathe three times when drinking, and say: 'It is more thirst-quenching (*arwā*), more healthy (*amrā'*), more health-giving (*abrā'*).'[208]

Drink (*sharāb*) in the language of the legislator and Jurists is water. The explanation of breathing during drinking is distancing the cup from his mouth and blowing onto the outside of it, after which he would again drink. Similarly this is made even more obvious in other *ḥadīth*: 'When one of you drinks, then let him not blow into the cup, but move the vessel away from his mouth.'[209]

In this way of drinking there are several points of wisdom and important benefits: and the Prophet ﷺ drew attention to their totality, in his words: 'It is more thirst-quenching and more healthy and more health-giving.' 'More thirst-quenching' means it is stronger, more complete and beneficial, in quenching thirst; 'more health-giving' is the superlative formed from 'health' (*bur'*) which signifies healing (*shifā'*), meaning it heals from the fierceness and malady of thirst, because it meets the heat of the stomach at intervals; so the second time quietens what the first could not, and the third what the second could not. Moreover, it is healthier for the heat of the stomach, and gives it more protection against cold, should it attack it when drunk at once and at one moment.

Moreover, it does not quench thirst if it is drunk at once because it confronts the heat of thirst only during one instant, and then leaves, while its fierceness and strength are not yet extinguished. Even if the intensity of the heat is broken slightly, its thirst is not completely quenched, as opposed to when the heat is broken and thirst quenched slowly and gradually.

Moreover, it has the healthiest result, and is less harmful than drinking one's drink in one draught. For one fears lest it extinguishes the innate heat, by the intensity of its cold, and its large amount. Or it might weaken the innate heat, which might lead to corruption of the temperament of the stomach and liver, and to serious diseases, especially among inhabitants of hot countries such as the Hijāz and Yemen and similar places, or during hot seasons, like the heat of summer. Indeed, drinking in one draught is very dangerous for them, because the innate heat is weak in the inner parts of these people, specially during those hot seasons.

His saying 'More healthy' (*amrā'*) is the superlative of 'healthful', (*marī'*) of food and drink when it enters the body and mixes with it easily, bringing pleasure and benefit. Similarly: Take it and *consume it with pleasure and benefit*... (IV:4) Pleasure in its result, benefit in its taste.

It is also said that this means it is swifter to move down from the gullet (*marī'*), because it is easy and light upon it, as opposed to a large quantity which does not move easily down the gullet.

Among the damage caused by a single gulp is that one fears an attack of coughing for the path of the water might be blocked because of the large amount coming upon it and thus could cause choking. If one breathes slowly and then swallows, one is safe from that. Among its advantages are that when the person drinks the first time, the hot smoky vapour which was upon the heart and liver rises up at the arrival of the cold water upon it, and the constitution evacuates it; but if he drinks in one draught the descent of the cold water and the rising of the vapour coincide; so they meet each other and are in conflict. Thence come coughing and choking, and the drinker gains no pleasure from drinking, nor is it healthy, nor is his thirst quenched completely.

ʿAbd-Allāh b. al-Mubārak, al-Bayhaqī and others report from the Prophet ﷺ: 'When one of you drinks, let him suck up the water thoroughly, and not gulp it down, for a liver ailment is the result of gulping.'

Liver ailment (*kubād*) is pain of the liver. It is known from experience that the arrival of water all at once upon the liver gives it pain and weakens its heat. The reason for that is the contrast between the heat of the liver and the quality and quantity of the cold water. If it were to arrive gradually, a little at a time, it would not conflict with its heat nor weaken it. This is similar to pouring cold water onto a cauldron while it boils; pouring a little at a time does it no harm.

Al-Tirmidhī reported in his *Jāmiʿ*, from the Prophet ﷺ: 'Do not drink in one breath, as camels drink, but in two or three; mention the Name of God, when you drink, and give praise when you finish.'[210]

To say the *basmalah* at the beginning of the food and drink, and to praise God at the end, is mightily effective in its benefit and wholesomeness and repelling harm. The Imām Aḥmad said: 'When food combines four things, then it is complete: When the Name of God is spoken at the beginning, and God is praised at the end, when many hands are stretched over it and when it is lawful.'

(d) *Drinking vessels*

Muslim relates in his *Ṣaḥīḥ* from *ḥadīth* of Jābir b. ʿAbd-Allāh, saying: I heard the Messenger of God ﷺ say: 'Cover the water container (*inā'*) and tie up the water-skin (*siqā'*). For during the year there is one night on which a pestilence (*wabā'*) descends; if ever it passes by a container which is not covered or a water-skin not tied, some of that illness falls into it,'[211] This is something not attained by the knowledge of physicians. Nevertheless it is known to many intelligent people through experience.

Al-Layth b. Saʿd, a *ḥadīth* narrator, said: The non-Arabs among us are on their guard against that one night in the year during the month of *Kānūn al-awwal* (December).

It is reliably reported from the Prophet ﷺ that he ordered the covering of the water container, even by spreading twigs over it. Now in laying twigs over it there is a wise reason, that one does not forget to cover it but becomes accustomed to this, even with twigs; also, that the intention was to prevent small creeping creatures from falling into it, by letting them pass over the twigs as a bridge.

It is reliably reported from him that he ordered that when one secures the water container one should utter the Name of God; indeed to mention the Name of God when covering the container repels Satan from it, and tying it up repels vermin from it. Therefore he ordered the Name of God to be mentioned in these two places, for these two reasons.

Bukhārī relates in his *Ṣaḥīḥ*, from *ḥadīth* of Ibn ʿAbbās, that the Prophet ﷺ forbade anyone to drink from the mouth of the water-skin.[212]

This contains several points of good manners, among which are: (1) that repeated breathing of the drinker into it will impart to it an offensive smell and distasteful odour, that might disgust; (2) that he might be harmed by taking in an overwhelming amount of water; (3) that it might contain some animal which he did not notice, which would injure him; (4) that the water might contain dust or something else which he can not see while drinking this way and might swallow; (5) that drinking in this way fills the belly with air, so that it has no space to accept its proper portion of water; or it repletes the belly, or damages it; and for many other good reasons.

One may ask: What do you do about the narrative reported by al-Tirmidhī that the Messenger of God ﷺ called for a container (*idāwa*) on the day of Uḥud, and he said: 'Loosen the mouth of the water container', then he drank from its mouth? And we should reply: We are content here with al-Tirmidhī's comment, that this *ḥadīth* does not have a sound chain of transmission and ʿAbd-Allāh b. ʿUmar al-ʿUmarī is classed as weak, on account of his memorization. And I do not know if he heard from ʿIsā, or not. He means here ʿIsā b. ʿAbd-Allāh, from whom he related this *ḥadīth* on the authority of a man from the Anṣār.

In the *Sunan* of Abū Dāwūd, from the *ḥadīth* of Abū Saʿīd al-Khudrī: The Messenger of God ﷺ prohibited drinking from the broken gap (*thulma*) in the cup and blowing onto the water.[213] This is among the good manners by which the drinker's own interests are achieved. To drink from the gap of the cup has several bad results: (1) any dust, or anything else, on the surface of the water collects at the gap rather than at the unbroken side; (2) this may cause distress to the drinker, and he cannot drink well from the broken gap; (3) dirt and offensive odours collect at the gap, and cleaning cannot reach there, as it does reach the unbroken side; (4) that the broken gap is the place of all that is unpleasant in the cup, and is the worst place in it. So one must avoid it and keep to the unbroken side; for in any thing, what is debased contains no good. One of the ancestors saw a man buying a low quality object, and said: Do not do that! Do you know that God had taken away blessing from all that is of low quality. (5) There can be a crack or jagged edge in the gap, which would wound the drinker's mouth. There is yet further harm.

As for blowing into the water, this gives it an unpleasant odour from the mouth of the one who blows, and this causes disgust, especially when he has bad breath. In short, the breath of the one who blows mixes in with the water.

Therefore, the Messenger of God ﷺ combined the prohibition of breathing into the container and of blowing into it in the *ḥadīth* related and confirmed by al-Tirmidhī from Ibn ʿAbbās, saying: The Messenger of God ﷺ forbade breathing or blowing into the water container.

One may ask: What do you do about the *ḥadīth* of Anas, contained in the two books of the *Ṣaḥīḥ*, that the Messenger of God ﷺ used to blow three times into the water container?

We should reply: We accept it and readily admit it; there is no opposition between this *ḥadīth* and the former. Its purpose is that he used to blow three times into his drink of water; the word 'water container' is used because it is the receptacle for a drink. This is similar to the expression which occurs in the sound *ḥadīth*: That Ibrāhīm, the son of the Messenger of God ﷺ, died 'at the breast', meaning while still suckling before the age of being weaned.[214]

The Prophet ﷺ used to drink milk (*laban*), sometimes pure (unmixed), and sometimes mixed with water. To drink sweet milk (unfermented) in these hot countries—both pure and unmixed—is very beneficial to preserve health, to moisten the body and rinse the liver; especially so when this milk is obtained from animals that have pastured on artemisia, achillea, lavender, and other herbs. For their milk is classified as a food yet also it is included with drinks and medicines.

In the *Jāmiʿ* of al-Tirmidhī, from the Prophet ﷺ, it says: 'When one of you eats any food, then let him say: 'O our God! Bless it for us, and nourish us with goodness from it!' When he is given milk to drink, let him say: 'O our God! Bless it for us, and increase us by it. Indeed only milk among food and drink brings sufficiency.'[215] Al-Tirmidhī said: This is a sound *ḥadīth*.

It is recorded in the *Ṣaḥīḥ* of Muslim: 'He would have some drink set aside at the beginning of the night, and would drink from it when he arose in the morning of that same day, and in the night following, and the next day and the next night and the morrow until the afternoon. If anything remained of it, he gave it to the servant to drink, or ordered it to be poured away.'[216]

This drink set aside is water in which dates had been cast to sweeten it, and it is both food and drink, and is very beneficial in the increasing of strength and preservation of health. And he did not drink it after three days, lest its fermentation might have made it intoxicant.

CHAPTER

35

Way of life[1]

(a) *Clothing*

THE GUIDANCE of the Prophet ﷺ on clothing was among the most complete and the most useful for the body. He always recommended the lightest of clothing, and the easiest to put on and remove. Mostly he would wear the *ridā'* (loose cloak) and *izār* (lower garment); these are lighter for the body than other sorts of clothing. He used to wear the *qamīṣ* (shirt), which indeed was his favourite garment.

His guidance concerning clothing, expressed through what he himself wore, is the most beneficial of all to the body. He did not wear his sleeves very long nor wide, but the sleeve of his *qamīṣ* reached to the wrist, not passing the hand, so as to inconvenience the wearer or prevent easy and energetic movement. Nor did it come too short, leaving the hand exposed to heat and cold.

The hem of his *qamīṣ* and *izār* would reach half way down the calf of the leg; it did not go beyond the heels, so as to hinder or burden him from walking, as if he was tied up. Nor was it shorter than the calf muscle, leaving it exposed to harm from heat and cold.

His turban (*ʿamāma*) was not large, such as to cause harm to the head or weaken it and expose it to debility and to mishap, as can be seen to occur in those who wear such headgear. Nor was it small, such as to be unable to protect the head from heat and cold, but medium, between large and small. He used to make the end of it come round beneath his chin. This has numerous benefits, for it protects the neck from heat and cold, and keeps it steady especially when riding a horse or camel, and in attack or flight. Many people wear it tucked in, rather than putting it around the chin. But what a difference between these two methods, concerning usefulness and adornment! For when you consider this way of wearing it, you find it one of the most useful of costumes, and most effective for protecting bodily health and vigour, and least likely to burden or distress the body.

1 Various regulations and guidance concerning everyday life, conduct and habits: clothing, *malbas*, dwelling place, *maskan*, sleep and waking, *nawm wa-yaqẓa*.

He almost always used to wear shoes when on a journey, because the feet need to be protected from the heat and cold, and sometimes also when at home.

The colours of clothing which he liked best were white and stripey (*ḥibra*) which means without nap and striped. It was not his custom to wear red, nor black, nor dyed nor shiny cloth. As for the red festive garment which he wore, it was the Yemeni cloak containing black, red and white, like the green festive garment. He wore the one and the other. This has already been sufficiently established, likewise the error of saying that he wore dark red.

(b) *The dwelling place*

Since the Prophet ﷺ knew that he was always journeying and that this world is the resting place of a traveller, where he stays for the duration of his life before he moves on to the next world, it was not his custom, nor that of his Companions and those who followed him, to pay much attention to dwelling places, their construction, their elevation, ornamentation or spaciousness. Rather, the best halting-places of the traveller should protect him from the heat and cold, and secure privacy and prevent creeping animals from entering. There should be no risk of its collapsing because of its weight, nor should vermin settle there because of its spaciousness; nor should it be affected by harmful airs and winds because of its height. It should not be below ground, injuring its inhabitant, nor rise very high above it, but medium. Those are the most moderate and beneficial dwellings, the least subject to heat and cold. Nor do they constrict the dweller so that he feels oppressed, nor are they excessively large, to no purpose, so that vermin shelter in their empty areas. There was no privy indoors which could have offended the dweller by its smell, but the odour within was of the most pleasant kind. The Prophet used to love perfume, and was never without it. His scent was one of the sweetest, and its fragrance one of the best perfumes. There was in the house no privy whose smell could be detected. There is no doubt that this is one of the most balanced and most beneficial of dwellings, the most suitable for the body and for preservation of health.

(c) *Sleep and waking*

Whoever looks carefully at the Prophet's ﷺ pattern of sleep and waking will find this the most balanced and most useful to the body, the organs and the faculties. He used to sleep for the first part of the night, awaken at the beginning of the second half, get up and clean his teeth with *siwāk* and perform *wuḍū'*, then pray, whatever God enabled him to do. Thus would the body, the limbs and the faculties take their share of sleep and repose, and their share of exercise, with ample reward. This is the greatest well-being for the heart and body, for this life and the hereafter.

He never took more than the due amount of sleep that was needed, nor did he deny himself as much as was necessary. He used to do this in the most perfect way, so he would sleep, when need called him to sleep, on the right side, remembering God, until his eyes grew heavy for him, while his body was not filled with food nor drink. His side did not have direct contact with the ground, nor did he use a raised bed, but he had a bed of leather stuffed with fibre. He used to rest on the pillow and sometimes put his hand beneath his cheek.

In the following section we shall elaborate on sleep, and what is beneficial and what is harmful of it.

Sleep is a state of the body which is followed by a sinking of the innate heat and the faculties to the interior of the body to seek repose. It is of two types: natural and unnatural.[2] The natural kind is when the effect of the psychical faculties, those of sensation and voluntary movement, becomes restricted. When these faculties are restrained from moving the body, it becomes relaxed and the moistures and vapours, which are normally dissolved and dispersed through movements and wakefulness, gather together in the brain, where they all originate. Thus the brain becomes inactive and relaxes. This is natural sleep. Unnatural sleep comes about through some accident of illness. That means that the moistures overpower the brain, too strongly for wakefulness to be able to disperse them; or many moist vapours rise up, as may occur as a consequence of repletion with food or drink, and make the brain heavy and slack, so that it becomes oblivious, and the psychical faculties cease to carry out their actions, and sleep occurs.

Sleep has two great benefits: (1) it causes the limbs to be still and gives them repose from fatigue which occurs to them, so they relieve the senses (*ḥawāss*) from the exertion of wakefulness, and put an end to trouble and tiredness; (2) it facilitates digestion of food and coction of the humours. For the innate heat, during sleep, moves vigorously to the interior of the body, as to assist this process. Therefore its exterior is cooled, and the sleeper needs a great deal of covering.

The most beneficial way to sleep is upon one's right side because the food will be properly settled in the stomach in this way. If the stomach is a little more inclined to the left, then one can change over slightly to the left side for a short while to hasten the digestion, because of the stomach's inclination towards the liver. Then settle on the right side so that the food may flow down more swiftly from the stomach.

Thus one should rest on the right side at the beginning and end of sleep. Excessive sleeping upon the left side is harmful to the heart because of the organs leaning towards it, causing matters to flow down to it.

The worst sleep is upon the back. But simply lying down thus for repose, not sleeping, does no harm. Worse still is to sleep stretched out, face down. In the

2 Sleep: the natural type of sleep is explained by the movement of moistures and vapours into the brain, together with relaxation of the body. In unnatural sleep it is again the moistures which 'overpower' the brain, but through some 'unnatural' cause.

Musnad, and the *Sunan* of Ibn Māja, from Abū Umāma we read: The Prophet ﷺ passed by a man sleeping in the mosque, sprawled out on his face, and he pushed him with his foot, saying: 'Get up (or: sit up), for this is a hellish sleep'.[217]

Hippocrates said in the *Prognostics*:[3] If the patient sleeps on his stomach, when his habit in health is not to do so, that indicates some confusion of the intelligence, and pain in the regions of the stomach. The commentators on his book say: Because he contradicted his good habit, and moved to this bad position, with neither apparent nor hidden reason.

Moderate sleep enables the natural faculties to carry out their actions, and it gives repose to the psychical faculty, increasing the essence of its carrier even to the point that its relaxing effect might prevent the dissolution of the spirits.

Sleep by day is bad; it produces moist illnesses and catarrhs, spoils the colour, produces inflammation of the spleen, slackens the nerves, makes the appetite lazy and weak, except in summer, at a time of noon heat. The worst sort is sleep in the first part of the day and after the afternoon prayer. ʿAbd-Allāh b. ʿAbbās saw one of his sons sleeping in the early morning and said to him: Get up! Would you sleep at the hour when worldly sustenance is being apportioned?

It has been said that sleep in the daytime has three causes: natural disposition, stupidity, and folly. From natural disposition: the sleep of the mid-day heat, which is a characteristic of the Messenger of God ﷺ. From stupidity: sleep in the early morning which distracts one from the business of this life and the next. From folly: sleep in the afternoon. One of the ancestors said: If anyone sleeps after the afternoon prayer, and then his intelligence is snatched away, let him blame no one but himself.

And the poet said: Nay! Indeed naps before noon bring the young man confusion, and in the afternoon, madness.

Sleep in the morning hinders one's sustenance, for that is the time in which created beings seek their livelihood, and it is the time when sustenance is apportioned. So sleep means deprivation, except for some unforeseen circumstance or in case of necessity. It is very harmful to the body because it slackens it and because it corrupts the superfluities which ought to be dissolved by exercise, so this sleep brings about aches, fatigue and weakness. If this is prior to natural evacuation, movement and exercise, and busying the stomach with something, then that is a chronic disease, bringing about all kinds of other diseases.

Sleep in the sun stirs up latent diseases. It is bad for anyone to sleep part in the sun and part in the shade. Abū Dāwūd has related in his *Sunan*, from *ḥadīth* of Abū Hurayra, who said: The Messenger of God ﷺ said: 'When one of you is in the sun, and the shade withdraws from him, so that part of him is in the sun and part in the shade, then let him get up.'[218] In the *Sunan* of Ibn Māja and others, from *ḥadīth* of Burayda b. al-Ḥusayb, it says: 'The Messenger of

3 Hippocrates, *Prognostics*. Loeb, III. 13.

God ﷺ forbade one to sit between the shade and the sun.'[219] So that is a clear indication of the prohibition of sleeping thus.

In the two books of the *Ṣaḥīḥ*, from al-Barā' b. ʿĀzib, the Messenger of God ﷺ said: 'When you are going to bed, make your *wuḍū'* as for prayer, then lie down upon your right side. Then say "O God! I submit my soul to You, and I turn my face towards You. I have entrusted my affair to You, I take You as my support, in longing and in fear towards You. I can go to none but You for refuge, nor escape from You. I believe in Your Book which You have revealed, and Your Prophet whom You have sent." Make these your last words. If you should die that night, then you die in the original natural state.'[220]

In the *Ṣaḥīḥ* of Bukhārī from ʿĀ'isha it is related that when the Messenger of God ﷺ prayed the two *rakʿas* of the dawn prayer—that is, those which are supererogatory—he would lie down upon his right side'.[221]

It has been said that the wisdom concerning sleeping on one's right side is that the person shall not be immersed in his sleep, for the heart inclines to the left side, so if he sleeps on his right side, the heart seeks its resting place on the left side, and that prevents the sleeper from becoming settled and sinking into heavy sleep. This is the contrary when he sleeps on his left side, which is the heart's usual place, and thereby would attain complete repose; so the person would sink deeply in his sleep, feel heavy and would miss the benefits of his religious and worldly life.

Since the sleeper is almost like a dead man—for sleep is the brother of death—therefore sleep is impossible to befall the Living One who never dies, praised be He. Nor do the people of Paradise ever sleep there. The sleeper needs one to guard his soul and protect it from any troubles which might occur to it, and also guard his body from misfortunes of troubles. His Lord and Creator, the Most High, is the one who alone can take charge of that. The Prophet ﷺ taught that the person going to sleep should utter words of entrustment, refuge, longing and fear, that he might thereby call to his aid the full guardianship of God and His protection for his soul and body. The Prophet ﷺ guided him as well to recall his faith, and sleep in that state, and let his final words be ones of faith. It could be that God would summon him during his sleep, and so if his last words were of faith, he would enter Paradise.

This guidance as to sleep serves the best interests of heart, body and spirit, in sleep and waking, for this life and the next. The blessings and peace of God be upon the one through whom his community obtained all that is good.

His words 'I commit my soul to You' mean: I have made it submissive to you, as the slave submits to his master and owner.

The directing of his face to Him indicates his complete absolute attention given to his Lord, and sincerity of intention and will towards Him, and his admission of humility, lowliness and docility. The Most High said: *If they should dispute with thee, say: I have submitted myself (lit. my face) to God, and (so have) those who follow me* (III:20). He mentions the face since it is the noblest part of the human being, and the seat of all the senses. Also *wajh* (face) contains the meaning of turning (*tawajjuh*) and intention. Similarly, the meaning of the words in the statement: 'Lord of the servants, to Him do intentions (*wajh*) and work turn.'

Entrusting (*tafwīḍ*) of the affair to Him means returning it to God, praised be He. Entrusting brings about peace and tranquillity of the heart, and contentment with what He decrees and chooses for him, over and above what the servant likes and is pleased with. Entrustment is one of the highest stations of servanthood (*ʿubūdiyya*) free of ulterior motives, and it is one of the stations of the élite, in contradiction to those who oppose this.

Now taking Him, praised be He, as support (lit. taking Him as a shelter to his back) contains the strength of reliance upon Him, confidence, leaning on Him, and complete trust (*tawakkul*) in Him. Whoever leans his back against a secure pillar does not fear any fall.

As the heart has two powers, power of desire and power of fear, and the servant is seeking for his benefit, fleeing from what would harm him, thus he joined the two matters in this entrustment and directing of himself, and said: 'in longing and in fear towards You.'

He praised his Lord, saying that there is no other refuge for the servant, nor is there any other to rescue him from his Lord. For He it is to whom the servant goes for refuge in order to save him from himself. As is found in the other *ḥadīth*: 'I take refuge with Your pleasure from Your anger, and with Your pardon from Your punishment, and I take refuge with You from You.'

For it is He, praised to Him, who protects His servant, and saves him from His harshness which comes about by His will and power; from Him come both trial and assistance, and from Him comes that from which deliverance is sought, and with Him is recourse in deliverance. He it is to whom one resorts so as to be saved from that which comes from Him, and with Him is refuge sought from that which comes from Him. He is the Lord of all, and nothing exists save by His will. *If God were to afflict thee, there is none that can remove the affliction but He* (VI:17). And: *Say: who can save you from God, if He wished to do you harm, or (can stop Him) if He wished to show you mercy?* (XXXIII:17).

He finished the supplication by acknowledging faith in His Book and His Messenger, who is the angel of deliverance and victory in this life and the next. This is the guidance given by his custom in sleep.

If he did not say: I am a Messenger, then his very guidance would speak in witness.

The Messenger of God ﷺ used to waken at the shout of the crier, that is, the cockerel. He would utter praise of God the Most High and pronounce the glorification (*takbīr*), and say 'There is no god but God' (*tahlīl*) and make supplication. Then he would clean his teeth with a *siwāk*, get up to perform his *wuḍū'*, then stand for prayer in the presence of his Lord, speaking in intimate dialogue with Him, uttering His praise, hoping in Him, longing and fearful.

What kind of protection for the health of heart, body, soul and powers, for the blessings of this life and the next, could be higher than this?

(d) *Exercise*

As for the management of activity and stillness, that is, exercise, we shall relate details to establish the conformity of his guidance in this matter, to the most perfect, praiseworthy and correct. So we say: It is well-known that the body, during its entire existence, is in need of food and drink. Now the food does not in its entirety become part of the body, but after digestion has occured there must always remain something left over. If this builds up as time passes, it collects in both quantity and quality. By its quantity it is harmful, since it obstructs and weighs down the body and causes the illnesses of retention (*iḥtibās*). If it is evacuated by medicines, it harms the body for most of them are poisonous, and would also expel what is good and useful. By its quality it is also harmful, since it might cause heat or cold through its natural quality, or through decay, or it might weaken the innate heat through its coction.

Obstruction of the superfluities will inevitably cause damage, whether they are left or evacuated. Movement is the most potent factor in preventing their generation, for it warms the limbs, and causes their superfluities to flow so that they do not collect together over a period of time. Thus, lightness and energy are restored to the body, it is made receptive for food, the joints are made firm and the sinews and ligaments are strengthened. One is safe from all the illnesses caused by matter and most of the diseases caused by the temperaments, when a moderate amount of exercise is employed, at the proper time, and the rest of the life style is correct.

The time for exercise is after the food has descended and digestion is complete. Moderate exercise is that in which the skin becomes reddened and increases, and the body becomes moist. But the sort in which the sweat pours down is excessive. Any limb which has much exercise becomes strong, and especially according to the type of that exercise. Rather is that the case with every faculty, for if a man concentrates much on learning by heart his memory is strengthened, and if he thinks a good deal, his cogitative faculty is strengthened. For every limb there is a special type of exercise. For the chest, it is recitation, beginning with what is said silently, proceeding to recite aloud gradually. Exercise of the hearing comes by hearing voices and speech, gradually, so one proceeds from the lighter to the heavier; and such is the case with the tongue, in speaking. So too the exercise of the sight; and exercise of walking, proceeding a little at a time.

As for horseback riding, archery, wrestling and running races, these are exercise for the whole body, and remove chronic illnesses, like leprosy, dropsy and colic.

Exercise for souls consists of study and education, of joy and happiness, patient endurance, firmness, courage and action; of generosity, doing good, and such things, whereby souls are trained. Among the greatest sorts of exercise for the soul is that of patience, love, bravery and beneficence, and the souls continue to be trained thereby, little by little, until these characteristics become well-established dispositions.

When you consider carefully his guidance in that, you find it to be the most perfect guidance for the preservation of the health and faculties, and prospering here and in the future life.

Apart from what the prayer contains regarding the preservation of sound faith and happiness in both worlds, it also includes some of the best qualities for maintaining the body's strength and health and dissolving its humours and superfluities. Likewise standing (in prayer) by night is among the most beneficial means to preserve health, and most able to prevent many of the chronic illnesses, and one of the most activating elements for the body, spirit and heart.

It is reported in the two books of the *Ṣaḥīḥ*, from the Prophet ﷺ, that he said: 'The devil ties three knots on to the nape of the neck of any one of you, when he sleeps; on each knot he beats out: You have a long night over you, so sleep. Then, if the man awakens and remembers God, one knot is undone, and if he makes *wuḍū'*, the second knot is undone; and if he prays, all his knots are undone, and he becomes energetic and happy of soul. Otherwise, he becomes evil of soul, and lazy.'[222]

In the fast prescribed by the *sharīʿa* there are means of preserving health, and exercise for body and spirit, such as cannot be rejected by anyone of sound intellect.

As for the struggle (or holy war—*jihād*), and the all-inclusive movements comprised in it, this is among the greatest means of strength and preservation of health, for firmness of the heart and body and warding off their superfluities, for putting an end to worry, anxiety and grief—this is something which is known only to whoever partakes in it. Similarly for pilgrimage and perfomance of rituals, and racing on horseback with arrows, and walking when on business or going to meet brethren, and fulfilling what is due to them, and visiting those of them who are ill, and following the funeral processions of their dead; and walking to mosques, for Friday prayer and congregations, the movement of *wuḍū'* and *ghusl* and other such things.

The minimum benefit therein is exercise that assists in the preservation of health and repelling superfluities. As for the significant benefits for which it was prescribed, as means to attain good things of this world and the next, and repelling their evils, that is another matter altogether.

So you have learnt that his guidance is above every other guidance, in medicine for the body and the heart, preserving their health, and warding off their sicknesses. There is no more to be added over and above that for whoever has followed his guidance.

Through God comes success.

CHAPTER

36

The Prophet's guidance on sexual intercourse (*jimāᶜ*)

(a) *General considerations and marriage*

CONCERNING sexual intercourse (*jimāᶜ*) and marriage (*bāh*), the guidance of the Prophet ﷺ is the most complete through which health is preserved, pleasure and the soul's gladness are complete, and the aims, for which it was instituted are attained.

Sexual intercourse was originally created for three matters, which are its primary aims: (1) preservation of progeny and the continuation of the human species, so as to complete the total of persons which God has decreed to be in the world; (2) expulsion of the fluid (*mā'*) which if restricted and retained would harm the entire body; and (3) fulfilment of desire, attainment of pleasure and enjoyment of God's bounty. This last, alone, is the benefit which will remain in Paradise; for there is no procreation there, nor any bodily retention to be evacuated by the descent of fluid.

The outstanding physicians consider that sexual intercourse is among the most laudable ways of preserving health. Galen said: Predominant over the substance of semen are fire and air. Its temperament is hot and moist, because of its being formed from pure blood by which the primary organs are nourished.

When there is an excess of semen, know that it should not be emitted save in the seeking of offspring, or else to expel that which is congested. If it remains long congested, it generates grave illnesses, such as delusions, madness, epilepsy and others. And its expulsion may cure many of these illnesses. If it remains a long while restricted, it becomes corrupt and changes to a poisonous quality which brings about grave illnesses such as have been mentioned. That is why the constitution repels it when it becomes plentiful in the body, without intercourse.

Some of the Ancestors have said that a man must commit himself to three things: (1) he must not neglect walking so that if he needs to walk, then he is able to do so; (2) he must not refrain from eating, for his intestines would grow narrow; (3) he must not leave aside intercourse, for if a well is not emptied, its water ceases.

Muḥammad b. Zakariyyā (al-Rāzī) said: If a man refrains from sexual intercourse for a long while, the powers of his nerves become weak, and their vessels become blocked, and the male organ will contract. He said: I have seen a group who had renounced this due to some kind of asceticism; their bodies grew cold, their movements were difficult, and distress afflicted them without reason; their appetite and digestion were impaired.

Among its benefits are lowering the gaze, self-restraint and the ability to refrain from what is forbidden, which the woman may also attain. So it brings benefit to the soul in present and future life, and it brings benefit to the woman. Therefore the Prophet ﷺ engaged in it frequently and with delight, and he would say: 'Of this world of yours, women and perfume are beloved to me'.[223] In the Book of Asceticism (*Kitāb al-zuhd*) of the Imām Aḥmad, concerning this *ḥadīth*, there is a subtle addition: 'I can endure patiently the lack of food and drink, but not the lack of women.'

He encouraged his community to marry saying: 'Marry, for I would rival other nations as to your number.'[224] And the Prophet ﷺ said: 'The best of this community have the most women.'[225] And the Prophet ﷺ said: 'Indeed I marry, I eat meat, I sleep, I fast and I break my fast. The one who does not follow my way of life (*sunna*) is not one of my followers.'[226] And he said: 'O you band of young men, whoever of you is able to marry, let him marry; for this is better for lowering the gaze and guarding chastity. Whoever cannot, let him fast, as fasting diminishes his sexual power.'1[227] When Jābir married a widow, the Prophet ﷺ said to him: 'Wherefore not a virgin, that you may dally with one another?'[228]

Ibn Māja related in his *Sunan*, from *ḥadīth* of Anas b. Mālik: The Messenger of God ﷺ said: 'Whoever wishes to meet God pure and purified, let him marry free women.'[229] Also in his *Sunan*, from *ḥadīth* of Ibn ʿAbbās (*marfūʿ*) that he said: 'We consider nothing equal to marriage for those who love one another'.[230]

In the *Ṣaḥīḥ* of Muslim, from *ḥadīth* of ʿAbd-Allāh b. ʿUmar, it says: The Messenger of God ﷺ said: 'This world is but a passing delight, and the best of its enjoyment of this world is a righteous woman.'[231]

He used to encourage men of his community to marry fine women who were virgins, and of religious inclination. In the *Sunan* of al-Nisāʾī from Abū Hurayra, it reads: The Messenger of God ﷺ was asked: 'Which women are best?' He replied: 'One who gladdens his sight and obeys his command, and who does nothing he disapproves of concerning herself or his wealth.'[232] And in the two Books of the *Ṣaḥīḥ*, on his authority also, from the Prophet ﷺ, who said: 'A woman is taken in marriage on account of her wealth, her noble

1 Sexual intercourse, *jimāʿ*; sexuality or sexual potency, *bāh*. The *ḥadīth* gives an exhortation to marry.

descent, her beauty and her religion. So obtain one who is religious, and you will prosper.'[233]

He would encourage marriage with a fertile woman, and he disliked one who did not bear children. As we find in the *Sunan* of Abū Dāwūd, from Maᶜqil b. Yassār: A man came to the Prophet ﷺ and said: 'I have obtained a woman of high birth and beauty, but she does not bear. Should I marry her?' He replied: 'No.' The man came to him a second time, and he forbade him. Then he came to him a third time, and he said: 'Marry a woman affectionate and fruitful, for I would rival other nations as to your number!'[234]

In al-Tirmidhī, from the same source (*marfūᶜ*), we read: 'Four things form the way of life of the prophets: marriage, the toothbrush (*siwāk*), perfuming, and henna.'[235] It is related in the *Jāmiᶜ* with (in the fourth word) *nūn* and *yā'*. I have heard Abū al-Ḥajjāj al-Ḥāfiẓ say: The correct version is: that it is circumcision (*khitān*) and that the *nūn* dropped from the margin. Thus was it related by al-Maḥāmilī, from the shaykh Abū ᶜĪsā al-Tirmidhī.

Among the necessary preliminaries of intercourse is that a man must fondle the woman and kiss her, and kiss heavily. The Messenger of God used to fondle his womenfolk, and kiss them. Abū Dāwūd related in his *Sunan*: he used to kiss ᶜĀ'isha and kiss heavily.[236] It is related from Jābir b. ᶜAbd-Allāh that the Messenger of God ﷺ discouraged intercourse without foreplay.

The Messenger of God ﷺ would have intercourse with all his womenfolk, and he would only perform one complete ablution (*ghusl*); and sometimes he would perform *ghusl* after he had intercourse with each one of them. Muslim related in his *Ṣaḥīḥ*, from Anas: the Prophet ﷺ would go around to all his womenfolk, with only one *ghusl*.[237] Abū Dāwūd related in his *Sunan*, from Abū Rāfiᶜ, a client of God's Messenger ﷺ protected by an oath of allegiance (*mawlā*) that the Messenger of God ﷺ visited all his women in one night, and for each one of them he performed *ghusl*. I said: 'O Messenger of God ﷺ, had you performed but one *ghusl*!' He said: 'This is purer and better.'[238]

It is prescribed for one engaging in intercourse, that when he wishes to repeat this before performing *ghusl*, then he should perform *wuḍū'* between the two sexual acts. Thus Muslim related in his *Ṣaḥīḥ*, from *ḥadīth* of Abū Saᶜīd al-Khudrī, that the Messenger of God ﷺ said: 'When any one of you comes to his woman, then wishes to repeat this, let him perform *wuḍū'*.'[239]

Performance of *ghusl* and of *wuḍū'* after intercourse is able to bring energy and well-being, and it compensates for whatever has been dissolved by intercourse. It brings perfect purity and cleanliness, and gathers the innate heat to the interior of the body after its dispersal through intercourse, and brings about cleanliness which God loves, the opposite of which He hates. This is the finest and subtlest arrangement for sexual intercourse, whereby health and the faculties are preserved.

(b) *Lawful and forbidden sexual intercourse*

The most beneficial intercourse is that which takes place after digestion, and when the body's state is one of moderation in heat and cold, dryness and moisture, emptiness and repletion. Any harm occurring when the body is replete is simpler and less severe than harm occurring when it is empty. Equally the damage is less when the body is moist than when dry; and when it is hot, less than when it is cold. It is fitting for intercourse to take place only when the appetite is strong, and complete dispersal takes place, not through exertion nor any erotic thoughts.

It is not fitting that one should summon up or over-exert the appetite for sexual intercourse, or force oneself to it. Rather a man should hasten to it, when the quantity of semen incites him, and desire for it is strong. Let him beware of intercourse with an old woman, or one too young—the like of whom should not be so taken, and for whom there is no appetite. Nor a woman who is sick, or of ugly appearance, or hateful. For intercourse with such women enfeebles the powers and weakens intercourse in a particular way.

Those physicians are mistaken who say that intercourse with a previously married woman is more beneficial than with a virgin, and better able to preserve the health. This is by an unsound analogy, and some would even caution against it. This is contrary to what most intelligent people would say and what is agreed upon according to nature and by law. For in sexual intercourse with a virgin there is a special characteristic, and a complete attachment between her and the one who has intercourse with her. Her heart is filled with love for him, and her affections are not divided between him and others: all of which does not apply to an experienced woman.

For the Prophet ﷺ said to Jābir: 'Then have you not married a virgin?'

God, praised be He, included in the perfection of the women of Paradise, those of dark eyes, who had not been touched previously by anyone and will only be touched by those to whom they are assigned of the people of Paradise.[2]

ʿĀ'isha said to the Prophet ﷺ: 'What is your opinion? If you were to pass by bushes which had been grazed, and bushes which had not been grazed, at which of them would you pasture your camel?' He replied: 'At that at which had not been grazed.'[240] She meant that he had taken no virgin as wife save her.

Intercourse with the woman with whom one is truly in love has very little weakening effect on the body, while it will also cause a large quantity of semen to be expelled. But intercourse with one who is hateful disturbs the body and weakens the powers, and will cause but a small amount of semen to be expelled.

Intercourse with a menstruating woman is unlawful by nature and by law. For it is very harmful, and physicians without exception warn against it.

2 Reference to the houris: 'none hath touched them ...' Qur'ān LV: 56, 74.

The best position for intercourse is for the man to be on top of the woman, stretched out over her, after foreplay and kissing. Thereby is the woman called a 'bed', as the Prophet ﷺ said: 'The child is to the bed.'[241] This is part of the man's complete guardianship over the woman, as the Most High said: *Men are protectors and maintainers of women* (IV : 34). And as the poet said:

> 'When I desired her, she was a bed that supported me.
> And when I was finished, an attendant who flattered.'

And the Most High said: *They are your garments and you are their garments* (II : 187). The most perfect and abundant garments are of this kind, for the man's bedspread is a garment for him, and also the woman's blanket is a garment for her. This excellent form is taken from this verse, and thereby the metaphor of clothing is a good one to express the spouses' relationship to one another.

There is another aspect, namely that she may wrap herself around him at times, and thus be like a garment on him. The poet said: 'When the bedfellow folded his side, then she bent herself and was to him a garment'.

The worst position is for the woman to be on top, and that he has intercourse with her lying on his back. For this is contrary to the natural form in which God made the man and woman, or rather the species of male and female. One evil aspect is that the semen cannot all come out, except with difficulty, and sometimes some remains within the organ, where it will decompose and corrupt and so become harmful.

Also, sometimes moistures may flow from the woman's private parts to the male organ; and moreover the womb in such a position is not able to contain all the fluid, nor retain it, nor envelop it, sufficiently for the formation of offspring.

Moreover the woman is passive both by nature and by law. If she should be the active partner, she contravenes the demands of nature and the law. The People of the Book used to approach women only upon their sides, and used to say that this was easier for the women.

The Quraysh and the Anṣār would sleep with their women flat on the back of the head, for which the Jews reproached them. Then God, the Exalted and Glorious, revealed: *Your women are as a tilth unto you: so approach your tilth when or how you will* (II : 223).

In the two Books of the *Ṣaḥīḥ*, from Jābir, we read: The Jews used to say: When the man comes to his wife from behind, into her forepart, the child will be cross-eyed. Then God, the Exalted and Glorious, revealed: *Your women are as a tilth unto you: so approach your tilth when or how you will.*'[242] In the words of Muslim: 'If he wishes, lying prostrate (*mujabbiya*), and if he wishes, not prostrate: however, in both positions, in one and the same place (*ṣimām*).'[243] 'Prostrate' means turned (*munkabba*) upon her face, and the 'place' means the vulva, which is the place of 'tilth' and childbearing.

As for the 'rear' (*dubur*), anal intercourse, that is never permitted by any of the prophets. If anyone attributes permission for entering the wife in the rear to one of the ancestors, he is mistaken.

In the *Sunan* of Abū Dāwūd, from Abū Hurayra, it is related that the Messenger of God ﷺ said: 'Cursed is the man who enters a woman in the rear'.[244] In the words of Aḥmad and Ibn Māja: 'God does not look upon a man who enters his woman in her rear parts.' In the words of al-Tirmidhī and Aḥmad: 'Whoever approaches a woman menstruating, or enters his woman in her rear, or went to a fortune-teller and believed what was said, he committed unbelief in what was sent down to Muḥammad.'[245] And in words of Bayhaqī: 'If anyone has anal intercourse, whether with a man or a woman, he committed unbelief.'

In the *Muṣannaf* of Wakīᶜ, Zamᶜa b. Ṣāliḥ related to me, from Ibn Ṭāwūs, from his father, from ᶜAmr b. Dīnār, from ᶜAbd-Allāh b. Yazīd, that ᶜUmar b. al-Khaṭṭāb quoted the Messenger of God saying: 'Indeed God is not ashamed of the truth. Do not enter your women in their hinder parts (*aᶜjāzihinna*) (or, that he said once: their rears (*adbārīhina*)).

And in al-Tirmidhī, from Ṭalq b. ᶜAlī, we read: The Messenger of God ﷺ said: 'Do not enter women in their hinder parts; for God is not ashamed of the truth.'[246]

In the *Kāmil* of Ibn ᶜAdiyy, from his *ḥadīth*, on authority of al-Maḥamilī, from Saᶜīd b. Yaḥya al-Umawiyy, it says: Muḥammad b. Ḥamza told us, from Zayd b. Rafīᶜ, from Abū ᶜUbayda, from ᶜAbd-Allāh b. Masᶜūd, (*marfūᶜ*): 'Do not enter your women in their hinder parts.'

We have related from *ḥadīth* of al-Ḥasan b. ᶜAlī al-Jawharī, from Abū Dharr, (*marfūᶜ*): 'Whoever enters either men or women in the rear has committed unbelief.'

Ismāᶜīl b. ᶜAyyāsh related, from Shurayk b. Abī Ṣāliḥ, from Muḥammad b. al-Munkadir, from Jābir (*marfūᶜ*): 'Be ashamed before God, for indeed God is not ashamed of the truth; do not come to your woman in their rear parts (*hushūsh*).' This was related by al-Dārquṭnī, in this way, and his words were: 'God is not ashamed of the truth. Entering women in their rear parts is not permitted.'

Al-Baghawī said: Hudba related to us, from Hammām, that Qutāda was questioned about one who entered his woman in her hinder parts, and said: ᶜAmr b. Shuᶜayb related to me, from his father, from his grandfather, that the Messenger of God said: 'That is the lesser form of sodomy.'[247] Imām Aḥmad said, in his *Musnad*: ᶜAbd al-Raḥmān related to us, from Hammām, who informed us on the authority of Qutāda, from ᶜAmr b. Shuᶜayb, from his father, from his grandfather—and then mentioned this. In the *Musnad* also, from Ibn ᶜAbbās: This verse was revealed: *'Your women are as your tilth,'* concerning individuals of the Anṣār, who came to the Messenger of God ﷺ and asked him; and he said: 'Come to her in any way, if it is in the vulva.'[248]

In the *Musnad* also, from Ibn ʿAbbās: ʿUmar b. al-Khaṭṭāb came to the Messenger of God ﷺ and said: 'O Messenger of God, I am almost destroyed.' He asked: 'What has destroyed you?' He replied: 'I changed my stopping place [ie. I changed the position during intercourse] yesterday.' The Prophet ﷺ did not reply; then God revealed to His Messenger: '*Your women are as a tilth for you . . . when and how you will.* Come from before or behind, but avoid the menstruating woman, and the rear parts.'[249]

In al-Tirmidhī, from Ibn ʿAbbās, (*marfūʿ*): 'God does not look upon a man who enters a man or woman in the rear.'[250]

We have related from *ḥadīth* of Abū ʿAlī al-Ḥasan b. al-Ḥusayn b. Dūmā, from al-Barā' b. ʿĀzib (*marfūʿ*): 'Ten people of this community have committed unbelief in the All-Mighty God: the murderer, the sorcerer, the cuckold or pimp, the one who has anal intercourse with a woman, one who refuses to give the alms tax (*zakāt*), one who has the means but dies without having gone on pilgrimage (*ḥajj*), the wine-drinker, the one who causes sedition among the Muslims, the one who trades in arms with the people who are engaged in war against Muslims, and the one who marries a woman forbidden to him.'[251]

ʿAbd-Allāh b. Wahb said: ʿAbd-Allāh b. Lahīʿa told us, from Mishraḥ b. Hāʿān, from ʿUqba b. ʿĀmir, that the Messenger of God said: 'Cursed is the one who enters women from their privy parts' meaning their rear parts.

In the *Musnad* of al-Ḥārith b. Abī Usāma, from *ḥadīth* of Abū Hurayra, and Ibn ʿAbbās, who both said: The Messenger of God preached to us before his death, and this was his last sermon in Madīna before he joined the Lord, the Glorious; and therein he warned us, saying 'If anyone has anal intercourse with his woman, or with a man or a youth, then at the gathering on the day of Resurrection his stench will be more horrid than a corpse, and the people will suffer from his bad stench until he enters the fire; and God makes void his recompense: he will receive from Him nothing as his due. He will enter a coffin of fire and will be shut in with nails of fire.' Abū Hurayra said: 'This is for one who does not repent.'

Abu Nuʿaym al-Iṣfahānī mentioned, from *ḥadīth* of Khuzayma b. Thābit (*marfūʿ*): 'God is not ashamed of the truth. Do not enter women by their hinder parts.'

Al-Shāfiʿī said: My uncle Muḥammad b. ʿAlī b. Shāfiʿ informed me that ʿAbd-Allāh b. ʿAlī b. al-Sā'ib told him from ʿAmr b. Uḥayḥa b. al-Jallāḥ, from Khuzayma b. Thābit: A man asked the Prophet ﷺ about entering women in their rear parts, and he said: 'It is permitted.' When the man turned to go, he called him back, and said: 'What exactly did you say? In which of the two openings (*khurba*) (or: in which of the two orifices (*khurza* and *khuṣfa*)). If you mean from her rear, into her front part, yes. But if from behind her, into her rear, no. Indeed God is not ashamed of the truth. Do not enter women in their rear parts.'[252]

Al-Rabīʿ said: al-Shāfiʿī was asked: 'What is your opinion?' he replied: 'My uncle is trustworthy, and so is ʿAbd-Allāh b. ʿAlī, and he spoke well of al-Anṣārī–meaning ʿAmr b. al-Jallāḥ. And Khuzayma is one of those whose trustworthiness is not doubted. So I do not allow this, nay, I forbid it.'

My comment: Because of the confusion and obscurity of this report, it was thus possible to transmit wrongly that the ancestors and imāms permitted intercourse in the rear part, while in reality they permitted only approaching a woman from behind as long as it was a means of having intercourse in the vulva, but not into the rear parts. The prohibition was thus obscure to one who heard these two explanations, or at best did not realise there was any difference between the two. In short, this is what the ancestors and imāms permitted, but a mistake was made concerning this, of the worst and most despicable sort.

For the Most High said: *Go to them in that way* (lit. from where) *God has ordered you* (II: 222). Mujāhid said: I asked Ibn ʿAbbās about the Most High's words: *go to them in that way God has ordered you.* And he said: 'Go to her where you have been ordered to withdraw, meaning during menstruation. And ʿAlī b. Ṭalḥa reported, from him that he says: 'In the vulva, so do not deviate to aught else.'

The verse shows that anal intercourse is forbidden, for two different aspects:

1. It is permitted only to enter her in the 'tilth', which is the place for childbearing; not in the private parts which are the place of harm. The place of tilth is meant in His words: *in that way God has ordered you.* The Most High has said: *So come to your tilth when or how you will* (II: 223). And coming to her in her front part, from behind, is inferred from the verse also. For He said: *When or how you will,* that is, from where you wish: from in front, or from behind. Said Ibn ʿAbbās: *and come to your tilth* means the vulva.

2. If God had forbidden intercourse in the vulva, on account of harm which could occur temporarily (ie. during menstruation), then what can be said concerning the hinder parts which are necessarily the place of harm, with the added harm of running the risk of not being able to have children and the imminent danger of women's rear parts being used as pretext for young boys' rear parts.

Furthermore, the woman has rights over the husband concerning intercourse. Anal intercourse neglects her rights, and her desire is thus not fulfilled, nor her object attained. Also, the rear is not shaped for that action, nor created for it; only the vulva was so prepared. Those who deviate from it, to the rear, are departing entirely from God's wisdom and His law.

In addition, it harms the man, and therefore the intelligent physicians, philosophers and others have forbidden it. For the vagina has a special property to draw the fluid which is restricted within, and thus give ease to the man through its release. Intercourse in the rear does not help to draw all the fluid, nor is all the restricted fluid released, as it runs counter to what is natural.

Also it is harmful from another aspect, which is that it causes very fatiguing movements, as it is contrary to nature.

Moreover, the rear part is the site of uncleanness and excrement, so intercourse thus compels a man to face towards this and have intercourse in such a place.

Furthermore, it is very harmful to the woman, for it is a strange way of proceeding, very unnatural and completely in contradiction to nature. It leads to stress and anxiety, and resentment between both parties. It removes dignity and light from the face, restricts the breast, destroys the light of the heart, brings to the face an alienation which becomes one of its characteristic expressions, recognised by one with even the least discernment. It inevitably arouses fierce aversion and mutual enmity, and estrangement between the two parties. It causes grievous deterioration to all aspects of their life after which no improvement can be expected, unless God wishes, then through repentance and sincerity. It takes away the partners' good qualities, and clothes them with the opposite, and similarly takes away the love between them, bringing in its place hatred and malediction.

It is one of the greatest causes for good fortune to cease and afflictions to occur. It brings about imprecation and detestation from God, and makes Him turn away from the one who commits it, and cease to regard him. So what good can be hoped for after that? And from what sort of evil can he then be secure? How can any servant live after incurring God's curse and hatred, when He has turned away and does not regard him? It completely drives away all modesty which is the life of the heart. When the heart has lost this, then it approves of what is odious, and thinks odious what is good. Then its corruption has become deep-rooted.

It changes nature away from the original state in which God created it, and sends man away from his own characteristics to such for which God did not create a single one of the animals. Rather it is nature inverted; when nature is reversed, then the heart, action and guidance are reversed; then man finds pleasant such actions and attitudes as are in fact contemptible, and he undermines his state, actions and his speech involuntarily.

This brings about such insolence and rashness as naught else does. It makes him the heir of meanness, ignominy and vileness as naught else does. It clothes the servant with the garment of detestation and hatred, and people's contempt and scorn, and they clearly despise him.

So God's blessing and peace be upon that one in whose guidance, and the following of whose message lies felicity of this world and the next; while a complete loss of this world and the next lies in contradicting his guidance and his message.

Harmful intercourse is of two kinds: harmful according to the revealed law and harmful according to nature.

The one that is harmful according to the law[3] is prohibited intercourse. Herein are degrees, some more serious than others. That which is conditionally prohibited is lighter than what is intrinsically prohibited. Examples of the former include prohibition of intercourse during the state of *iḥrām* (conditions necessary for a person on *ḥajj* or *ʿumra*), fasting, *iʿtikāf* (seclusion, while fasting in a mosque), and the prohibition of having intercourse with the woman whose husband committed *ẓihār* (a prohibited formula of divorce) before his payment of the penalty; also the prohibition of intercourse with a menstruating woman and other similar cases. Because this prohibition is only temporary; there is no set penalty (*ḥadd*) for this type. Intercourse which in no way can become permitted is of two kinds: one includes intercourse with a *maḥārim* (persons with whom marriage is forbidden). This is among the most harmful sorts of intercourse, and is punishable by death penalty, according to one group of scholars, such as Aḥmad b. Ḥanbal and others. On this we have a well-traced established *ḥadīth*. There is also intercourse which can become lawful, like intercourse with a foreign woman. If she has a husband, then in intercourse with her two rights are to be observed: a right pertaining to God, and a right pertaining to the husband. If she is forced, then in this there are three rights; if she has a family and relatives, to whom disgace would attach, there are four rights; if she is one forbidden to him, there are five. The harmfulness of this type is according to the degrees of its illegality.

Intercourse unlawful according to nature is also of two types: one harmful by its quality, as has been described, and another harmful by its quantity, like excessive indulgence in it, for this weakens the strength, injures the nerves, brings about tremor, palsy and trembling, dims the sight and other faculties, stifles the innate heat, dilates the vessels and renders them susceptible to harmful superfluities.

The most beneficial time for intercourse is after food in the stomach has been digested, and at a moderate time, not in hunger, for that weakens the innate heat, nor in repletion, for that brings about obstructive illnesses; not in fatigue, nor after the bath, nor evacuation, nor any psychological agitation such as anxiety, worry or grief, nor intense joy.

The best time is after part of the night has passed, coinciding with the digestion of food. Then he performs *ghusl* or *wuḍū'*, and sleeps afterwards; thus are his powers restored to him. He must beware of movement and exercise afterwards, for this is very harmful.

(c) *Treatment for infatuation*

This is an illness of the heart, contrary to other diseases in its essence, cause and

3 Lawful: the meaning appears to be that the unlawfulness caused by contravening a law of ritual cleanliness is less severe than that pertaining to contravention of natural law, eg. forbidden degrees of consanguinuity.

treatment. When it has taken root and become settled, its medication is hard for the physician, and the search for its treatment wearies the patient.

God, praised be He, spoke of it in His Book only concerning two groups of people: of women and lovers of young boys. He spoke of it about the wife of ʿAzīz with regard to Joseph. And He spoke of it about the people of Lot. The Most High said, telling of them when the angels came to Lot: *The people of the city came in joy. Lot said: These are my guests so do not disgrace me. But fear God, and shame me not. They said: Did we not forbid thee to entertain anyone? He said: There are my daughters, if you must so act. Indeed, by thy life (O Prophet) they are, in their intoxication, straying* (XV:67–72).

Some do not give the Messenger of God ﷺ his due respect, and they say that he was tested with regard to Zaynab bint Jaḥsh. They claim that when he saw her and said: 'Glory to One Who overturns hearts!' she took his heart, and he set out to say to Zayd b. Ḥāritha: 'Keep hold of her.' However God revealed to him: *Behold! thou didst say to one who had received the grace of God and thy favour: Retain thy wife, and fear God. But thou didst hide in thy heart that which God was about to make manifest; thou didst fear thy people, but it is more fitting that thou shouldst fear God.* (XXXIII:37). These people claim that this is a question of infatuation; one of them has composed a book on this type of love, in which he mentions the love (*ʿishq*) of prophets, and he includes this incident. The one who says this simply shows he is ignorant of the Qur'ān and the prophets, and is reading into God's words what they cannot bear, and attributes to God's Messenger ﷺ that from which God declared him innocent. For Zaynab bint Jaḥsh was married to Zayd b. Ḥāritha, whom the Messenger of God ﷺ had adopted as a son. So he was called Muḥammad's son. Zaynab was somewhat proud and superior. He consulted God's Messenger ﷺ about divorcing her, and God's Messenger ﷺ replied: 'Hold on to your wife, and fear God,' keeping secret the fact that he would marry her if Zayd divorced her. He feared the gossip of the people, who would say that he married his son's wife, for Zayd was called his son. This was his secret, such was his fear of the people. Therefore God, praised be He, mentioned this verse, recounting therein His favours to him, in which He did not reproach him, and told him that it was not fitting for him to fear the people in a matter which God had made lawful for him, and that God is more worthy to be feared. So he should not be distressed concerning what God had made lawful for him, on account of the people's gossip. God told him that He, praised be He, betrothed him to Zaynab, after Zayd renounced his desire for her. This was so that his community might follow his example, and a man might marry the former wife of his adopted son, though not the wife of his natural son. Thus, He said in the verse of banning (*taḥrīm*): *Wives of your sons proceeding from your loins* (IV:23). The Most High said: *Muḥammad is not the father of any of your men* (XXXIII:40), and He said earlier: *Nor has He made your adopted sons your sons* (XXXIII:4).

So consider how God defended His Messenger ﷺ, and the way in which He refuted the false claims of those who attacked him. Through God comes success.

Yes, the Messenger of God ﷺ loved his wives, and the most beloved of them all to him was ʿĀʾisha. His love for her, or for any other, did not reach the highest point, which was for his Lord. On the contrary, it is reliably reported that he said: 'Were I to take any one of the people of the earth as a close friend (*khalīl*), I would take Abū Bakr as a close friend.'[253] And in another narrative: 'Indeed your master is the close friend of the Merciful.'

Love for images is a trial only for hearts which are empty of love for God the Most High and are turned away from Him, seeking compensation elsewhere. If the heart is filled with love of God and with longing to meet Him, it ousts the illness of loving images. Therefore the Most High said, concerning Joseph: *Thus, that We might turn away from him evil and shameful deeds. For he was one of Our servants, sincere and purified* (XII:24), indicating that sincerity is a means for warding off infatuation and such evil and vileness as might spring from it and result as a consequence. For turning away the consequence turns away the cause.

Therefore some of the ancestors said: Infatuation is the movement of an empty heart; meaning empty of all else but the beloved. The Most High said: *But the heart of Moses' mother became a void; she was almost going to disclose him* (XXVIII:10); that is, empty of all else but Moses because of her excessive love for him and her heart's attachment to him. Infatuation has two components: finding perfection in the one loved and desire to be joined with that one. When either of these is absent, then there is no infatuation.

The sickness of infatuation has thwarted the efforts of many intelligent people; some of them have spoken of it in terms which we shall avoid mentioning for the sake of accuracy. We say: the wisdom of God, the Glorious, concerning His creation and His command, has so ordained that there occurs compatibility and harmony between like and like; that a thing should be attracted to what is suitable and related to it by constitution, and should flee from what is opposite and contrary to it by constitution. So the inner significance of accord and union, in the upper and lower world, is one of proportion, similarity and compatibility. The inner significance of disharmony and separation is due to the absence of similarity and conformity. The perfection and command is thus ordered. Like leans towards like, and moves towards it, while the opposite flees and escapes from its opposite.[4] The Most High has said: *He it is Who created you from a single person (*nafs*), and made his mate of like nature in order that he might dwell with her* (VII:189). Praised

4 Those who are of like qualities are inclined to each other, but those who have dissimilar qualities differ; or, according to their mutual knowledge when created before this life, so they will relate to one another in this life.

be He, He attributed a man's dwelling contentedly with his wife to her being of his own kind and essence. The reason for this contented dwelling, which is love, is her being as a part of him. That indicates that the reason is not beauty of form, nor compatibility in aim and will, nor in character and guidance, even though these too are among the causes of contentment and love.

It is confirmed in the *Ṣaḥīḥ*, from the Prophet ﷺ, that he said: 'Spirits are armed forces. Such of them as know one another are in unity, such as do not know one another are at variance.'[254] In the *Musnad* of Imām Aḥmad, and elsewhere, it is said concerning the cause of this *ḥadīth* that a woman in Mecca caused people to laugh, and she came to Madīna and stayed with a woman who caused people to laugh. The Prophet ﷺ said: 'Spirits are armed forces . . .' (and the rest).

God's revealed Law (*sharīʿa*), praised be He, has established that judgement of one thing is similar to judgement of its like; and the Law never makes a distinction between two exactly similar cases, nor does it bring together two opposing ones. If anyone thinks differently, this is due either to his insufficient knowledge of the Law, or to shortcomings in the knowledge of similarity and disparity, or to his relating to His Law that regarding which no authority has been revealed, but rather it is from the opinions of men. By His wisdom and justice did His creation and His Law appear; by justice and the scales did creation and the Law arise. This means regarding as equal similars and making a distinction between different things. This is how it has been established in this world and will be so on the day of Resurrection. The Most High said: *Gather together the wrong-doers and their wives, and the things they worshipped other than God, and lead them to the way to hell!* (XXXVII: 22–3).

Umar b. al-Khaṭṭāb said, and after him Imām Aḥmad: 'Their wives are their peers and equals.' The Most High said: *When their sons are paired like with like*(LXXXI: 7), that is: one who performs a deed will be joined with his like and peer. Those who have mutual love, in God, will be joined in Paradise, and those who have mutual love in obeying Satan will be joined in Hell. A man is with whoever he loves, whether he wishes it or not. In the *Ṣaḥīḥ* of al-Ḥākim and others, from the Prophet ﷺ: 'If a man loves any group of people, he will be gathered up with them (in the next world).'[255] Love (*maḥabba*) is of many kinds. The best and noblest is love in God, for God; for it necessarily entails the love of that which God loves and entails the love of God and His Messenger ﷺ. Another is love of harmony in a Sufi order or religion, or a school of law (*madhhab*) or a religious sect, or relationship or craft, or a common purpose. Then is love caused by desire to obtain some aim from the loved one, whether from his honour, his wealth, his teaching or his guidance, or fulfilling some desire through him. This is conditional love, which ceases with its cause; the one who loves you for the sake of some matter turns away when it is achieved.

Concerning love that stems from harmony and compatibility between the lover and the beloved: that is an intrinsic love, and it only ceases when some contingency causes it to cease. The love of infatuation (*ʿishq*) is of this kind, for it is spiritual preference and total mutual emotional absorption. From no other kind of real love can occur such delusions and emaciation, preoccupation and bewilderment.

It may be asked: If the cause of infatuation is what you have mentioned, namely union and spiritual affinity, then why does it not always exist from both sides, but so often you find it only on the side of one of the lovers? If its cause were emotional union and spiritual absorption, then love would be shared by the two.

The reply is that the cause may not have its effect on the one loved because some condition is not fulfilled or because of some impediment. The absence of love from the side of the other must inevitably be from one of these three causes: (1) some defect in the love; that it is conditional love, and is not intrinsic. There does not have to be complete sharing in conditional love, but it may be accompanied by aversion on the part of the beloved; (2) some impediment existing in the lover, which prevents the beloved from loving him, whether in his physical constitution, or his character traits or his moral conduct, his behaviour, his appearance, or anything else; (3) some impediment existing in the beloved, hindering him from sharing with the lover in his love. Were it not for that impediment, the beloved would show a love for his lover similar to the other's love for him.

When these impediments are not present, and love is intrinsic, then it can only be shared equally. Were it not for the impediment of pride, envy, superiority, and enmity among the unbelievers, the Messengers would be more dear to them than their own selves, their families and their property. When this impediment leaves the hearts of their followers, their love for the Messengers is above their love for themselves, family and property.

In short, infatuation is classed among the illnesses, and can be treated. Its treatments are of various kinds. If it be such that it is within the law and within the capacity of the lover to be joined with his beloved, then that is his treatment. As is confirmed in the two Books of *Ṣaḥīḥ*, from *ḥadīth* of Ibn Masʿūd: the Messenger of God said: 'O group of young men! Whoever of you is able to marry, let him take a wife; whoever cannot, let him fast (which will diminish his sexual powers) for it is a protection.'[256] He thus indicated two treatments for the lover: basic, and compensatory. He commanded him the essential, which is the treatment laid down for this illness (marriage); therefore he should not deviate from it to aught else so long as he finds it possible.

Ibn Māja related in his *Sunan*, from Ibn ʿAbbās, from the Prophet ﷺ, who said: 'We have seen naught equal to marriage for those who love one another.'[257] This is the meaning which God the Glorified advised, shortly after the verse in which He made lawful marriage to free women and maidservants in case of need, in His words: *God wishes to lighten your difficulties, for man was created weak* (IV:28). The mention of His lightening, praised be He, in this place, and His words concerning the weakness of human species, are an indication of man's being too weak to control this appetite. The Exalted One lightened it by permitting him good women, two or three or four, and permitting him those he wished among those he owned; He permitted him to marry slave girls, if he so needed, as treatment for this appetite, and as alleviation for this weak disposition, and as a mercy to him.

(d) *Treatment through despair*

If the lover finds no means to be joined with the beloved, either because it was not decreed, or because it was not legally possible, this being the incurable illness, then one treatment is to let his soul realise despair. For when the soul despairs of anything, it is at peace from it, and pays no attention to it.

If this sickness of infatuation does not cease with despair, then the nature has become much distorted, and another treatment should be sought, which is the treatment of his intellect. He should know that attachment of the heart to that which he cannot hope to obtain is a kind of madness. For such a person is like someone who is madly in love with the sun, and whose spirit is attached to the idea of climbing up to it and accompanying it in orbit round the heavens. Such a person, in the opinion of all intelligent people, would be classed among the mad.

If union is not possible on legal grounds, while on the other hand there is nothing to indicate that it is impossible within the decree of God, then his treatment is to consider it as that which is not possible by decree. For if anything is not permitted by God, the servant's treatment and deliverance are dependant on avoiding it. Let him realise that he is deprived, restrained, with no way of reaching it, and that union with his beloved is of the same sort as other impossible things.

If the 'soul commanding' to evil does not respond, then let him abandon his aim for one of two motives: either out of fear, or by (considering) the loss of a beloved whom he loves more and who is more useful and better for him, and can bring more lasting pleasure and happiness. When the intelligent person compares the attainment of a beloved who will swiftly pass away with the loss of a loved one who is greater and more lasting, more useful and more pleasant, the disparity appears clearly to him. So do not sell the pleasure of eternity, which has no risk attached, for the pleasure of an hour, which is turned into pain and which in reality is no more than dreams, or fleeting imagination. Pleasure passes, the result remains; desire ceases, and misery remains.

Secondly, a calamity might befall him which might be more troublesome to him than the departure of his beloved; or rather, the two matters are combined, that is, the loss of what is dearer and the suffering of what is more painful. If he becomes certain that the result of allowing himself to indulge in the union with the beloved would be to suffer these two consequences, it will definitely be easier to abandon his beloved, and he would realize that endurance of such a loss is a lesser evil. His intelligence, his religion, his virtue and his humanity command him to bear the lesser harm which is turned quickly to pleasure and happiness and joy, to ward off these two mighty forms of damage; while his ignorance and vain desire, injustice, heedlessness and rashness would command him to prefer his beloved which is essentially ephemeral, bringing to him whatever it brings. The sinless one is the one whom God preserves.

If his soul does not accept this medicine and does not submit to this treatment, then let him consider the ill deeds of his worldly life, brought about by this desire, and the benefits from which it hinders him. It is the most likely to bring about the evils of this world, and to vitiate his true interests. It intervenes between the servant and that guidance which is the foundation and the support of his true welfare.

If his soul does not accept this medicine, then let him recall the unpleasant characteristics of the one loved, and all that might be a motive for avoiding the beloved. For if he looks for these characteristics and reflects on them, he finds them to be many times the good qualities which are a motive for his love. Let him question his neighbours about such of these as are hidden from him; for just as good qualities are the motive for love and desire, so evil qualities are the motive for hatred and aversion. So let him compare the two motives, and let him chose the easiest and most effective amongst these as a way of escape from his beloved. Let him not be among those deceived by the outward sign of beauty on the body of a leper; let his sight pass beyond beauty of form to perceive evil of action; and let it pass from fineness of appearance and body, to the vileness of inner quality and the heart.

If all of these medicines prove ineffective there remains for the sufferer naught but sincerely taking refuge with the One Who answers the afflicted when he calls on Him. Let him cast himself into His presence, at His door, asking His help, in humiliation, lowliness and abandonment.

When he is guided to do so, then he has knocked upon the door of success; he should be virtuous and conceal his troubles and neither celebrate the renown of the beloved, nor yet seek to show up his faults among the people, thus exposing him to harm; for then he would be a wrongdoer and oppressor.

Let him not be deceived by the *ḥadīth* falsely attributed to God's Messenger ﷺ, related by Suwayd b. Saʿīd from ʿAlī b. Mushir from Abū Yaḥyā al-Qattāt, from Mujāhid, from Ibn ʿAbbās, from the Prophet ﷺ. It is related also on the authority of Ibn Mushir from Hishām b. ʿArwa, from his father, from ʿĀ'isha, from the Prophet ﷺ; it is also related by al-Zubayr b. Bakkār, from ʿAbd al-Mālik b. ʿAbd al-ʿAzīz b. al-Mājishūn, from ʿAbd al-ʿAzīz b. Ḥāzim, from Ibn Abī Najīḥ, from Mujāhid, from Ibn ʿAbbās, from the Prophet ﷺ, that he said: 'If anyone is deeply in love, is restrained, and then dies, he is a martyr.' In another narrative: 'If anyone is deeply in love, but conceals this, and is restrained and endures patiently, God pardons him and brings him into Paradise.'

This *ḥadīth* is not truly from the Messenger of God ﷺ, and cannot possibly be his words. For martyrdrom is a high rank in God's sight, comparable to the rank of righteousness; and it has its own actions and states which are a condition for reaching it. Martyrdom is of two kinds: general and particular. The particular: martyrdom in the path of God. The general is that there are five sorts mentioned in the *Ṣaḥīḥ*, and infatuation is not one of them. For how could infatuation—which is 'assigning partners' (*shirk*) in love, and being empty of God, and giving possesion of the heart and spirit and love to aught else—how could this be a means of attaining the rank of martyrdom? This is impossible. For the corruption which love of forms wreaks on the heart is above all other corruption. Rather, it is the strong drink of the spirit, which intoxicates it and impedes it from the remembrance and love of God, from taking delight in secret conversation with Him and finding intimacy with Him, and entails the subjugation of the heart to other than him. For the heart of the infatuated person is enslaved by the beloved; for infatuation is the kernel of servanthood, which is the perfection of lowliness, love, humility and glorification. How can the heart's servitude to other than God be one of the means of attaining the degree of the most excellent and the leaders of those who profess God's unity, and the foremost of the saints? Were the chain of transmission of this *ḥadīth* as clear as the sun, it is yet mistaken and imaginary. There is no record of the Messenger of God ﷺ mentioning infatuation in any true *ḥadīth* whatsoever.

Infatuation can be lawful or unlawful, so how can it be imagined that the Prophet ﷺ would declare every lover who conceals his love and restrains himself to be a martyr? Do you think one who loves a woman belonging to another, or loves young boys or prostitutes, will by his love attain the rank of martyrdom? Is this aught else but contradiction of what is known of the Prophet's ﷺ religion? Love is one of the illnesses for which God, praised be He, has provided remedies, by law and within the decree. Treatment for it may be either obligatory, if it is an unlawful love, or encouraged. When you reflect on the illnesses and afflictions which the Messenger of God ﷺ judged to be as martyrdom for his Companions, you will see that these are illnesses for which there is no treatment, like the one suffering from plague or an abdominal complaint, the one castrated, burned or drowned, the death of a woman killed by her unborn child. These are trials from God, for which the servant can do naught, and for which there is no treatment, and of which the causes are not unlawful deeds, and are not followed by corruption of the heart, and worship of aught beside God, such as results in infatuation.

If this is not sufficient to invalidate the attribution of the *ḥadīth* to God's Messenger ﷺ, then follow the specialists of *ḥadīth*, those learned in *ḥadīth* and its weaknesses; it is not recorded of any single specialist among them that he testified to its soundness nor even its acceptability. How indeed, seeing that they reproached Suwayd for this *ḥadīth*, and on account of it they charged him with terrible things, and some of them thought it lawful to attack him because of that? Abū Aḥmad b. ʿAdīyy said in his *Kāmil*: This is one of the *ḥadīth* for which Suwayd is held in reproach. Similarly, Bayhaqī said: It is one of these for which he is reproached. Ibn Ṭāhir said likewise in *al-Dhakhīra;* and it is mentioned by al-Ḥākim in the *History of Nishapur*. He said: I am astonished at this *ḥadīth*. It is related only from Suwayd, yet he is trustworthy. It is mentioned by Abū al-Faraj b. al-Jawzī in *Kitāb al-Mawḍūʿāt*; and Abū Bakr al-Azraq traces it in the first place on the authority of Suwayd; when he was blamed for it, he dropped the mention of the Prophet ﷺ, and it did not go beyond Ibn ʿAbbās.

It is altogether unacceptable to place this one among the *ḥadīth* of Hishām b. ʿArwa, from his father, on the authority of ʿĀ'isha, from the Prophet ﷺ. And whoever has the least familiarity with *ḥadīth* and their weaknesses will not stand for this at all, nor suffer that it might be from the *ḥadīth* of Ibn al-Mājishūn, from Ibn Abī Ḥāzim, from Ibn Abī Najīḥ, from Mujāhid, from Ibn ʿAbbās, traced back. There is speculation as to its soundness when traced back as far as Ibn ʿAbbās.

The people had charged Suwayd b. Saʿīd—the narrator of this *ḥadīth*—with terrible evil, and Yaḥyā b. Maʿīn reproached him for it, and said: 'This one is vile and lying; had I a horse and a spear, I would fight him.' Imām Aḥmad said: 'Disregarded as to *ḥadīth*.' Said al-Nisā'ī: 'He is not trustworthy.' Said al-Bukhārī: 'He had become blind, and *ḥadīth* not his own were attributed to him.' Said Ibn Ḥibān: 'He brings problems, on the authority of the trustworthy ones, so one must avoid his narratives.' The best word spoken of him is from Abū Ḥātim al-Rāzī: 'He is truthful, but with much that is counterfeit.' Then, the words of al-Dārquṭnī: 'He is reliable; yet when he grew old, sometimes a *ḥadīth* would be read to him containing something to be rejected, yet he permitted it.' So it is a shortcoming on Muslim's part to use his *ḥadīth*, seeing this is his state. But Muslim related such of his *ḥadīth* as corresponded with others and was not narrated solely by him, and was neither disclaimed nor irregular; but this does not apply to this *ḥadīth*. God knows best.

CHAPTER

37

Preservation of health by scents

A SWEET scent is the nourishment of the spirit, and the spirit is the instrument of the faculties, and the faculties increase with scent; for it is beneficial for brain and heart and the other internal organs, and makes the heart rejoice, pleases the soul and revitalizes the spirit.[1] It is the truest of all for the spirit, and the most suitable for it; for there is a close relationship between scent and the good spirit. Scent was one of those things beloved in this world to the one who was the most fragrant of all the purely scented ones, may God's blessings and peace be on him.

In the *Ṣaḥīḥ* of Bukhārī we read that 'he ﷺ used not to refuse scent.'[258] And in the *Ṣaḥīḥ* of Muslim, from the Prophet ﷺ: 'If one is offered a sweet scent (*rayḥān*), let him not refuse it; for indeed it is sweet scented and light to carry.'[259] And in the *Sunan* of Abū Dāwūd and Nisā'ī, from Abū Hurayra, from the Prophet ﷺ: 'If anyone is offered scent (*ṭīb*) let him not refuse it, for it is light to carry, sweet of scent.'[260]

In the *Musnad* of al-Bazzār, from the Prophet ﷺ, it says: 'Indeed God is pure, He loves purity; clean, He loves cleanliness; noble, He loves nobility; generous, He loves generosity. So cleanse your courtyards and open courts, and be not like the Jews, who collect refuse within their houses.'

Ibn Abī Shayba remarked that the Prophet ﷺ had a supply of ground perfume (*sukka*, generally as made of musk and *rāmik*, a black pitch-like substance), from which he used to perfume himself.

And it is reliably reported of him that he said: 'God demands this duty of every Muslim, that he should perform *ghusl* every seven days; and if he has perfume, then he should apply this.'[261]

Perfume has this special characteristic that the angels like it, but the demons flee from it; for what the demons like best is an unpleasant, putrid smell. Good spirits love a beautiful scent, while evil spirits like an evil smell. Every spirit is attracted to what is suitable to it: evil females to evil males, and the reverse; goodly females to goodly males and the reverse. Even though this refers to men

1 A sweet scent, or fragrance, *rā'iḥa ṭayyiba*, is food for the spirit, *rūḥ*.

and women, it also includes words and deeds, food and drink, clothing and scents; either through the general sense of its words or its meaning.

CHAPTER

38

Preservation of health of the eye

ABŪ DĀWŪD related in his *Sunan,* from ʿAbd al-Raḥmān b. al-Nuʿmān b. Maʿbad b. Hawdha al-Anṣārī, from his father, from his grandfather, that the Messenger of God ﷺ ordered scented antimony at the time of going to sleep, but said: 'Let the one fasting avoid it.'[262] Abū ʿUbayda said: Scented (*murawwaḥ*) means scented with musk.

In the *Sunan* of Ibn Māja and elsewhere, from Ibn ʿAbbās: The Prophet ﷺ had a *koḥl* container from which he would apply *koḥl* three times in each eye.[263] And in al-Tirmidhī, from Ibn ʿAbbās: The Messenger of God ﷺ when using *koḥl* would apply it three times to the right eye, beginning and ending with this one, and to the left eye twice.

Abū Dāwūd related, on his authority: 'If anyone uses *koḥl,* let him apply this an uneven number of times.' It is uncertain whether the 'uneven number' refers to both the eyes together—so that this should be three times in one and twice in the other, considering the right eye to be preferred and more suitable to begin with; or refers to each eye, so that this should be three times in the one and three times in the other. These are two opinions expressed within Imām Aḥmad's school of Law and others.

Koḥl is able to preserve the health of the eye, to strengthen and cleanse the perceptive faculty; it can deal gently with bad 'matter' and remove it, and some of its varieties give adornment.

Using it when going to sleep is especially good: for the eye takes in the *koḥl* and after that rests from movement which could be harmful to it, and the constitution itself is thus of help to the eye. Here, antimony has unique properties.

In the *Sunan* of Ibn Māja, from Sālim, from his father (*marfūʿ*): 'See that you use antimony. It clears the sight and makes the hair grow.'[264] And in the Book of Abū Nuʿaym: 'It can cause hair to grow, it removes uncleanness and clarifies the sight.'[265] In the *Sunan* of Ibn Māja also, from Ibn ʿAbbās (*marfūʿ*): 'Your best *koḥl* is antimony: it cleanses the sight, and makes the hair grow.'[266]

MEDICINE OF THE PROPHET

PART TWO

Simple Drugs and Foods

Some of the simple drugs (adwiya) *and foods* (aghdhiya), *as mentioned by the Prophet* ﷺ, *arranged in alphabetical order (according to the Arabic)*[1]

Hamza

1. *Ithmid* (Antimony)

THIS is the stone of the black *koḥl*,[2] brought from Isfahan, which is the best. It is also brought from the Maghreb. The best is quick to break up, its pieces are shiny, and its interior is smooth, containing no impurities.

Its temperament is cold and dry. It is beneficial for the eye, and strengthens it and firms its muscles, preserves its health, and disperses excess flesh in its ulcers and causes them to scar over. It cleanses the eye's impurities and clears it. It dispels headache, when used as *koḥl* with thin liquid honey. When pounded and mixed with a little fresh fat and spread on the site of a burn, no scars will occur, and it is beneficial for the blistering caused by burns. It is the best of *koḥls* for the eye, when a little musk is added to it, especially for old people and those whose sight has grown weak.

2. *Utrujj* (Citrus medica L. Rutaceae. Citron)

It is confirmed in the *Ṣaḥīḥ* that the Prophet ﷺ said: The believer who recites the Qur'ān is likened to the *utrujj*: its taste is good, its scent is good.[267]

The *utrujj* has many benefits. It is composed of four elements: peel, flesh, acid pulp, and seeds. Each one of these has its own temperament: the peel is hot and dry, the flesh hot and moist, the pulp cold and dry, the seeds hot and dry.

Among the uses of the peel are that it keeps away moth when placed among clothes; its scent rectifies any corruption of the air and pestilence. It sweetens

1 See EI², s.v. *'adwiya'*. Traditionally, simples were often classed together with foods, especially as the transition from treatment by regulation of diet to the use of medicines was meant to be gradual, cf. Chapter 1.

2 See Chapter 38.

the breath when kept in the mouth, and it dissolves winds. When added to food, like spices, it aids the digestion.

Ibn Sīnā says: When drunk, and its peel used as a poultice; the juice of its peel is beneficial for bites of vipers, and the burnt peel, as an embrocation, is good for vitiligo.

Its flesh softens the heat of the stomach, is beneficial to those of a bilious temperament and checks hot vapours. Al-Ghāfiqī says: Eating its flesh is beneficial for haemorrhoids.

Its pulp (*ḥummāḍ*) is costive, breaks the yellow bile, soothes hot palpitation, and it is beneficial for jaundice, when drunk or used as an eye salve. It breaks bilious vomiting, awakens the appetite for food, restrains the constitution and is useful for bilious diarrhoea. The juice of its pulp quietens sensuousness in women, is useful as an embrocation for freckles and dispels tetter. That is deduced from its action on colour: when it falls on clothing, the juice removes its colour. It has a power to refine, cut and cool; it extinguishes the heat of the liver, strengthens the stomach, restrains the sharpness of the yellow bile, removes the distress this causes, and it quenches thirst.

Its seeds have a dissolving and dessicative power. Ibn Māsawayh said: The special property of its seeds is to act against lethal poisons, when one drinks the amount of two *mithqāl*, shelled, in warm water, and also, when cooked, as an embrocation. When it is pounded and put on the place of a bite, it is of benefit. It softens the constitution and sweetens the breath. Most of this efficacy is found in its peel.

Another said: The special property of the seeds is to be of benefit against scorpion bites, when two *mithqāls* weight, peeled, is drunk in warm water. The same is true when it is pounded and put on the place of a sting.

Another said: Its seeds are good for all kinds of poisons and beneficial for the sting from all kinds of vermin.

It is said that one of the Chosroes [kings of pre-Islamic Persia] was angry with a group of physicians and ordered them to be imprisoned, giving them a choice of only one food which they could have. So they chose the *utrujj*. They were asked: 'Why did you choose that one, instead of another?' They replied: 'Because now it has a scent, and its sight is delightful. Its peel is of good scent, its flesh is fruit; its pulp is a condiment; its seeds are an antidote; and it contains oil.'

So it is right that something which has such benefits should be likened to the summit of existence, that is, of the believer who recites the Qur'ān. Some of the ancestors liked to gaze on it because of the joy which the sight of it could bring.

3. *Aruzz* (Oryza sativa L. Gramineae. Rice)

Concerning rice[3] there are two spurious *ḥadīth* attributed to the Messenger of God ﷺ: (1) 'Were it a man it would be clement'; (2) 'everything which the

3 Rice was introduced during the Islamic era.

earth brings forth has both illness and healing, except rice; for it contains healing and no illness.' We have mentioned these simply to draw attention to them and give warning that they should not be attributed to him.

Rice is hot and dry. It is the most nourishing of grains after the wheat, and has the most excellent humour. It gently firms the belly, it strengthens and tans the stomach, and remains in it. The physicians of India claim that it is the most excellent and beneficial of foodstuffs when cooked with cow's milk. It has an effect on fertility of the body and increases semen; it contains plenty of nourishment, and cleanses the complexion.

4. *Arz* (Cedrus libani A. Rich. Coniferae. Cedar)

This is the *ṣanawbar* (pine). The Prophet ﷺ mentioned it: 'The believer is likened to the young sown corn which the winds stir; they leave them standing one time, make them bend at another. And the hypocrite is likened to the cedar; it remains standing upon its root, until it is torn up all at once.'[268] Its kernel is hot and moist, containing a power of coction, of softening and of dissolution; it has a sharpness which is removed by soaking in water. It is hard to digest but contains much nourishment. It is good for cough and for cleansing moistures of the lung; it increases semen, and brings about indigestion. Its antidote is the seed of the bitter pomegranate.

5. *Idhkhir* (Cymbopogon schoenanthus Spreng. Gramineae. Lemon-grass)

It is confirmed in the *Ṣaḥīḥ* that the Prophet ﷺ once said in Mecca: 'None may uproot its vegetation.' About this al-ʿAbbās asked: 'Except the *idhkhir*, O Messenger of God? for it is for their graves and for their houses.' And he said: 'Except the *idhkhir*.'[269]

Idhkhir is hot in the second degree and dry in the first; gentle, opening obstructions and the 'mouths' of veins; diuretic, emmenagogue; it breaks up stones, dissolves hard inflammations in the stomach, liver and kidneys, when drunk and used as a poultice. Its root strengthens the bases of the teeth and the stomach: it quietens nausea and restrains the belly.

Bā'

1. *Biṭṭīkh* (Citrullus (vulgaris) lanatus (Thunb.) Mansf. Cucurbitaceae. Watermelon)

Abū Dāwūd and al-Tirmidhī related from the Prophet ﷺ that he used to eat watermelon with fresh dates (*ruṭab*), saying: 'The heat of the one repels the cold of the other.' Concerning watermelon there are a number of *ḥadīth*, the only valid one being this single *ḥadīth*.

The kind of watermelon meant here is the green variety. It is cold and moist, containing a cleansing power. It is swifter in descending from the stomach than the large and small cucumbers (*qiththā'* and *khiyār*). It quickly changes to whatever humour it meets in the stomach. One suffering from fever would benefit from eating it; if, on the other hand, he suffers from a chill, its effect is reversed by adding a little ginger or similar. It should be eaten before food, so that something is taken afterwards; otherwise it causes nausea and vomiting. Some of the physicians have said: Before food, it acts as a cleanser of the belly and eradicates any illness.

2. *Balaḥ* (from Phoenix dactylifera L. Palmae. Fresh dates)[4]

It is related by al-Nisā'ī and by Ibn Māja in their *Sunan*, from *ḥadīth* of Hishām b. ʿUrwa, from his father, from ʿĀ'isha, who said: The Messenger of God ﷺ said: 'Eat *balaḥ*, with *tamr*, for when Satan regards the son of Adam eating these two, he says: the son of Adam has remained until he has eaten the new with the old.'[270] In another narrative: 'Eat *balaḥ* with *tamr*, for Satan is grieved when he sees the son of Adam eating them and says: The son of Adam has lived until he has eaten the new with what is old.' Al-Bazzār narrated this in his *Musnad*, and these are his words.

My comment: the particle used here, *bi*, has the meaning of *ma*ʿ (ie. eat this accompanied by that).

Some physicians in Islam have said: The Prophet ﷺ ordered *balaḥ* to be eaten with *tamr*, and not *busr* with *tamr*, simply because *balaḥ* are cold and dry, while *tamr* are hot and moist, so each one of them contains a corrective to the other. This does not apply to *busr* with *tamr*; for each of them is hot, although the heat of *tamr* is greater. It is not fitting, from the medical point of view, to combine two hot or two cold substances, as has already been discussed.

This *ḥadīth* draws attention to this accurate principle of the medical profession and to the importance of observing the necessary steps to neutralise the adverse qualities of foods and drugs, one by another, and it respects the medical law whereby health is preserved.

Balaḥ contain cold and dryness. They are beneficial for the mouth, gums and stomach, but because of their harshness they are bad for chest and lung. Slow in the stomach, they give little nourishment. In relation to the date palm, they are like *ḥiṣrim* (sour grape) in relation to the vine. Both of them generate winds, rumblings in the stomach, and distension, especially when water is drunk afterwards. This adverse effect can be remedied by eating the fruit with *tamr* or with honey and butter.

4 See also *tamr, ruṭab, jummār, ʿajwa.*

3. *Busr* (from Phoenix dactylifera L. Palmae. Unripe dates)

It is confirmed in the *Ṣaḥiḥ* that when Abū al-Haytham b. al-Tayhān received the Prophet ﷺ, Abū Bakr and ʿUmar as guests, he brought them a cluster (*ʿadhq*); this refers to a cluster of dates, just as *ʿunqūd* refers to a bunch of grapes. He asked him: 'Have you not selected for us its *ruṭab* (ripe dates)?' And he replied: 'I wish you to pick out its *busr* and its *ruṭab*.' [271]

Busr are hot and dry, their dryness being greater than their heat. They dry up moisture, tan the stomach, restrict the belly and are beneficial for the gums and mouth. The most beneficial are those which are brittle and sweet. Eating them in quantity, and eating *balaḥ*, can bring about obstruction in the intestines.

4. *Bayḍ* (Eggs)

Al-Bayhaqī mentions in *Shaʿb al-Īmān* a narrative (*marfūʿ*) that one of the prophets complained to God, praised be He, of weakness, so He ordered him to eat eggs. There is speculation as to whether this *ḥadīth* is confirmed.

Fresh eggs should be chosen in preference to old ones, and hens' eggs are preferable to those of other birds. They are moderate, slightly inclining to cold.

Ibn Sīnā said: Its yolk is hot and moist, and it generates healthy laudable blood. It gives mild nourishment, and when soft is quick to descend from the stomach.

Another said: Egg yolk soothes pain, it smoothes the throat and trachea; it is beneficial for the throat and cough, ulcers of the lung, kidney and bladder; it disperses roughness, especially when taken with oil of almond; and it cocts and softens what is in the chest and relieves sore throat.

White of egg, dropped into a severely inflamed eye, cools it and quietens the pain. Smeared on burns as soon as they occur, it prevents blistering. Applied to the face, it prevents sunburn. Mixed with frankincense and smeared on the forehead, it is useful for catarrh.

Ibn Sīna mentions eggs among cardiac drugs, then says: 'Although it is not a drug in the strict sense of the word, it can be included among those items which effectively strengthen the heart. I am here referring to the yolk, for it combines three qualities: its ability to change into blood swiftly; its slight amount of superfluity; and the fact that the blood generated therefrom is similar to the blood which nourishes the heart, being light and making its way to it swiftly. Therefore it is the most suitable remedy with which to eliminate the common run of illnesses which dissolve the essence of the spirit.'

5. *Baṣal* (Allium cepa L. Liliaceae. Onion)

Abū Dāwūd related in his *Sunan*, from ʿĀ'isha, that she was asked about onions, and replied: 'The last item of food which the Prophet ﷺ ate contained onions.'[272]

It is confirmed from the Prophet ﷺ, in the two books of of the *Ṣaḥīḥ*, that he prevented anyone eating them from entering the mosque.[273] Onion is hot in the third degree and contains superfluous moisture. It is beneficial for 'changing of the waters', repels the hot wind, brings forth the appetite, strengthens the stomach, arouses sexual appetite, increases semen, improves the complexion, cuts phlegm, and cleanses the stomach.

Its seeds dispel leukoderma. When applied as an ointment is very effective against alopecia. With salt, it removes warts. If sniffed by one who has drunk a laxative medicine it prevents vomiting and nausea and dispels the smell of the medicine. Its juice used as a sternutatory clears the head.

Onion juice dropped into the ear can be used for treating hardness of hearing and for ringing noises, for pus and water occurring in the ears. Used as a *koḥl*, it is beneficial for water running down in the eyes. Mixed with honey its seeds are used as *koḥl* for leucoma.

Cooked onion is most nutritious. It is beneficial for jaundice, cough and harshness of the chest. It is diuretic and softens the constitution. For the bite of a non-rabid dog, a compress made from its juice mixed with salt and rue is beneficial. Used as a suppository, it opens the 'pores' of haemorrhoids.

Against onion can be said that it causes migraine and makes the head ache, generates winds, and darkens the sight. Eating it in quantity brings about forgetfulness, spoils the intellect and changes the scent of the mouth and breath, offending one's companions and the angels. But by cooking the onion these harmful effects are eliminated.

In the *Sunan* it is related that the Prophet ﷺ ordered the one who ate onion, and also garlic, to suppress adverse effects by cooking. Its odour is dispersed by chewing leaves of rue.

6. *Bādhinjān* (Solanum melongena L. Solanaceae. Aubergine)

In a fabricated *ḥadīth* attributed to the Messenger of God ﷺ it is said that the aubergine is for that for which it is eaten. These words are unworthy to be attributed to anyone of intelligence, let alone any of the prophets.

The aubergine is of two kinds: white and black. There is disagreement as to whether it is cold or hot. In fact it is hot. It generates black bile and haemorrhoids, obstructions, cancer and leprosy. It spoils and darkens the complexion and harms the mouth by a putrid odour.

The white variety, which is oblong, is free of those effects.

Tā'

1. *Tamr* (from Phoenix dactylifera L. Palmae. Dates)

It is confirmed in the *Ṣaḥīḥ*, from the Prophet ﷺ, that whoever starts his day with seven dates (or: with seven dates of al-ʿĀliya) will not be harmed that day by poison nor witchcraft.[274] It is confirmed that he said: 'In a house where there are no dates its people will be hungered'.[275] It is confirmed that he ate dates with butter, dates with bread, and dates on their own.

Dates[5] are hot in the second degree. There are two opinions as to whether they are moist in the first, or dry in the first degree.

They strengthen the liver, soften the constitution, clear sore throat, and they are aphrodisiac, especially with pine kernels. For people who are not used to eating dates—like those who live in cold countries—they cause obstructions, harm the teeth, and stir up headache. This can be warded off by eating them with almonds and poppy.

They are among the most nourishing of fruits for the body, by virtue of the hot moist essence they contain. To eat them on an empty stomach kills worms. For despite their heat they contain a power as an antidote. If taken continuously on an empty stomach they dry up and weaken the substance of the worms, so they reduce or kill them. They are a fruit, a food, a medicine, a drink and a sweetmeat.

2. *Tīn* (Ficus carica L. Moraceae. Figs)

Because there were no figs in the land of Ḥijāz and in Madīna, there is no mention of them in the *sunna*. For the land where they grow is incompatible with a land where date palms grow. Nonetheless, God in His Book the Qur'ān swears by the fig tree,[6] for the multiplicity of its benefits and uses. And the correct opinion is that the one referred to in the oath is the fig tree which we know.

The fig is hot. Concerning its moisture and dryness there are two opinions. The best is the white variety with ripe peel, which cleanses the gravel of kidney and bladder, and gives protection from poisons.[7] It is more nourishing than all other fruit, being beneficial for harshness of the throat, chest and trachea. It cleanses the liver and spleen, clears the phlegmatic humour from the stomach, and nourishes the body well. Yet it encourages lice when eaten in very large amounts.

Dried fig is nourishing and beneficial to the nerves, and is recommended along with walnut and almond. Galen said: 'When eaten with walnut and rue before taking lethal poison, it is beneficial and guards from harm.'

5 See Chapter 18.

6 'By the fig tree . . .' the opening words of *Sūra* 95, *al-Tīn*.

7 Protection from poisons: the fig was an ingredient of early versions of the Antidote.

It is related from Abū al-Dardā' that when the Prophet ﷺ was given as a present a tray of figs, he said: 'Eat'. And he ate from them and said: 'If I were to say that any fruit descended from Paradise, I should say these. For the fruit of Paradise has no stones. So eat from them: for they put an end to haemorrhoids and are beneficial for gout.' There is room for speculation as to the validity of this.

The flesh of the fig is best. It makes the fevered thirsty, quietens the thirst caused by salty phlegm, is beneficial for chronic cough, is diuretic, opens obstructions of liver and spleen, and is suitable for kidneys and bladder. Eating figs on an empty stomach is exceedingly beneficial in opening up the alimentary passages, especially when combined with almond and walnut. Eating them with heavy foods is very bad.

The white mulberry (*tūt*) has similar properties, but it is less nourishing, and more harmful to the stomach.

3. *Talbīna*

It has already been mentioned that this is broth of ground barley. We have mentioned its benefits and the fact that it is more beneficial to the people of Hijāz than broth of whole barley.[8]

Thā'

1. *Thalj* (Snow)

It is confirmed in the *Ṣaḥīḥ*, from the Prophet ﷺ, that he said: 'O my God, cleanse me from my sins with water, snow and ice.'[276] The legal point in this *ḥadīth* is that illness is treated by its opposite. For sins contain such heat and burning as is opposed by snow, ice and cold water.

It is not said that hot water is more effective in removing dirt. For cold water has the property, not found in hot water, of firming and strengthening the body. Sins bring about two effects: defilement and weakening. So the aim is to treat them with what purifies and strengthens the heart. Thus his mention of cold water, snow and ice is an indication of these two matters.

Snow is most truly cold, and those are mistaken who say it is hot. The doubt is caused by the fact that animals are generated in snow. Yet this does not indicate that it is hot, for animals are also generated in cold fruit and in vinegar. The fact that it causes thirst is due to heat arising from it, not to any heat within itself.

It harms the stomach and nerves. It calms toothache caused by excess heat.

8 See Chapter 24 b, and under *sha'īr*.

2. *Thūm* (Allium sativum L. Liliaceae. Garlic)

Garlic is close to onion. In the *ḥadīth* it says: Whoever eats these two, let him kill them by cooking. [277] The Prophet ﷺ was given as a present some food containing garlic, and sent it to Abū Ayyūb al-Anṣārī, who said: 'O Messenger of God, you dislike it and yet you send it to me?' He replied: 'I speak in secret to One to whom you do not speak.'[278]

It is hot and dry in the fourth degree; it heats strongly, and is a very effective dessicant for those who are chilled, and for those of phlegmy temperament, and for one who is about to succumb to palsy. It dries semen, opens obstructions and dissolves thick winds; it helps digestion, cuts thirst, loosens the belly, and is diuretic. It is a substitute for *tiryāq* (antidote) in cases of vermin bite and all cold inflammations. Pounded and used as a poultice it is beneficial for serpent bite or scorpion sting, drawing out the poison from them, warming the body and increasing its heat; it cuts the phlegm, dissolves distention, clears the throat, preserves the health of most people. It is beneficial for 'changing of the waters' and chronic cough. Garlic is eaten raw, cooked or grilled. It is beneficial for pain of the chest arising from cold, and it expels leeches from the throat. When it is pounded with vinegar, salt and honey, then placed on a decayed tooth, it breaks it up and makes it fall out. Placed on a painful tooth, it calms the pain. If the amount of two *dirham* is pounded and it is taken with honey water, it expels phlegm and worms. It is used as an embrocation with honey to treat leukoderma.

Among the adverse effects of garlic are that it causes headache and harms the brain and eyes, weakens the sight and the sexual powers, causes thirst, arouses the yellow bile, and leaves a strong smell on the breath. This can be counteracted by chewing leaves of rue.

3. *Tharīd*

It is confirmed in the two books of the *Ṣaḥīḥ* that the Prophet ﷺ said: 'The excellence of ʿĀ'isha over other women is like the excellence of *tharīd* over other food.'[279]

Tharīd is a thick soup based on bread and meat. Now bread is the best of foods, and meat the chief of condiments. So when they are combined, there is nothing better.

There is disagreement as to which of them is more excellent. The truth is that man's need for bread is greater and more general, whereas meat is nobler and more excellent, for it is nearer to the substance of the body than anything else, and it is the food of the people of Paradise. The Most High said to those who sought herbs, cucumbers, garlic (*fūm*), lentils and onions: *Do you then seek to exchange that which is better for that which is worse?'* (II:61). Many of the ancestors consider that *fūm* means wheat (*ḥinṭa*). Therefore, the verse is a proof to the effect that meat is better than wheat. God, exalted be He, knows best.

Jīm

1. *Jummār* (from Phoenix dactylifera L. Palmae)

This is the heart of the date-palm. It is confirmed in the two books of the *Ṣaḥīḥ*, from ʿAbd-Allāh b. ʿUmar, who said: When we were with the Messenger of God ﷺ, sitting down, the *jummār* of a date palm was brought, and the Prophet ﷺ spoke the *ḥadīth*: 'Among trees there is one like the Muslim man; its leaves do not fall.'[280]

The *jummār* is cold and dry in the first degree. It seals over ulcers, is beneficial for spitting of blood, for looseness of the belly, predominance of yellow bile, and agitation of the blood. It is not of evil chyme. It is of slight nutritional value and is slow to digest. All of the tree has beneficial qualities. Therefore the Prophet ﷺ likened it to the Muslim man because it is so good and useful.

2. *Jubn* (Cheese)

In the *Sunan*, from ʿAbd-Allāh b. ʿUmar, it says that when at Tabūk the Prophet ﷺ was brought some cheese, and he called for a knife, pronounced the Name of God and cut it.[281] Abū Dāwūd relates this. The Companions used to eat it in Syria and Iraq.

The moist unsalted cheese is good for the stomach and passes easily into the organs; it increases the flesh and softens the belly in a moderate way. Salted cheese is less nutritious; it is bad for the stomach and harmful to the intestines. Old cheese restricts the belly, as does grilled cheese, and is good for ulcers and prevents diarrhoea.

Cheese is cold and moist. Grilling it makes it more appropriate to its temperament. Fire rectifies and moderates it, refines its essence, and sweetens its taste and odour. Old salty cheese is hot and dry. Grilling rectifies it, too, for it refines its essence and breaks its sharpness, the fire drawing from it certain hot, dry constituents appropriate to it. The salted kind causes emaciation and generates stones of the kidneys and bladder, and it is bad for the stomach. The addition of refining ingredients is worse because these cause it to reach the stomach.

Ḥā'

1. *Ḥinnā'* (Lawsonia inermis L. Lythraceae. Henna)

Ḥadīth concerning the excellence of henna, and the mention of its benefits, have already been given (see pp. 63, 183) and need not be repeated here.

2. *Al-ḥabba al-sawdā'* (Nigella sativa L. Ranunculaceae. Nigella, black cumin)

It is confirmed in the two books of the *Ṣaḥīḥ*, from *ḥadīth* of Abū Salma, from Abū Hurayra, that the Messenger of God ﷺ said: 'Take note of this black grain (*al-ḥabba al-sawdā'*), for it contains healing for every illness except the poisonous'[282] ('poisonous' means 'death').

Nigella is *shūnīz* in the Persian language.[9] It is the black cumin, also called Indian cumin. Al-Ḥarbī related from al-Ḥasan: It is the seed of *khardal* (mustard); al-Harawī said: It is the green grain, the fruit of the *buṭm* (terebinth). Both of these explanations are imaginary. The correct one is that it is the *shūnīz*.

It has very many benefits. His words 'healing for every illness' are like the words of the Most High: *Destroying everything by the command of its Lord* (XLVI:25). That is, everything which can be destroyed and its like. It is beneficial for all cold illnesses. It is relevant for hot dry illnesses in an incidental way, for when a little of it is taken with cold, moist medicines, it brings their powers to the illness and speeds up the effect.

Ibn Sīnā and others have specified saffron in camphor pastilles, because it is swift to reach the trouble and take effect. There are similar cases to this, known to the skilful people of the art. One must not underestimate the usefulness of hot properties in the treatment of hot illnesses. For you will find these in many medicines, including the astragalus, and those ophthalmic medicines which are composed with it, such as sugar, and others among the hot simples. Ophthalmia is a hot swelling, as the physicians agree. In the same way hot sulphur is useful in the treatment of scabies.

Shūnīz is hot and dry in the third degree; it disperses distension, expels round worms, is beneficial for vitiligo, for quartan fever and for phlegmatic fever; it opens obstructions, dissolves winds, and dries up the liquid and moistures of the stomach. If it is crushed and kneaded with honey, and drunk with hot water, it dissolves stones which form in the kidneys and bladder. It is diuretic, emmenagogue, galactagogue, when drunk for several consecutive days. If warmed with vinegar, and used as embrocation on the belly, it kills round worms. When kneaded with juice of colocynth, moist or cooked, it has a stronger effect in

9 *Shūnīz* is not Nigella, but *Papaver somniferum* L. (poppy), also known as *khashkhāsh* in Arabic. Nor is Nigella the same as *khardal, Sinapis alba* L., Cruciferae, or the *buṭm*. IQ reports both these opinions but discards them.

expelling worms. It cleanses, cuts, and dissolves; and it expels cold catarrh, when pounded, tied in a cloth and sniffed continuously.

Its oil is beneficial for ophiasis and for warts and moles. When a *mithqāl* of it is drunk with water, it is beneficial for difficult respiration and tightness of the breath. A poultice with it is beneficial for cold headache. When seven grains of it are soaked in human milk, and it is given as a sternutatory to one suffering from jaundice, it brings most effective relief.

Cooked with vinegar and used as a mouth wash, it is beneficial for toothache caused by cold. Crushed and used as a sternutatory, it is beneficial during the early stages of water occurring in the eye. When used as a poultice with vinegar, it clears away pustules and ulcerated scabies, and dissolves chronic phlegmatic and hard inflammations.

Shūnīz is also beneficial for facial paralysis, if its oil is used as a sternutatory. When the amount of half to one *mithqāl* is drunk, it is beneficial for the sting of tarantulas. When the seeds are crushed till soft and mixed with oil of terbeinth seeds, and three drops are instilled into the ear, it is beneficial for cold occuring in that place. It is also useful in the treatment of wind and obstruction.

Fried seeds, pounded till soft, and soaked in oil, relieve catarrh accompanied by much sneezing, when three or four drops are instilled into the nose. Burnt seeds, mixed with wax melted with oil of iris or oil of henna, are used as an embrocation for ulcers coming out on the legs, after they have been washed with vinegar. This treatment removes the ulcers.

Crushed with vinegar, the seeds are used as embrocation on vitiligo and black leukoderma, as well as thick lichen; it is beneficial and cures the ailment.

Two *dirham* of the powder of *shūnīz* swallowed with cold water every day before the sufferer has succumbed to hydrophobia will save the life of one bitten by a mad dog. When used as a fumigant, it expels vermin.

When astragalus is melted in water, and spread on the inside of the palate, and *shūnīz* sprinkled on, this is one of the good dry medicaments; it is amazingly useful for haemorrhoids. The benefits of *shūnīz* are many times what we have mentioned. The dosage is two *dirham* when taken by mouth. Some claim that it is lethal in large quantities.

3. *Ḥarīr* (Silk)

It has already been related[10] how the Prophet ﷺ permitted to Zubayr and to ʿAbd al-Raḥmān b. ʿAūf to wear silk, because they both had itch. We have also mentioned its uses and its temperament, so there is no need to repeat it here.

10 See Chapter 12 a and b.

4. *Ḥurf*[11] (Lepidum sativum L., Nasturtium officinale R. Br. Cruciferae. Cress)

Abū Ḥanīfa (al-Dīnawarī) said: This is the grain which is used for medicinal purposes, the *thuffā'*, about which there is reported a narrative from the Prophet ﷺ. The plant is called *ḥurf*, and the common people call it 'grain of *rashād*'.' Abū ʿUbayd Said: *Thuffā'* is *ḥurf*.

My comment: The *ḥadīth* which he indicated, narrated by Abū ʿUbayd and others, from the *ḥadīth* of Ibn ʿAbbās, is that the Prophet ﷺ said: 'What is in the two most bitter means of healing? *Thuffā'* (cress) and *ṣabir* (patience or aloe).'[283] And this is narrated by Abū Dāwūd in *al-Marāsīl*.

Cress is hot and dry in the third degree. It warms and softens the belly, expels worms and round-worms, dissolves inflammations of the spleen, awakens the appetite for sexual intercourse, cleanses ulcerated scabies and tetter.

When made into a poultice with honey, it dissolves inflammation of the spleen. Cooked with henna, it expels superfluities in the chest. Drinking it is beneficial for bites and stings of vermin. When used as a fumigation in any place, it removes vermin. It prevents hair loss. When mixed with gruel of barley and vinegar, and used as a poultice, it is beneficial for sciatica, and dissolves hot inflammations when these are at their end.

Used as a poultice with water, it causes boils to coct, and it is beneficial for lassitude in all the limbs; it is aphrodisiac and increases the appetite for food. It is beneficial for asthma, difficulty in breathing, thickness of the spleen; it clears the lungs and is emmenagogue. When drunk or used as a clyster it is beneficial for sciatica and pain in the hip socket, causing superfluities to come out; and it clears any sticky phlegm in the chest and lung.

If the measure of five *dirham* is crushed and drunk in hot water, it purges the constitution, dissolves winds, and is beneficial for the pain of colic caused by cold. When crushed and drunk, it is beneficial for vitiligo.

If cress is applied to vitiligo and on white leukoderma with vinegar, it is beneficial. This is also the case with headaches arising from cold and from phlegm. When fried and drunk, it restrains the constitution, especially when left whole, because its stickiness is dissolved by frying. When its juice is used to wash the head, it removes impurities and sticky moistures.

Galen said: Its power is like that of mustard seed. Therefore it is used for warming the pains of the thigh known as *nasā* (sciatica) and pains of the head, and all illnesses which call for warming; it warms, just as the mustard seed warms. It can also be mixed into medicines given to sufferers from asthma, as it is well-known that it reduces the thick humours very strongly, just as the mustard seed does; for it is like it in every respect.

11 Also known as *thuffā'*. Another name, *rashād*, is more commonly used today, and is given as the name used by 'the common people' by Abū Ḥanīfa, *Plants*, No. 154 and 276, p. 83 and 131.

5. *Ḥulba* (Trigonella foenum-graecum L. Leguminosae. Fenugreek)

It is reported of the Prophet ﷺ that he visited Saᶜd b. Abī Waqqāṣ in Mecca, and said: 'Summon a physician for him!' So al-Ḥārith b. Kalada was called, and he looked at Saᶜd and said: 'There is nothing wrong with him. Make up a mixture for him of *ḥulba* with moist *ᶜajwa* dates; let them be cooked into a broth.' That was done, and he was cured.

Ḥulba is hot in the second degree, dry in the first degree.

When cooked with water it softens the throat, chest and belly, and relieves cough, hoarseness, asthma, and difficult breathing. It is aphrodisiac. It is good for wind, phlegm, and haemorrhoids, causing the chymes to descend which are compounded in the intestines. It dissolves sticky phlegm from the chest, and is beneficial for boils and sicknesses of the lung. For these illnesses it is taken in broths, with clarified butter (*samn*) and sugar (*fānīdh*).

When drunk with five *dirham* of valerian, it is emmenagogue. When cooked, and used for washing the hair, it makes it curly and removes lichen.

When ground to a flour, mixed with natron and vinegar, and used as a poultice, it dissolves inflammation of the spleen. A woman may sit in water in which fenugreek has been cooked, for this is beneficial for pains caused by inflammation of the uterus. When used as a poultice for hard inflammations having little heat, it is beneficial and dissolves them. Drinking its juice is beneficial for indigestion arising from winds, and it makes the intestines smooth.

Eaten cooked with dates (*tamr*) or honey or figs on an empty stomach it dissolves sticky phlegm arising in the chest and stomach and is beneficial for persistent cough.

It is beneficial for constipation, and releases the belly. When put on contracted fingernails it corrects them. Its oil, mixed with wax, is beneficial for fissure arising from the cold. Its benefits are many times those we have mentioned.

It is related by al-Qāsim b. ᶜAbd al-Raḥmān that the Messenger of God ﷺ said: 'Seek a cure with fenugreek.' Some physicians have said: 'If people knew its benefits, they would buy it for its weight in gold'.

Khā'

1. *Khubz* (Bread)

It is established in the *Ṣaḥīḥ* that the Prophet ﷺ said: 'On the day of Resurrection, the earth will be one loaf of bread, which the Almighty will turn over with His hand, as food for the people of Paradise.'[284]

Abū Dāwūd related in his *Sunan*, from *ḥadīth* of Ibn ᶜAbbās: The food most loved by the Messenger of God ﷺ was *tharīd* made with bread, and *tharīd* made with *ḥays* (dates, *samn*, and curd or bread).[285]

From the same source, from *ḥadīth* of Ibn ʿUmar: The Messenger of God ﷺ said: 'I would love to have white bread, made from brown wheat, served with *samn* and curds (*laban*).' A man got up from the group, fetched some and brought it. Then the Prophet ﷺ asked: 'In what was this *samn* kept?' He replied: 'In a lizard skin.' He said: 'Take it away.'[286]

Al-Bayhaqī related, from *ḥadīth* of ʿĀ'isha (*marfūʿ*): 'Give respect to bread. Part of this respect is that its condiment should not be waited for.' But it seems this *ḥadīth* cannot be fully traced back, nor attributed; nor can the preceding narrative.

Now the *ḥadīth* concerning the prohibition of cutting bread with a knife is groundless, and does not come from the Messenger of God ﷺ. The story was initially about the prohibition of cutting meat with a knife; that too is not sound.

Said Muhannā': I asked Aḥmad about the *ḥadīth* of Abū Maʿshar, from Hishām b. ʿUrwa, from his father, from ʿĀ'isha, from the Prophet ﷺ: 'Do not cut meat with a knife, for that is something the non-Arabs do.' He replied: It is not sound, and is not recognised; the *ḥadīth* of ʿAmr b. Umayya is the contrary of this, and the *ḥadīth* of al-Mughīra. By the *ḥadīth* of ʿAmr b. Umayya he means: 'The Prophet ﷺ used to make an incision in sheep's meat;' and by the *ḥadīth* of al-Mughīra: 'When he received him as a guest, he would order a side of meat and it would be roasted; then he took a large knife and began to make incisions.'[287]

The best type of bread is that which is well kneaded and has risen properly. Bread from the stove (*tannūr*) is the best sort; after that, bread from the oven (*furn*); then bread made on hot ashes (*malla*) ranks third. The best bread is made from fresh wheat (*ḥinṭa*).

The most nutritious type is bread from semolina flour (*samīd*) being the slowest to digest because of the small amount of bran. Then comes bread of white flour, (*ḥuwārī*), then bread made of coarsely ground flour (*khashkār*).

The best time for eating a loaf of bread is at the end of the day on which it was baked. Soft bread is gentler on the stomach, and more nutritious and moistening, and it moves down more swiftly. Dry bread has the opposite properties.

Bread from wheat (*burr*) is by temperament hot in the middle of the second degree, near to the mean in moisture and dryness. The dryness is dominant over that part of it which the fire has dried, and moisture over the opposite.

Bread from fresh wheat (*ḥinṭa*) has a special characteristic of causing fatness very quickly. *Qaṭā'if* (shredded wheat with honey) generates a thick humour, while *fatīt* (crumbled bread) causes distension and is slow to digest. That made with curds is very nutritious, but causes obstructions and is slow to move down.

Bread of barley is cold and dry, in the first degree; it is less nutritious than wheat bread.

2. *Khall* (Vinegar)

Muslim relates in his *Ṣaḥīḥ*, from Jābir b. ʿAbd-Allāh: The Messenger of God ﷺ asked his family for condiments, and they replied: 'We have only vinegar.' So he called for this, and began to eat, saying: 'How good a condiment is vinegar.'[288] In the *Sunan* of Ibn Māja, from Umm Saʿīd, from the Prophet ﷺ: 'How good a condiment is vinegar! O God, bless vinegar. No house will be destitute where there is vinegar.'[289]

Vinegar is a combination of heat and cold, of which the latter is predominant. It is dry in the third degree, and has a strong dessicative power. It prevents matters from flowing down, and refines the constitution.

Wine vinegar is beneficial for inflamed stomach, calms the yellow bile, and repels the harm of deadly drugs. It dissolves milk and blood when these have solidified in the interior. It is beneficial for the spleen, tans the stomach, restricts the belly, quenches thirst, and prevents incipient inflammation. It helps the digestion, opposes phlegm, refines thick foods and thins the blood.

When drunk with salt, it is beneficial for one who has eaten deadly fungus. When made into a broth, it dislodges the leech which has attached itself to the root of the palate. When warmed and used as a mouth rinse, it is beneficial for toothache and strengthens the gums.

It is beneficial for whitlow when applied as an embrocation, and for itching, hot inflammations, and burns. It increases the appetite, sweetens the stomach, and is good for young people, and in the summer for the inhabitants of warm lands.

3. *Khilāl* (Toothpicks)[12]

Concerning this there are two unconfirmed *ḥadīth*. It is related from *ḥadīth* of Abū Ayyūb al-Anṣārī (*marfūʿ*): 'How good are those who use a toothpick! There is nothing harder upon the angels than pieces of food remaining in the mouth.' Included in the chain of transmission is Wāṣil b. al-Sā'ib. According to al-Bukhārī and al-Rāzī, this *ḥadīth* is unacceptable. While al-Nisā'ī and al-Azdī said that his *ḥadīth* is rejected. It is related from *ḥadīth* of Ibn ʿAbbās that ʿAbd-Allāh b. Aḥmad said: 'I asked my father about a shaykh from whom Ṣāliḥ al-Wuḥāẓī related *ḥadīth* (he was known as Muḥammad b. ʿAbd al-Malik al-Anṣārī). He said that ʿAṭā' told us from Ibn ʿAbbās that the Messenger of God ﷺ forbade one to use a toothpick of fibrous cane (*layṭ*) or myrtle (*ās*), and he said: "They give one the veins of leprosy." But my father said: I saw Muḥammad b. ʿAbd al-Malik, who was blind, fabricate the *ḥadīth* and lies.'

Finally, the use of *khilāl* is beneficial for the gums and teeth, preserving their good health, and it cures bad breath. The best is that which is taken from the

12 This can still be bought, eg. in Cairo, for use as a tooth cleaner.

bough of *al-akhila* (Ammi visnaga (L.) Lam. Umbelliferae), olive wood, and poplar. But to use a toothpick made from sugar cane, myrtle (*ās*), basil (*rayḥān*), and ocimum (*bādharūj*) is harmful.

Dāl

1. *Duhn* (Fatty matter)[13]

Al-Tirmidhī related in *Kitāb al-Shamā'il*, from *ḥadīth* of Anas b. Mālik: The Messenger of God ﷺ used to put a quantity of oil on his head, and would comb his beard a great deal, and would often use a head covering (*qināʿ*). His clothes were like those of a dealer in oil (*zayyāt*).

Oil stops up the pores of the body, and prevents any matter from being dissolved from it. When applied after washing in hot water, it beautifies and moistens the body. When used as a hair oil, it makes the hair long and beautiful. Oil is beneficial for measles, and repels most of the damage it can cause. In al-Tirmidhī, from *ḥadīth* of Abū Hurayra (*marfūʿ*), it says: Eat oil (*zayt*), and use it for oiling. We shall deal with this.

In hot countries, such as the Ḥijāz and its like, oil is one of the best means of preserving health and restoring the body. It is a necessity for these people. But the inhabitants of cold countries do not need it. Its continual use on the head contains some risk to the sight.

The most useful of the simple oils is oil (*zayt*), then clarified butter or ghee (*samn*), followed by sesame oil (*shīraj*).

Of the compound oils (*adhān*), some are cold and moist, like violet oil, which is beneficial for hot headache, and cures insomnia; it moistens the brain, and is beneficial for fissures and predominance of dryness and dessication. It is useful as an embrocation on scabies and dry itch. It facilitates the movement of the joints, and is restorative to those of hot temperaments in the season of summer.

Two void *ḥadīth* have been attributed to the Messenger of God ﷺ concerning violet oil: (1) 'the superiority of violet oil over other oils is like my superiority over other people;' (2) 'the superiority of violet oil over other oils (*adhān*) is like the superiority of Islam over other religions (*adyān*).'

Some oils are hot and moist, like oil of *bān* (Moringa aptera). This is not the oil of its flower, but an oil which is extracted from a dusty white seed, like the pistachio, rich in oily substances and fat. It softens hardness of the nerves; it is beneficial for spots (*barash*), freckles (*namash* and *kalaf*) and leukoderma, evacuates thick phlegm, softens dry sinews and warms the nerves.

Concerning *bān* there is a false invented *ḥadīth* which has no basis: 'Oil yourselves with *bān*, for it will put you in good favour with your womenfolk.'

Among the benefits of *bān* are that it cleanses the teeth and makes them shine by removing plaque. Anyone who rubs his face and head with it will not

13 For detailed discussion, see *Albucasis*.

be afflicted by measles nor fissures. When it is rubbed on the loins and male member and surrounding area, it is beneficial for cold of the kidneys and for the dripping of urine.

Dhāl

1. *Dharīra* (Acorus calamus L. Araceae. Calamus, sweet flag)

The following is established in the two books of the *Ṣaḥīḥ*, from ʿĀ'isha: 'I perfumed the Messenger of God ﷺ with *dharīra*, with my own hand, at the Farewell Pilgrimage, before and during the state of *iḥrām*.'[290]

We have already spoken of *dharīra* (powdered scent), its uses and its nature, so there is no need to repeat all this.

2. *Dhubāb* (Flies)

It has already been stated, in the accepted *ḥadīth* from Abū Hurayra, that the Prophet ﷺ ordered that when flies fell into food they should be fully immersed in it, for the sake of the healing property found in the wing. For it is like the antidote to the poison which is in the other wing. We have mentioned there the uses of flies.

3. *Dhahab* (Gold)

It is related by Abū Dāwūd and al-Tirmidhī that when the nose of ʿArfaja b. Asʿad was cut off, on the day of al-Kulāb, and he made himself a nose of paper which then began to go putrid on him, the Prophet ﷺ ordered him to make himself a nose of gold.[291] But there is only this one *ḥadīth* concerning ʿArfaja.

Gold is the adornment of this temporal life; it is the talisman of existence, and makes the soul glad, strengthens people's backs, and is God's secret on His earth. Its temperament includes all the qualities, and it contains a gentle heat, which enters into all the electuaries (*maʿjūnāt*) which are gentle and refreshing. It is most moderate and the noblest of minerals.

Among its special properties is that when it is buried underground, the earth does not harm it nor diminish it in any way. When gold filings are mixed with medicines, these are beneficial for weakness of the heart, and tremors (*rajafān*), arising from the black bile. It is beneficial for premonitions (*ḥadīth al-nafs*), for grief and anxiety, for upsets and for love sickness. It fattens and strengthens the body, dispels pallor (*ṣafār*), and improves the complexion. It is beneficial for leprosy and all pains and illnesses caused by the black bile. For its special property, it is included in medicaments for alopecia and ophiasis, drunk or as an embrocation. It clears and strengthens the eye, and is beneficial for many of its illnesses, and it strengthens all organs.

Keeping it in the mouth removes bad breath. If anyone has a malady requiring cautery, and gold is used for the cautery, the place will not blister, and it will heal swiftly. If a little of it is used as an eye salve, it strengthens and clears the eye. If gold is used for the centre stone of a seal ring, and it is heated to cauterise the front parts of a dove's wing, the bird will know its own dove-cote and will not stray away from it.

It has an amazing property in strengthening souls, which is the reason for the permission of its use during war and in the army.

Al-Tirmidhī has related, from *ḥadīth* of Burayda al-ʿIṣrī: 'The Messenger of God ﷺ entered on the day of victory (*fatḥ*) and his sword had gold and silver upon it.'[292]

People lust after gold, and when they obtain it, it makes them forget all they love in this world.

The Most High has said: *Fair in the eyes of men is the love of what they covet: women and sons, heaped up hoards of gold and silver, branded horses, cattle and well-tilled land* (III:14).

In the two books of the *Ṣaḥīḥ*, from the Prophet ﷺ, it is said that if the son of Adam had a valley of gold, he would desire a second; if he had a second, he would desire a third. But nothing fills his belly save dust: God pardons the one who repents.[293]

Moreover, gold is the worst obstacle preventing humankind from gaining the great victory on the day of recall, and it is the greatest cause of disobedience to God. For through it the bonds of relationship are severed, blood is shed, the forbidden is declared licit, rights are hindered; and God's servants oppress one another. It causes men to desire this world; it makes them mean about the next life and what God has prepared therein for His friends. For how many rights have been denied for its sake and false claims recognized. How many oppressors were assisted thereby, and how many oppressed people were subjected. How good are the words of Abū Qāsim al-Ḥarīrī concerning gold:

Woe be to it, a deceiver, a hypocrite, yellow two-faced, like the hypocrite. It appears with two descriptions to the eye of the beholder, adornment of the one desired, and the colour of the desirer.
Among the people of the truth, love of it urges people of the truth to dare the anger of the Creator.
Without it, the right hand of the thief would not be cut off, nor would any injustice be manifest from an evildoer,
Nor a miser shrink back from one who knocks [a beggar], nor the one given an extension complain of the delay of the hindrance.
Nor would one seek refuge from the one who envies and strikes, and its evil effect on created beings;
indeed nought will help you in times of hardship, save fleeing like the runaway slave.

Rā'

1. *Ruṭab* (from Phoenix dactylifera L. Palmae. Fresh dates)

God the Most High said to Maryam: *And shake towards thee the trunk of the palm-tree; it will let fall fresh ripe dates upon thee; so eat and drink and cool thine eye* (XIX: 25–6).

In the two books of the *Ṣaḥīḥ*, from ʿAbd-Allāh b. Jaʿfar, it says: I saw the Messenger of God ﷺ eating cucumber (*qiththā'*) with fresh dates.[14][294] And in the *Sunan* of Abū Dāwūd, from Anas: The Messenger of God ﷺ used to break his fast with some fresh dates, before he prayed; if there were none, then with dried dates (*tamarāt*). If there were none of these he would take a drink of water.[295]

Ruṭab have the same constitution as water: hot and moist, they strengthen the cold stomach, to which they are appropriate. They are aphrodisiac, they enrich the body, are suitable for those with cold temperaments and are very nourishing.

They are more suitable than any other fruit for the people of Madīna and other such places, where it is their own fruit, and are among the most beneficial for the body. If someone is not accustomed to them they will hasten putrefaction in his body and, thence, will generate blood which is not desirable; if he eats a large amount, this will lead to headache and black bile, and harm his teeth. This can be counteracted with oxymel (*sakanjabīn*) and similar items.

Concerning the Prophet ﷺ and his breaking his fast with *ruṭab*, or *tamr*, or water, this has a very subtle explanation. Fasting clears the stomach of food; the liver finds nothing to attract and to send on to the faculties and organs. Sweet substances are the quickest to reach the liver being what it likes best, especially *ruṭab*; so it eagerly accepts them, and thus both the liver and the faculties benefit thereby. Next come *tamr* because of their sweetness and nutriment. If not these, then broth of water, which extinguishes the burning of the stomach and the heat of fasting, and then the stomach is prepared for food and accepts it with good appetite.

2. *Rayḥān* (Sweet-smelling plants)

God The Most High said: *If he be of those nearest to God, there is for him rest, and mercy* (rayḥān) *and a garden of delights* (LVI: 88–9), and *Corn, with leaves and stalk, and sweet-smelling plants* (rayḥān) (LV: 12).

In the *Ṣaḥīḥ* of Muslim, from the Prophet ﷺ, it is said: If anyone is offered *rayḥān*, let him not refuse it. For it is light to carry, sweet of scent.[296]

In the *Sunan* of Ibn Māja, from *ḥadīth* of Usāma, from the Prophet ﷺ, it is

14 *Hadīth* concerning *ruṭab* and *qiththā'*: see Chapter 18, n. 1.

quoted that he said: 'Is there one who will work for Paradise, for no thought can encompass Paradise. By the Lord of the Kaʿba, it is light which shines like pearls, sweet scent (*rayḥāna*) which trembles, a fortified castle, a river which never ceases, ripe dates, a beautiful comely wife, many festive garments, dwelling for ever in a safe house, fruit and green plants, beautiful sounds and a blessing, in a place lofty, magnificent.' They said: 'Yes, O Messenger of God, we are those who will work for it.' He replied: 'Say: If God the Most High wills.' Said the people: 'If God wills.'[297]

The word *rayḥān* is used to indicate any plant with a sweet scent. The people of each region have some particular plant which is known as such. The people of the west specify it by the word *ās*, which is the type the Arabs know of as *rayḥān*. The people of Iraq and Syria specify it as *ḥabaq*.

As for *ās* (myrtle), its temperament is cold in the first degree, dry in the second. Withal, it is composed of opposite powers, the most plentiful being the cold earthy essence. It contains something hot and gentle. It is a strong dessicant for the head. Its constituents are close to one another in power, this being a costive restrictive power, from within and without together.

It checks bilious diarrhoea and dispels hot moist vapour; sniffed, it makes the heart rejoice greatly. Smelling it, or strewing it in the house, wards off pestilence (*wabā'*).

Its use locally cures inflammations in the two veins of the kidneys. Its leaves may be pounded, fresh, and then beaten with vinegar, and put on the head to stop nosebleed. When its dry leaves are crushed and dusted onto ulcers containing moisture, this is beneficial for them. It strengthens weak organs, when used as a poultice, and is beneficial for whitlows. Similarly it is good when powdered on pustules and ulcers in the hands and feet.

When the body is rubbed with it, this cuts down sweat, dries excess moistures, and dispels odour from the armpits. To sit in its cooked liquid is beneficial for the protrusion of anus or uterus, and for flaccidity of the joints. When poured onto broken bones which have not healed, it is beneficial.

It cleanses scurf, moist ulcers and pustules of the head, retains falling hair and blackens the hair. When its leaves are pounded and a little water is poured on them, then mixed with a little oil or rose oil and used as a poultice, this is appropriate for moist ulcers, itching and erysipelas, and severe inflammations, skin eruptions and haemorrhoids.

Its seeds are beneficial for haemoptysis, coming from the chest and lung, and they tan the stomach. Because of its cleansing properties it is not harmful to the chest and lungs. Its special characteristic is to assist looseness of the belly accompanied by cough. This is a rare quality in medicines. It is diuretic, beneficial for inflammation of the bladder, bites of tarantula and scorpion. To use its root as a toothpick is dangerous, so one must beware of this.

The Persian *rayḥān*, called *ḥabaq* (basil), is hot, according to one opinion. Smelling it is beneficial for hot headaches, when water is sprinkled on it; it has the contingent effect of cooling and moistening. According to another opinion it is cold. There are two opinions as to whether it is moist or dry. The truth is that it includes the four constitutions.

It brings on sleep. Its seeds restrict bilious diarrhoea and calm stomach trouble, strengthen the heart, and are beneficial for atrabilious diseases.

3. *Rummān* (Punica granatum L. Punicaceae. Pomegranate)

The Most High said: *In the two (gardens) are fruit and dates and pomegranates* (LV:68).

It is related from Ibn ʿAbbās (both shortened and with a full chain of transmission) that every pomegranate you have is pollinated from a seed from the pomegranates of Paradise.[298] The shortened version is similar. Ḥarb and others have mentioned, from ʿAlī, that he said: 'Eat the pomegranate with its flesh, for it tans the stomach.'

Sweet pomegranate is hot and moist, good for the stomach, which it strengthens by virtue of its gentle costiveness. It is beneficial for the throat, chest and lung, and helps a cough. Its juice softens the belly and gives the body slight but excellent nourishment. It is swift to dissolve because of its fineness and subtlety. It generates slight heat in the stomach, and winds; therefore, it aids the sexual powers and is not suitable for the fevered. It has a wonderful characteristic that when eaten with bread, it prevents it from putrefying in the stomach.

The sour kind is cold and dry, costive and gentle. It is beneficial for an inflamed stomach; it is more diuretic than the rest of the pomegranates. It calms the yellow bile, cuts short diarrhoea, prevents vomiting, refines the superfluities, extinguishes the heat of the liver, strengthens the organs. It is beneficial for bilious palpitation and for pains occurring to the heart and the mouth of the stomach. It strengthens the stomach, repels superfluities from it, damping down yellow bile and blood.

Its juice can be extracted with its flesh, and cooked with a little honey until it becomes like an ointment; if used as a *koḥl*, it removes yellowness from the eye, and cleanses it of thick moistures. Smeared on the gums, it is beneficial for decay in that region. When its juice is extracted with its flesh, this releases the belly and causes the bilious putrid moistures to descend, and it is beneficial for protracted tertian fevers.

Medium-tasting pomegranate (ie. between sweet and sour) is midway in its constitution and action; it is slightly more inclined towards the gentleness of the sour kind.

Seeds of the pomegranate with honey can be used as an embrocation on whitlow and foul ulcers, and its stems (pericarps) used for wounds. They say that whoever eats three flowers (*junbudh*) of the pomegranate each year will be secure from ophthalmia all year long.

Zā'

1. *Zayt* (Olive oil)

The Most High said: . . . *lit from a blessed tree, an olive neither of the east nor of the west, whose oil would well-nigh give light even if no flame touched it* (XXIV:35).

Al-Tirmidhī and Ibn Māja report, from *ḥadīth* of Abū Hurayra, that the Prophet ﷺ said: 'Eat olive oil (*zayt*) and anoint yourselves with it, for it is from a blessed tree.'[299] Al-Bayhaqī and Ibn Māja also have from ʿAbd-Allāh b. ʿUmar that the Messenger of God ﷺ said: 'Eat olive oil with your bread, and oil yourselves with it, for it is from a blessed tree.'[300]

Olive oil is hot and moist in the first degree, and it is mistaken to say that it is dry.

The characteristic of olive oil corresponds to the type of olives from which it comes. That which is pressed from ripe olives is the most moderate and the best; oil taken from unripe olives contains cold and dryness. That pressed from red olives is midway between the two other oils. Oil pressed from black olives will warm and moisten moderately, and it is beneficial for poisons, loosens the belly, and expels worms. Oil from old olives has a greater strength to warm and dissolve. That which is pressed out with water is less hot and gentler, more effective and beneficial. All of its types soften the skin and delay whitening of the hair.

Liquid of the salty olive prevents blistering of burns and strengthens the gums. Its leaves are beneficial for erysipelas and itching, foul ulcers and skin eruptions, and prevent sweating. Its benefits are many times greater than we have mentioned.

2. *Zubd* (Butter)

Abū Dāwūd related in his *Sunan*, from the two sons of Busr, those known as Sulamī: The Messenger of God ﷺ came to visit us, and we set before him butter and dates (*tamr*). For he used to like butter and dates.[301]

Butter is hot and moist, containing many benefits: it has a power of cocting and dissolving, and it heals inflammations which occur in the side of the ear and the two veins of the kidneys, inflammations of the mouth, and other inflammations which occur in women and children's bodies; this is when it is used alone. When taken as an electuary (*luʿiq*), it is beneficial for haemoptysis sited in the lung, and it cocts inflammations occurring there.

It has a laxative effect and calms the nerves and severe inflammations occurring from black bile and phlegm, and it is beneficial for dryness occurring in the body.

It can be rubbed onto children's gums, at the place where teeth should come through, to assist the formation and the growth of their teeth. It is beneficial for cough arising from cold and dryness. It dispels tetter and roughness in the body and softens the constitution. But it reduces the appetite for food and dispels the desire for sweet things like honey and dates.

The fact that the Prophet ﷺ combined butter and dates showed wisdom, for this means the rectification of one by the other.

3. *Zabīb* (from Vitis vinifera L. Vitaceae. Raisins)[15]

Two *ḥadīth* are related concerning raisins, neither of them sound: (1) 'How good a food are raisins! They sweeten the breath and melt the phlegm;' (2) 'How good a food are raisins! They remove fatigue, strengthen nerves, extinguish anger, clarify the complexion, and sweeten the breath.' Here too there is no sound attribution to the Messenger of God ﷺ.

The best raisins are large-bodied, plump in their substance and flesh, thin-skinned, with their pips removed, small berried (or: with small pips). The body of raisins is hot and moist in the first degree, their seeds are cold and dry, for they are like the grapes from which they come. The sweet ones are hot; the sour are costive and cold; the white are more costive than others. Their flesh when eaten is suitable for the trachea and beneficial for cough and pains of the kidney and bladder. They strengthen the stomach and soften the belly.

The kind with sweet flesh are more nourishing than grapes, but less nourishing than dried figs. They have a cocting, digestive power, costive, and dissoluent, in moderation. In sum, they strengthen the stomach, liver and spleen, and are beneficial for the pain of throat, chest, lung, kidney and bladder.

They are best eaten without their pips. They provide sound nourishment and do not cause obstruction as dates (*tamr*) do. When eaten with their kernel (*ʿajm*), they are more beneficial to the stomach, liver and spleen. When their flesh is attached to partly dislodged nails, they come out more quickly. The sweet kind, and the seedless, are beneficial to people of moistures and phlegm. They are good for the liver because of their special properties.

They are also of use for the memory. Al-Zuhrī said: 'If anyone wishes to learn *ḥadīth* by heart, let him eat raisins.'

And al-Manṣūr used to repeat, from his grandfather ʿAbd-Allāh b. ʿAbbās: 'Their pips are a malady (*dā'*); their flesh is a remedy (*dawā'*).'

4. *Zanjabīl* (Zingiber officinale. Zingiberaceae. Ginger)

God The Most High said: *They will be given to drink therein a cup mixed with ginger* (LXXVI: 17).

Abū Nuʿaym mentioned in the Book of Prophetic Medicine, from *ḥadīth* of Abū Saʿīd al-Khudrī: The King of the Byzantines sent God's Messenger ﷺ a

15 See also *ʿinab* and *karm*.

present of a jar of ginger; so he gave each person a piece to eat and gave me a piece.'

Ginger is hot in the second degree, moist in the first. It is warming, aids digestion and has a moderate softening effect on the belly. It is beneficial for obstructions of the liver caused by cold and moisture, and for clouded sight arising from moisture, both when eaten and when used as *koḥl*. It encourages sexual intercourse and it dissolves the thick winds arising in intestines and stomach.

In sum, it is good for the liver and stomach, when these are cold in temperament. When two *dirham* of it are taken with sugar in hot water, it evacuates sticky mucous superfluities. It occurs in the electuaries (*maʿjūnāt*) which dissolve and melt the phlegm.

The medium-tasting sort is hot and dry; it is aphrodisiac, increases semen, warms the stomach and liver, helps the digestion, dries up phlegm which is dominant in the body, and increases the power of the memory; it is appropriate for cold of the liver and stomach and it stops moisture of the stomach which arises from eating fruit. It sweetens the breath. Through it, any harm from heavy cold food is avoided.

Sīn

1. *Sannā*

This has already been discussed, as has *sannūt*.[16] There are seven opinions as to its identity: (1) honey; (2) *robb* of the *ʿakka* (skin) of the *samn*, bringing out black lines on the *samn*; (3) a grain resembling cumin, but which it is not; (4) Kirmānī cumin; (5) dill (*shibitt*); (6) dates (*tamr*); (7) fennel (*rāzyānaj*).

2. *Safarjal* (Cydonia vulgaris pers. Rosaceae. Quince)

Ibn Māja relates in his *Sunan* the *ḥadīth* of Ismāʿīl b. Muḥammad al-Ṭalḥī from Shuʿayb b. Ḥājib, from Abū Saʿīd, from ʿAbd al-Malik al-Zubayrī, from Ṭalḥa b. ʿUbayd-Allāh: I entered the presence of the Prophet ﷺ, who had in his hand a quince. He said: 'Take this, O Ṭalḥa, for it rests and relaxes the heart.'[302] This is related by al-Nisā'ī through another narration: I came to the Prophet ﷺ who was with a group of his Companions, and he was holding in his hand a quince, which he was turning over. When I sat down before him, he held it out to me, then said: 'Here you are, Abū Dharr, for it strengthens the heart, refreshes the soul, and dispels heaviness of the chest.'

Other unsound *ḥadīth* are related about the *safarjal*, of which these are an example.

16 For *sennā* and *sannūt*, see Chapter 11.

Quince is cold and dry, varying in this respect in accordance with the variation in its taste. All are cold, costive, and good for the stomach.

The sweet variety is less cold and dry, and closer to the mean. The sour variety is more costive, drier and colder. All of them quench thirst and stop vomiting, are diuretic, restrict the constitution, are beneficial for ulcers of the intestines, haemoptysis and cholera. They are beneficial for nausea. They prevent the rising of vapours, when taken after food. When washed the burnt ashes of its branches and leaves act like zinc.

Taken before food quinces are costive, whereas after food they have a laxative effect on the constitution, and hasten the descent of heavy substances. In large quantities they are harmful to the nerves, cause colic and extinguish the yellow bile generated in the stomach.

When roasted they are lighter and less rough. If the centre is scooped out and its pips removed, then filled with honey and the whole fruit coated with dough and put onto hot ashes, it is extremely beneficial.

The best fruits are those which are eaten roasted or cooked with honey. Their seeds are beneficial for hoarseness of the throat and trachea, and for many illnesses. Their oil prevents sweating and strengthens the stomach. *Robb* (concentrate) made from it strengthens the stomach and liver, and it fortifies the heart and refreshes the soul.

Now the meaning of 'relaxing the heart' is that it gives it rest. And it is said: 'It opens and expands it'. This meaning is derived from the Arabic *jumām al-mā'* which describes its expansion and its abundance. 'Darkness' (*ṭakhā'*) for the heart is like clouds covering the sky. Said Abū ʿUbayd: 'Darkness' indicates heaviness and covering. One may say: There is no darkness in the sky, meaning cloud and darkness.

3. *Siwāk* (Toothbrush)

In the two books of the *Ṣaḥīḥ*, from the Prophet ﷺ, it says: If it were not that I would make it difficult for my community, I would order them to use the *siwāk* before every time of prayer (*ṣalāt*).[303] And in these same sources it is quoted that when he arose after a night's sleep he would clean his mouth with the *siwāk*.[304] In the *Ṣaḥīḥ* of Bukhārī, his comments are that the Prophet ﷺ said: 'The *siwāk* is a means of purifying the mouth, pleasing to the Lord.'[305] In the *Ṣaḥīḥ* of Muslim it says that when he entered his house he would begin by using the *siwāk*.[306] There are many *ḥadīth* about this.

It is reliably reported concerning the Prophet ﷺ that he cleansed his teeth when close to death. Also it is true that he said: 'I have often spoken to you about *siwāk*'.

The best kind of *siwāk* is made from the wood of *arāk* (Salvadora persica L.) and similar. It should not be made from an unknown tree, for this might be poisonous. One must use it in moderation. Excessive use might cause one to remove the elegant shine of the teeth and make them susceptible to the vapours rising up from the stomach and impurities. When used in a moderate way, it cleanses the teeth, strengthens the centre of the tongue, frees the tongue, prevents cavities, sweetens the breath, cleanses the brain, arouses the appetite for food. The best way to use it is moistened with rose water.

Another most useful toothbrush is made from the roots of walnut. The author of the *Taysīr* said: They claim that when a *siwāk* made of walnut roots is used to clean one's teeth every fifth day, it cleanses the head, refines the senses, and fortifies the intellect.

The *siwāk* has many benefits: it refreshes the mouth, strengthens the gums, cuts phlegm, makes the sight clear, removes cavities, makes the stomach healthy, purifies the voice, assists the digestion of food, and facilitates the passages of speech, giving energy for recitation, invocation and prayer, repels sleep and pleases the Lord, delights the angels and increases one's good deeds. It is recommended at all times; it is confirmed at times of prayer and for ablution, on awakening from sleep, and when the odour of the mouth changes. It is recommended for a person breaking his fast and for one fasting at all times, because of the general nature of those *ḥadīth* concerning it, because the person fasting has need of it and finally because it pleases the Lord. God's pleasure is sought during the fast, more eagerly than it is sought when not fasting. Furthermore it purifies the mouth; and purity for the person fasting is one of the most excellent of deeds.

In the *Sunan*, from ʿĀmir b. Rabīʿa, it says: I saw God's Messenger ﷺ, more times than I could count, using the *siwāk* while he was fasting.[307] Bukharī relates that Ibn ʿUmar said: He would use the *siwāk* at the beginning and towards the end of the day.

People are agreed that the person fasting rinses his mouth as an obligation and as an approved action. Rinsing is more effective than the *siwāk*. God does not wish that one should approach Him with an unpleasant odour, nor is this the kind of act prescribed for devotion.

He only said: 'The fragrance of the altered breath (*khulūf*) is with God on the Day of Resurrection' as an encouragement to fast, not an encouragement to keep the odour. Rather, the one fasting has more need of the *siwāk* than the one not fasting. Also, the pleasure of God is greater than his finding pleasant the altered breath of the mouth of the one fasting. God's favour for the use of the *siwāk* is greater than preserving the altered breath of the one fasting.

Moreover, the *siwāk* does not prevent the scent of the altered breath, which it removes, from being acknowledged by God on the Day of Resurrection. Rather, the fasting person comes to that Day with the breath of his mouth sweeter than musk, as a sign of his fasting, even if he removed it with the *siwāk*. In the same way, the wounded man will come to the Day of Resurrection with the colour of his wound as the colour of blood, and its scent of musk. Yet he is commanded to remove it in this world.

Moreover, altered breath (*khulūf*) does not cease because of the *siwāk*, for its cause remains, this being the stomach's emptiness from food. Only its effect ceases, and that is, the congealing around the teeth and gums.

Moreover, the Prophet ﷺ taught his community what was approved for them during the fast and what was disapproved of. He did not classify the *siwāk* among the disapproved. For he knew that they frequently used the *siwāk*, for he had specifically pointed it out to them, with the most eloquent words, in general and specific terms. And they saw him clean his teeth when fasting, times without number; he knew that they would follow his example. He did not say to them at any time: 'Do not use the *siwāk* after noon time.' Delaying explanation beyond the time of need is prohibited. God knows best.

4. *Samn* (Clarified butter)

Muḥammad b. Jarīr al-Ṭabarī related, with his *isnād*, from *ḥadīth* of Ṣhuayb (*marfūᶜ*): Use cow's milk! For it is healing, and their *samn* is a medicine, their meat is a malady. He related it from Aḥmad b. al-Ḥasan al-Tirmidhī: We were told by Muḥammad b. Mūsā al-Nisā' ī, from Diffāᶜ b. Daghfal al-Sadūsī, on the authority of ᶜAbd al-Ḥamīd b. Ṣayfī b. Ṣuhayb, from his father, from his grandfather. But the contents of this *isnād* are not confirmed.

Samn is hot and moist in the first degree; it contains a slight cleansing power and subtlety, and it is able to disperse the inflammations occurring in soft bodies. It is stronger than butter (*zubd*) in its power of coction and softening. Galen said that he cured with it inflammations occurring in the ear and in the tip of the nose. When it is used as an ointment on the site of the teeth, these grow swiftly.

Mixed with honey and bitter almond, it cleanses the chest and lungs, and cleanses thick sticky chymes. However, it is harmful to the stomach, especially to someone whose temperament is phlegmatic.

Samn of cows and goats, when drunk with honey, counteracts deadly poisons and helps with the sting of serpents and scorpions. In the book of Ibn al-Sunnī, from ᶜAlī b. Abī Ṭālib, it says: *Samn* is the most excellent of all the means that people use for healing.

5. *Samak* (Fish)

It is related by Imām Aḥmad b. Ḥanbal and by Ibn Māja in his *Sunan*, from *ḥadīth* of ᶜAbd-Allāh b. ᶜUmar, from the Prophet ﷺ, that he said: 'Two items of dead meat and two of blood have been made lawful for us: fish and locusts, liver and spleen.'[308]

There are many kinds of fish.[17] The best are those of pleasing taste, good-smelling, of moderate size, with thin skin, and neither hard nor dry flesh,

17 See also *ᶜanbar*.

and those which live in fresh water running over the stones, feeding upon plants, not on anything polluted.

The best places for fish are in a river with good water. They generally shelter in stony places, then sandy areas, and fresh running water where there is no impurity nor mud, that is water which is in constant motion and flows rapidly and is open to the sun and winds.

Sea fish is excellent, laudable and subtle. The fresh sort is cold and moist, difficult to digest, generating much phlegm, with the exception of sea fish and that which follows its path. This generates a commendable humour. It makes the body fertile, increases semen and rectifies hot temperaments.

The best of salted fish is that which has been recently salted. It is hot and dry, and as its age increases, so do its heat and dryness. Of these, the eel (*sillūr*) is very sticky (it is also called *jirrī*). The Jews do not eat it. When it is eaten fresh, it loosens the belly. When salted, left to mature and then eaten, it purifies the trachea and improves the voice. When pounded and applied externally, it expels the secundine (*salā*) and superfluities from the interior of the body because of its power of attraction.

It is appropriate for one suffering from ulcers of the intestines to sit in liquid of the salted eel, at the outset of the illness. This draws the 'matters' to the exterior of the body. Used as a clyster it cures sciatica.

The best portion of a fish is that close to the rear of it. Fresh fat fish make the body well-nourished.

In the two books of *Ṣaḥīḥ*, from *ḥadīth* of Jābir b. ʿAbd-Allāh, it says: The Prophet ﷺ sent us with three hundred horsemen, our leader being Abū ʿUbayda b. al-Jarrāḥ. We came to the coastal plain and were afflicted with fierce hunger, until we were becoming almost deranged. Then the sea cast up for us a fish known as *ʿanbar*; we ate this for the duration of half a month and used its fat as condiment, until our bodies became firm. Abū ʿUbayda took one of its ribs, and put a man upon his camel, set it up, and he passed beneath it.[309]

6. *Silq* (Beta vulgaris L. Chenopodiacea. Beet)

It is related by al-Tirmidhī and Abū Dāwūd, from Umm al-Mundhir: The Messenger of God ﷺ entered, accompanied by ʿAlī; we had vines hanging. The Messenger of God ﷺ began to eat, and ʿAlī ate with him. Then the Messenger of God ﷺ said: 'Desist, O ʿAlī, for you are convalescing'. So I brought them beet and barley, and the Prophet ﷺ said: 'O ʿAlī, now take from this, for it is more suitable for you.'[310] Al-Tirmidhī said: This is a rare, but good *ḥadīth*.

Silq is hot and dry in the first degree. It is said to be moist in the first degree, and also to posses both qualities. It contains some refining coldness, some dissolving and opening faculty. The black sort is somewhat costive; it is beneficial for alopecia and for freckles, lichen and warts, when its juice is applied. It kills lice; it is used as an ointment with honey for tetter; it opens obstructions of liver and spleen. The black sort restricts the belly, especially in conjunction with lentils, for the two are bad. But with lentils the white sort softens; its juice is used as a clyster for diarrhoea; it is beneficial for colic, with *marī* (salt fish) and spices. It contains little nourishment, has bad chyme, burns the blood, and is rectified by vinegar and mustard. In large quantities it generates constipation and distension.

Shīn

1. *Shūnīz*

This is *al-ḥabba al-sawdā'*, which has already been discussed under the letter *ḥā'* above.

2. *Shubrum* (Euphorbia pithyusa L. Euphorbiaceae. Euphorbia)

Al-Tirmidhī and Ibn Māja relate in their books of the *Sunan*, from *ḥadīth* of Asmā' bint ʿUmays, that the Messenger of God ﷺ asked: 'What do you use as a purgative?' She said: 'Euphorbia'. He said: '*Ḥārr, yārr* (very hot!).'[311]

Euphorbia is a shrub, both small and large, about the height of a man or taller; its branches are red, streaked with white; in the heads of its branches are clusters of leaves; it has small blossoms, yellow to white, which fall and leave behind tiny twigs containing small seeds, like the terebinth in size, of red colour. It has roots covered by red bark. The parts used are the bark of its roots and the milky substance from its branches.

It is hot and dry in the fourth degree. It purges the black bile and the thick chymes, the yellow water and the phlegm. It causes discomfort and nausea. In large amounts it is lethal. For use, it must be soaked in fresh milk for a day and a night, and the milk must be changed two or three times during the day. It is taken out and dried in the shade, and is mixed with rose and tragacanth, and drunk with honey water or pressed grape juice. Dosage is between four and two *dāniq*, according to strength.

Said Ḥunayn: Milk of euphorbia [latex?] has no good qualities. I do not consider any dose at all would be good. For by its use, the itinerant doctors[18] have killed many people.

3. *Shaʿīr* (Hordeum vulgare L. Graminea. Barley)

Ibn Māja relates the following from *ḥadīth* of ʿĀ'isha who said: When any one of his family was indisposed, the Messenger of God ﷺ used to call for a broth

18 Itinerant doctors, *aṭibbā' al-ṭuraqāt* cf. Chapter 1, n. 5.

of barley to be made; then he would order them to drink the broth. He would say: 'Indeed it mends the heart of the sorrowful and relieves the heart of the sick, just as one of you removes dirt from her face with water.'[312] The meaning of 'mend' (*ratw*) is to firm and strengthen it; to 'relieve' (*sarw*) is to uncover and remove.

It has already been stated that this broth is water of boiled barley. It is more nourishing than *sawīq* (porridge) of barley. It is beneficial for cough and sore throat, and suitable for calming the fierceness of superfluities; it is diuretic, cleanses the stomach's contents, quenches thirst, extinguishes heat. It has a power to cleanse, refine and dissolve.

The recipe is as follows. Take a quantity of good, crushed barley, and five parts of pure water, put it all in a clean pot, cook it over a moderate fire until two fifths of it remain; then it is strained, and as much as is needed may be used with sweetener added.

4. *Shawīy* (Roast)

God the Most High said, regarding the hospitality of his friend Abraham: *He hurried and brought a roasted calf,* ʿijl ḥanīdh (XI:69). Now *hanīdh* means roasted on *raḍf,* hot stones.

In al-Tirmidhī, from Umm Salama it says that she brought to the Messenger of God ﷺ a roasted side of meat, and he ate of it; then getting up for prayer, he did not perform the *wuḍū'*.[313] Said al-Tirmidhī: This is a sound *ḥadīth*. Similarly, from ʿAbd-Allāh b. al-Ḥarth: We ate with God's Messenger ﷺ some roasted meat in the mosque. Similarly, from Mughīra b. Shuʿba: I was a guest one night with God's Messenger ﷺ, and he ordered a side of meat to be roasted. Then he took a large knife and began to cut pieces from the meat for me. Then Bilāl came to give the call for prayer, and he threw down the knife and said: 'Wherefore are his hands dusty?'

The most beneficial sort of roast is of a lamb one year old; then the delicate, fat calf. It is hot, moist, tending towards dryness, and generates plentiful black bile. It is one of the foods of the strong and healthy and those who take exercise. The meat cooked in water (*maṭbūkh*) is more beneficial and lighter on the stomach, and moister than baked or roasted meat.

The worst is that roasted in the sun; roasted on coals is better than that roasted on flames, which is the *ḥanīdh*.

5. *Shaḥm* (Fat)

It is confirmed in the *Musnad,* from Anas, that a Jew entertained the Messenger of God ﷺ and offered him barley and rancid fat (*ihāla sanikha*).[314] Now *ihāla* means melted-down fat and *sanikha* means rancid.

It is confirmed in the *Ṣaḥīḥ,* from ʿAbd-Allāh b. Maghfal: a bag of fat was hung up, on the day of Khaybar, and I took hold of it and said: 'By God, I shall not give any of this to anyone. So I turned, and there was the Messenger of God ﷺ, laughing, but he said nothing.'[315]

The best sort of fat is that which comes from an animal fully developed; it is hot and moist, but has less moisture than *samn*. Thus, if fat and *samn* are melted, the fat is quicker to solidify.

It is beneficial for hoarseness, and it softens and putrefies. Its damage is repelled by salted *laymūn* (lime fruit) and ginger. Fat of goats is the most costive of fats. Fat of the he-goat is the strongest in dissolving, and is beneficial for ulcers of the intestines. In that respect goose fat is stronger, and it is used for a clyster for abrasions and dysentery.

Ṣād

1. *Ṣalāt* (Ritual prayer)

God the Most High said: *And seek God's help with patient perseverance and prayer. It is hard, except for those who bring a lowly spirit* (II:45). And He said: *O ye who believe! Seek help with perseverance and prayer: for God is with those who patiently persevere* (II:153). And the Most High said: *Enjoin prayer on thy people, and persevere therein. We do not ask thee to provide sustenance, for We provide it; but the reward of the hereafter is for righteousness* (XX:132).

And in the *Sunan* it says: When something serious troubled the Messenger of God ﷺ he took refuge in prayer.[316] We have already noted how healing can be sought in prayer for most pains before they take root.

Prayer can bring about one's provision (*rizq*); it preserves health, wards off harm, repels maladies, strengthens the heart, brightens the face, gladdens the soul, removes langour, invigorates the limbs, reinforces the faculties, expands the breast, nourishes the spirit, illumines the heart, preserves well-being, protects against affliction, attracts blessing, keeps Satan at a distance, and brings one closer to the Merciful.

In short, it has a wonderful effect in the preservation of the health of body and heart and their faculties, and in repelling evil substances from them. If ever any two men are tested by frailty or malady or trial or affliction, the one who prays will receive a lesser portion, and the outcome for him will be sounder.

Prayer has a wonderful effect in warding off the evils of this life, especially when it is given its due and is properly performed, outwardly and inwardly. There is nothing equal to worship for warding off the evils of this life and the next and for attracting their benefits. The secret is that worship is a link to God the Glorious; in accordance with the servant's connection to his Lord the Glorious, the doors of good things (*khayr*) are opened to him, the causes of evil are cut off from him, and the materials of success are poured upon him by his

Glorious Lord. So health and well-being, accomplishments and wealth, rest and blessings, joys and pleasures—all these are made present and are swiftly brought to him.

2. *Ṣabr* (Patient perseverance)

Patience is half of faith; for this is a quality composed of patience and gratitude (*shukr*). As one of the ancestors (*salaf*) has said: Faith is in two halves: one half patience, one half gratitude. And the Most High said: *Indeed in that there are signs for each one who is patiently persevering and truly grateful* (XIV : 5).

Patience in relation to faith is like the head in relation to the body. It is of three types: (1) Patience concerning the obligations (*farḍ*) laid down by God, that one should not neglect them; (2) patience in abstaining from actions forbidden by Him, that one should not commit them; (3) patience concerning His judgements (*qaḍā'*) and decrees (*qadar*), that one should not resent them. Whoever perfectly fulfils these three degrees has perfected patience. For the pleasure of this world and the next, their blessings, and victory and conquest can only be reached over the bridge of patience, just as no-one reaches Paradise except by crossing over the Path. ʿUmar b. al-Khaṭṭāb said: We attained the best of life through patience.

If you reflect on the degrees of perfection acquired in the world, you will see that they are all dependent on patience. And if you reflect on imperfection, which one is blamed for possessing, you will see it all stemming from lack of patience. Thus courage and purity, goodness and love of others, all this is the patience of an hour.

> Patience is a talisman, upon the treasure of exaltedness,
> Whoever alights upon the talisman wins its treasure.

Most sickness of the body and heart arises simply from lack of patience. And there is naught like patience for preserving the health of hearts, bodies and spirits. For it is the great remedy, the mighty *tiryāq*, even if it were to contain only the company of God *for God is with the patient* (II : 153), and His affection for them for indeed *God loves those who are patient* (III: 146), and His giving victory to His people 'for victory comes with patience'; and that it is a good for the people of patience. *And if you show patience, that is indeed the best course for those who are patient* (XVI: 126), and that it is the cause of prosperity. *O ye who believe! persevere in patience, vie in perseverance, be ever vigilant, and fear God, that perchance you may prosper* (III: 200).

3. *Ṣabir* (Aloe vera L. Liliaceae. Aloe)

Abū Dāwūd related in the *Kitāb al-Marāsīl*, from *ḥadīth* of Qays b. Rāfiᶜ al Qaysī, that the Messenger of God ﷺ said: 'In what two bitter things lies healing? Aloe and *thuffā*.'

And in the *Sunan* of Abū Dāwūd, from *ḥadīth* of Umm Salma: the Messenger of God ﷺ entered my house at the death of Abū Salma. Now I had put aloes upon myself, and he asked: 'What is this, O Umm Salma?' I replied: 'It is but aloe, O Messenger of God, there is no scent in it.' He said: 'It lights up the face, so do not put it on except at night.' And he forbade it during the day.[317]

Aloe is very beneficial, especially the Indian variety; it cleanses the bilious superfluities in the brain and the optic nerves; when applied as ointment on the forehead and temples with rose water, it is beneficial for headache. It is beneficial for ulcers of the nose and mouth, and purges black bile and melancholy.

Persian aloe sharpens the intellect, strengthens the heart and cleanses the bilious and phlegmatic superfluities from the stomach, when two spoonfuls are drunk in water. It restores the jaded and spoiled appetite. When drunk in the cold, there is fear lest it purge blood.

4. *Ṣawm* (Fasting)

Fasting[19] is a protection (*junna*) from illnesses of the spirit, heart and body; its benefits are numberless. It has a wonderful effect in preserving health, melting the superfluities, restraining one from consuming things which could be harmful; this is especially so when it is moderate and practised at the best times according to the revealed Law and the body's natural need for it. Then indeed it contains such rest for the faculties and the organs as to preserve their powers. And it has a special property which causes its preference, which is its ability to make the heart rejoice, here and hereafter. It is the most beneficial thing for those of cold and moist temperaments, and it has a great influence on the preservation of their health.

It is included in spiritual and natural drugs. When the one fasting observes closely both the natural and legal conditions of fasting its benefit is great for heart and body, averting the foreign corrupting substances to which it is susceptible, and removes the evil substances acquired according to how closely these conditions are observed. It guards the one fasting from that from which he

19 *Ṣawm*, fasting, the obligatory fast of Ramaḍān, also optional fasting as a pious practise. Its aims are given as protection (*junna*) and defence (*wiqāya*) which is protection (*ḥimya*), a word also used for prophylactic diet (cf. Chapter 18 b). This sense of protection is not purely physical, and is consistent with the other aim, concentration of the heart and attention upon God (*ijtimāᶜ al-qalb wa-l-hamm*).

should be guarded, and helps him to achieve the aim, the secret, the final reason of the fast. For the aim of fasting is another matter beyond the abstention from food and drink. In regards to that matter fasting is specially set aside among all good deeds as the one dedicated to God, praised be He. For it is a defence and protection for the servant against what harms his heart and body, here and hereafter. God Most High said: *O you who believe! Fasting is prescribed for you as it was prescribed for those before you, that perchance you may be God-fearing* (II:183).

One of the two aims of fasting is protection and defence, which is of great benefit. The other aim is the consolidation of the soul's powers in the love of God and His obedience.

There has already been mention of some of the secrets of fasting under the guidance of the Prophet ﷺ for it.

Ḍād

1. *Ḍabb* (Lizard)

It is established in the two books of the *Ṣaḥīḥ*, from *ḥadīth* of Ibn ʿAbbās, that when a lizard was presented to the Messenger of God ﷺ he refrained from eating it. He was asked: 'Is it forbidden?' and he replied: 'No, but it is not found in my people's land, and I find that I dislike it.'[318] So it was eaten in his presence, and at his table, while he watched. And in the two books of the *Ṣaḥīḥ*, from *ḥadīth* of Ibn ʿUmar, it is reported that the Prophet ﷺ said: 'I do not declare it lawful, nor do I declare it unlawful.'[319] It is hot and dry, and an aphrodisiac. When pounded and put upon the place of a thorn, it draws it out.

2. *Ḍifdaʿ* (Frog)

The Imām Aḥmad said: The frog is not lawful in medicine, for the Messenger of God ﷺ forbade its killing. He means the *ḥadīth* which he relates in his *Musnad*, from *ḥadīth* of ʿUthmān b. ʿAbd al-Raḥmān: A physician mentioned a frog in a medicine, in the presence of the Messenger of God ﷺ, and he forbade killing it.[320]

Ibn Sīnā said: If a man eats blood of the body of a frog, his body becomes inflamed, his colour fades, and he emits semen until he dies. Therefore physicians have discontinued its use, out of fear of the harm it causes.

The frog is of two kinds: the water frog and the earth frog. Eating the earth frog is fatal.

Ṭā'

1. *Ṭīb* (Perfume)

It is reliably reported of the Messenger of God ﷺ that he said: 'Beloved to me in this world of yours are women and scent, and my delight is in prayer.'[321] The Messenger of God ﷺ made frequent use of scent. Unpleasant odour would trouble him, and he would find it unbearable.

Scent is the nourishment of the spirit, which is the instrument of the faculties. The faculties are doubled and increase with scent, just as they increase with food and drink, quietness and happiness, the company of those loved, the occurrence of pleasant matters, and the absence of the one whose absence brings happiness, whose encounter is heavy upon the spirit, and whose company causes distress and dejection; for indeed the company of the latter weakens the faculties and brings grief and concern. The effect of such company on the spirit is similar to that of fever on the body, and equal to that of unpleasant odour.

Thus among those things which God, praised be He, made the Companions to love is the abandonment of such characteristics while in the company of the Messenger of God ﷺ, because he would be offended thereby. *When you are invited, enter; and when you have taken your meal, disperse, not seeking familiar talk. Such behaviour annoys the Prophet, and he is ashamed of you, but God is not ashamed of the truth* (XXXIII: 53).

In short, scent was one of the things most beloved to the Messenger of God ﷺ. It has an effect on the preservation of health, and it repels many pains and their causes, due to the fact that the constitution is strengthened by it.

2. *Ṭīn* (Clay)

Among fabricated *ḥadīth*, of which nothing is confirmed, are found such as 'whoever eats clay, has helped to kill himself,' and 'O Ḥumayrā', do not eat clay, for it restricts the belly, makes the complexion pale, and removes the brightness of the face.'

Every *ḥadīth* concerning clay is of this unsound sort and has no origin from the Messenger of God ﷺ. Clay is bad and harmful and blocks the passages of the veins. It is cold and dry, strongly dessicative; it prevents looseness of the belly, brings about haemopthysis and ulcers of the mouth.

3. *Ṭalḥ* (?Musa paradisica, M. sapientium. Musaceae. Banana)

God The Most High said: *And (among) ṭalḥ trees (with fruits) ranged one above another* (LVI: 29). Most of the commentators say: It is the *mawz* (banana); and 'ranged' (*manḍūd*) means ranged one opposite another, like a comb. It is said that *ṭalḥ* is a tree with thorns, and ranged in the place of every thorn is fruit. Its fruit has been ranged, some upon others, and it is like the banana.

This explanation is more correct. Maybe those ancestors who mentioned the banana meant it by way of comparison, not as an identification. And God knows best.

It is hot and moist. It is best when ripe and sweet. It is beneficial for roughness of the throat and lung, and for cough, and ulcers of kidneys and bladder. It is diuretic, aphrodisiac and increases semen. It loosens the belly. If eaten before food it hurts the stomach and increases yellow bile and phlegm. Its harmful effect is remedied by sugar or honey.

4. *Ṭalᶜ* (from Phoenix dactylifera L. Palmae. Palm spathe)

God The Most High said: *Tall palm trees* (nakhl) *with branches* (ṭalᶜ) (*of fruit stalks, with dates) one above another* (naḍīd) (L:10). And He said: . . . *and date-palms with spathes near breaking* (haḍīm) (XXVI:148).

The spathe of the palm is that part of its fruit which shows when it first appears. Its covering is called *al-kufurrī*; and *naḍīd* is that which is ranged one part upon another. The word *naḍīd*[20] is used only so long as it remains in its covering; when it opens up, it is no longer called *naḍīd*. As for 'near breaking' (*haḍīm*), that is, packed closely in (*munḍamm*) to each other. It is similar to *naḍīd*, too. That is before the *kufurrī* splits away from it.

The spathe is one of two types: male and female. During the process of pollination (*talqīḥ*) something similar to wheat flour is taken from the male and placed in the female. This is fecundation (*ta'bīr*), which corresponds to the pollen (*liqāḥ*) between the male and female.

Muslim relates in his *Ṣaḥīḥ*, from Ṭalḥa b. ᶜUbaydallāh: I passed with the Messenger of God ﷺ across a date plantation, where he saw a group of people carrying out pollination, and asked what they were doing. They said: 'They are taking pollen from the male and putting it into the female.' He said: 'I do not think that is of any use.' They heard what the Messenger ﷺ said and stopped pollinating; consequently the crop was unsuccessful.

The Prophet ﷺ said: 'This is naught but opinion: if it is of benefit, then do it. For I am only a human like you, and opinion may be mistaken or may be correct. But I did not tell you this on the authority of God, the Glorious, and I shall not tell a lie against God.'[322]

The palm spathe is aphrodisiac and stimulates sexual intercourse. If a woman uses the flour of the spathe as a pessary before intercourse, this will greatly assist her to conceive. It is in the second degree of cold and dryness. It strengthens and lightens the stomach, and alleviates corruption of the blood with thickness and slow digestion.

Only those of hot temperament can tolerate it. If anyone uses it in quantity, then it is necessary to add to it a certain amount of hot electuaries (*jawārishāt*).

20 *Naḍīd*, arranged or piled up, cf. *manḍūd* in the previous entry; both from the root *nḍd*, signifying that which is carefully arranged, as are the fruits of the banana and the palm.

It restricts the constitution and strengthens the intestines. The *jummār* (palm core) acts in the same way, likewise *balaḥ* (fresh dates) and *busr* (unripe dates). Excessive use of the palm core harms stomach and chest, and it may sometimes bring about colic. It is rectified by *samn* or by such things already mentioned.

ʿAyn

1. *ʿInab* (from Vitis vinifera L. Vitaceae. Grapes)[21]

In the *Ghaylānīyyāt*, from *ḥadīth* of Ḥabīb b. Yasār, from Ibn ʿAbbās, it says: I saw God's Messenger ﷺ eating grapes, pulling them off the stalk.

Said Abū Jaʿfar al-ʿAqīlī: There is no foundation to this *ḥadīth*. My comment: Dāwūd b. ʿAbd al-Jabbār Abū Sulaym al-Kūfī said: Yaḥyā b. Maʿīn said he used to lie.

It is related of the Messenger of God ﷺ that he loved grapes and water-melon.

God, praised be He, has mentioned grapes in six places in His Book, recounting the bounties He has bestowed upon His servants, in this abode and in Paradise. They are among the most excellent and most beneficial of fruits, and can be eaten fresh or dry, green or ripe. They are classified as fruits, as food, as condiment, as medicine and as drink. Their constitution is the constitution of the pips: heat and moisture. The good ones are large and juicy. White grapes are recommended rather than black, when they are equally sweet. Those left two or three days after picking are preferable to those eaten the day they are picked, for the latter produce distension and loosen the belly. Those hung up until their skin shrivels are very nourishing and strengthen the body. Their nutritional value is similar to that of figs and raisins. When the grape pips are removed, they are more softening to the belly. Excessive amounts can cause headache. Any harm is warded off by the use of sour pomegranate. The benefits of grapes are that they purge the constitution, and the good ones are fattening and give excellent nourishment. They share with fresh dates and figs the distinction of being called 'the chief of fruits.'

2. *ʿAsal* (Honey)

The benefits of honey have already been listed. Said Ibn Jurayj: al-Zuhrī said: Take honey, for it is good for the memory. The best sort is the pure, the white, the least sharp, and the sweetest. That which is gathered from mountains and trees has a superiority over that gathered from beehives, as the excellence of its quality is in accordance with the bees' source of nectar.

21 Cf. *zabīb*, *karm*.

3. *ʿAjwa* (from Phoenix dactylifera L. Palmae. Pressed dates)

In the two books of the *Ṣaḥīḥ*, from *ḥadīth* of Saʿd b. Abī Waqqāṣ, from the Prophet ﷺ, it is related that he said: 'Whoever starts the morning with seven *ʿajwa* dates will be harmed that day neither by poison nor by magic.'[323]

And in the *Sunan* of al-Nisā'ī, and Ibn Māja, from *ḥadīth* of Jābir and Abū Saʿīd, from the Prophet ﷺ, it says: '*ʿAjwa* come from Paradise, and they heal poison; truffles are a type of manna, and their juice is healing for the eye.'[324]

It has been said that this refers to *ʿajwa* of Madīna. It is one of the types of date found there and is among the most beneficial of all those which grow in the Ḥijāz. It is a noble kind, compact, firm of body, strong, among the softest, best and most delicious of dates.

We have already mentioned dates (*tamr*), their constitution and their benefits, under the letter *tā'*, and have spoken of *ʿajwa* warding off poison and magic, so this need not be repeated here.

4. *ʿAnbar* (Ambergris)[22]

Mention has already been made above of the story in the two books of the *Ṣaḥīḥ*, from *ḥadīth* of Jābir, concerning Abū ʿUbayda, and how people ate of *ʿanbar* for half a month, and that they provided themselves from its flesh with dried meat for the journey to Madīna, and sent some to the Prophet ﷺ.

That is one of the indications that the permissibility of eating what the sea contains is not restricted to fish, but it includes all marine dead (*mayta*) creatures.

The objection raised is that the sea threw it forth alive, then it ebbed away from it and consequently it died. But it is lawful, they say; for its death was caused by the fact that it became separated from the water.

This is not sound. For they merely found it dead upon the shore and had not observed it coming forth from the sea alive, then the water ebbing away from it. Also, had it been alive, the sea would not have cast it onto the shore. It is well known that the sea casts out onto the shore only its dead creatures, not those which are alive.

Moreover, if the import of what they said were taken into account, that could not be a condition for its permissibility, for nothing is permitted while there is doubt about the reason for which it is permitted. Therefore, the Prophet ﷺ forbade eating game when the hunter finds it drowned in water because of the doubt surrounding the cause of its death, whether this was caused by weapons or the water.

As for the *ʿanbar* which is one of the types of perfume, it is among the most splendid kinds, after musk. It is a mistake to prefer it to musk and regard it as the

22 See under *samak* for the narrative of the fish cast up on the shore.

best of all the types of perfume. For it is confirmed that the Prophet ﷺ said concerning musk: 'It is the best of perfumes.' If God wills, we shall mention later the special properties and benefits which are peculiar to musk, that make this the perfume of Paradise. And the hills of musk which will be the seats of the righteous there, are made of musk, not *ʿanbar*.

The person who says that it does not suffer change with the passing of time, therefore it is similar to gold, has been misled; and this does not indicate that it is superior to musk. For by this one special property it does not contend with the many special properties which musk contains.

Its varieties are many, and its colours various, including white, grey, red, yellow, green, blue, black and variegated. The best is the grey, then the blue, then the yellow, and the least good is the black.

People have disputed as to its origin; some say that it is a plant which grows in the depths of the sea, swallowed by some of the sea creatures, and then spewed forth as excrement when they are sated; then the sea casts it onto the shore.

It is said too that it is dew which falls from heaven onto the islands of the sea, and the waves throw it onto the shore; or that it is the excrement of a sea creature, resembling a cow. However, others deny this, saying it is refuse from the sea, that is, foam.

Ibn Sīnā said: It is thought to come forth from a spring in the sea; the saying that it is sea foam, or excrement of an animal, is far from correct.

The temperament of ambergris is hot and dry. It strengthens the heart, brain, senses and organs of the body. It is beneficial for palsy and facial paralysis and illnesses caused by phlegm, for cold pains of the stomach, for thick winds, and for obstruction, when it is drunk or rubbed on externally. When used as fumigant, it is beneficial for catarrh, headache and cold migraine.

5. *ʿŪd* (Aquilaria malaccensis Lam. (A. agalocha). Aloe wood)

Indian *ʿūd* is of two kinds: (1) used medicinally, known as *kust*, or *qusṭ*, which will come under the letter *qāf*; (2) used in perfumes, called *al-aluwwa*.

Muslim relates in his *Ṣaḥīḥ*, from Ibn ʿUmar, that *al-aluwwa* was used without being moistened, for perfuming, *kāfūr* (camphor) being thrown in with it. He says: Thus was the Messenger of God ﷺ wont to perfume himself.[325] It is confirmed in the description of the delights of the people of Paradise that their perfuming vessels are of *al-aluwwa*.

The word for perfuming vessels (*majāmir*) is the plural of *mujmar*, meaning that which is used for the perfuming process with aloe wood or other substances. Aloe wood is of various types: the best is Indian, then Chinese, then Qamārī, then Mandalī. The best is the black and the blue, solid, compact, and greasy. The least good is the lightweight sort which floats on the water. It is said that it is a tree which is cut down and buried in the earth for a year, so the earth eats away the non-useful portions. What is left is *ʿūd al-ṭīb* (scented aloe wood) which the earth does not affect at all, while the bark and the non-scented parts are rotted away.

It is hot and dry in the third degree. It opens obstructions, breaks winds, disperses excess moisture, strengthens the intestines, invigorates and gladdens the heart, and is beneficial for the brain. It strengthens the senses, restricts the belly, and is beneficial for incontinence originating from cold of the bladder.

Ibn Samajūn said: *ʿŪd* is of many types, all contained in the name of *al-aluwwa*. It is used internally and externally, and is used as a fumigant alone or with other substances. Mixing it with *kāfūr* for fumigation has a medicinal significance, one rectifying the other. The purpose of fumigation is the purification of the essence of the air, as one of the six essential elements through which the preservation of the health of the body is achieved.

6. *ʿAdas* (Lens esculenta Moench. Leguminosae. Lentils)

There are *ḥadīth* concerning lentils, all of them falsely attributed to the Messenger of God ﷺ, for he said nothing whatever about them. Like the *ḥadīth*: 'Indeed seventy prophets have declared it blessed', and the *ḥadīth*: 'Indeed it refines the heart, makes tears abundant, and is the food of the righteous.' Now the finest and most correct saying about it is that it is the desired food of the Jews, which they preferred to manna and quails. (cf. II:61).

It is connected with garlic and onions in this reference. Its nature is that of the female. Cold and dry, it contains two opposing powers: it restricts the constitution, and loosens it. Its shell is hot and dry in the third degree; pungent, loosening the belly. Its antidote (*tiryāq*) is contained in its shell. Therefore, it is more beneficial whole than ground, lighter upon the stomach and less harmful. Its kernel is slow to digest for it is cold and dry. It generates black bile and has clearly a harmful effect on melancholy, and hurts the nerves and the sight. It also generates thick blood. It must be avoided by those with black bile, for if they eat them in quantity, then it causes evil illnesses such as delusions (*waswās*), leprosy and quartan fever. Its harmful effects are reduced by beet and spinach, and by adding a large amount of oil (*duhn*). The worst is that which is eaten in a solidified state. One should avoid mixing it with sweet things because it generates liver obstructions. Eating it in excess harms the sight because of its strongly dessicative properties; it brings on dysuria, causes cold inflammations and thick winds. The best kind is the white and plump lentils which cook in a short time.

As for the opinion of the ignorant, that it was the meal which Abraham set before his guests, that is a false lie; God speaks only of his hospitality with roast meat, that is, a calf (XI:69).

Bayhaqī reported from Isḥāq: Ibn al-Mubārak was asked about the *ḥadīth* which dealt with lentils 'that it was declared blessed on the tongues of seventy prophets.' He said: 'Not even by the tongue of one prophet, for it is naught but harmful and distensive: now who narrated such a thing to you?' They said: 'Salm b. Sālim.' 'On whose authority?' 'From you.' He exclaimed: 'And from me, too?!'

Ghayn

1. *Ghayth* (rain)

This is mentioned in several places in the Qur'ān. It is a beautiful name to hear and it is named for the spirit and the body. All rejoice to hear it mentioned, and hearts are glad at its arrival. Its water is the most excellent and most gentle of waters, the most beneficial and most blessed, especially when it comes from a thunder cloud and is collected in the mountain pools.

It is moister than other waters, because it has not spent much time on the ground, whereby it would gain from the earth's dryness, and no element of dryness is mixed with it. Therefore it changes and putrefies very fast because of its gentleness and the speed with which it can be affected.

As to whether the spring rain or winter rain is more gentle, there are two opinions: in support of winter rain, they say that the heat of the sun at that time is less, so it attracts only the gentlest of the sea's water, while the air is pure, and free of smoky vapours and the dust which mixes with the water. All this brings about its subtlety and purity and keeps it free from admixtures. Those who favour the spring rain say: the heat causes the thick vapours to dissolve and brings about mildness and fineness of the air. Therefore, the water is light, and its earthly components are few, and this coincides with the time when plants and trees have new life and the air is sweet.

Al-Shāfiʿī reported, from Anas b. Mālik: We were with the Messenger of God ﷺ when rain came upon us, so he held his garment close to him, and said: 'It has but recently come from its Lord.'[326]

We have already mentioned his guidance concerning prayers for rain (*istisqā'*), what is said about rain, and his seeking blessings from rain when it first comes.

Fā'

1. *Sūrat al-Fātiḥa*

The Opening Chapter of the Qur'ān,[23] also known as Mother of the Qur'ān, the 'Seven much-rehearsed' (*mathānī*), the complete healing, the effective remedy, the complete incantation, the key to wealth and prosperity, the preserver of strength, the repeller of trouble, anxiety, fear and grief; this is for whoever

23 Cf. Chapter 31 b on its use as an incantation. Here, however, IQ is concerned with its spiritual value, for general blessing, rather than as a cure.

knows its value, and gives it its due, and recites it well over his illness, and knows the way to seek healing and recovery thereby, and grasps the inner meaning whereby it is so.

When one of the Companions came to know of that, he used it as incantation for stings and recovered at once. The Prophet ﷺ asked him: 'How did you find out that it was an incantation?'

Whoever is granted success and assisted with the light of 'insight' will come to be acquainted with the secrets of this *Sūra*, and what it contains of the Unity of God, knowledge of the essence and names and attributes and actions, confirmation of the Law and the decree and the return, absoluteness of the Unity of Lordship and divinity, the perfection of confident trust, and entrustment [of affairs] to the One Who holds all command; to Whom belongs all praise in Whose hand is all good; to Whom the command returns; and to Whom the creatures turn in need, seeking His guidance which is the root of happiness in both abodes.

He will be given the knowledge of its essential concepts and how they relate to the attainment of blessings of both worlds, and how it wards off whatever would spoil them; that health, complete and absolute, and perfect bliss are dependent on it, conditional on the realization of such knowledge. Thus it will set him free of other medicines and spells, and by means of it will seek to open the doors to all good, and repel evil and its causes.

This is a matter which requires the creation of a different nature (*fiṭra*) and a different intellectual attitude (*ʿaql*) and a different faith (*īmān*). By God, you will find no corrupt doctrine, nor false innovation (*bidʿa*) that cannot be completely refuted and made null and void by the *Fātiḥa*, in the most direct, the truest and the clearest way. For all access to divine knowledge, the actions of the heart and the medicines for their ailments, the *Fātiḥa* contains the key and the place which indicates it. Nor will one find any way-station (*manzil*) of those travelling to the Lord of the Worlds, that does not begin and end in the *Fātiḥa*.

And, I swear to you, its importance is greater even than that. The servant who is certain, and takes refuge in it, and can understand the One who spoke by it and sent it down as a complete healing, and powerful protection, and clear light, and understands it and its requirements, as is fitting, will fall into no innovation, nor *shirk*; nor is he afflicted by any disease of the heart, except momentary pain.

Certainly the *Fātiḥa* is the greatest key to the treasures of the earth, as well as those of Paradise. However, not everyone can use this key successfully. If those seeking these treasures were to discover the secret of this *Sūra*, and realize its innermost meanings, and put teeth into this key, and knew how to open with it, they would acquire these treasures without impediment or hindrance.

We have not said this by chance nor by way of metaphor, but as the truth. However, God the Most High has an outstanding wisdom in hiding this secret from the souls of most of creation, just as He shows great wisdom in hiding the treasures of the earth from them. For treasures which are concealed have been subject to evil satanic spirits, which come between them and human beings, and which can be overpowered only by noble exalted spirits which vanquish them by their great quality of faith, from which they draw weapons which the devils cannot understand. Most human souls are not of this kind, so they cannot withstand nor overpower those spirits, nor do they take anything of their spoils. For 'whoever slays a man takes his spoils.'

2. *Fāghiya* (from Lawsonia inermis L.)

These are the blossoms of henna which are among the finest of scented herbs. Al-Bayhaqī related in his book *Shuʿab al-Īmān* ('branches of faith') from *ḥadīth* of ʿAbd-Allāh b. Burayda, from his father, (fully traced back): The chief of scented herbs, in this world and the next, is *fāghiya*. There is another narrative concerning it, from Anas b. Mālik, saying: The *fāghiya* was the herb most beloved of the Messenger of God ﷺ. God knows best the status of these two *ḥadīth*, for we do not testify anything about the Messenger of God ﷺ of which we cannot verify the authenticity.

Fāghiya is moderate in heat and dryness, with some costiveness. When placed in the folds of woollen clothing it preserves them from moth. It is an ingredient in ointments for paralysis and distension (*tamaddud*). Its oil (*duhn*) is a dissoluent to the limbs, and softens the nerves.

3. *Fiḍḍa* (Silver)

It is confirmed that the signet ring of the Messenger of God ﷺ was of silver, as was its centre stone. The pommel of his sword was of silver.[327] There is no attested statement whatsoever from him concerning the prohibition of clothing nor adornment of silver, in the same way that it is attested that he forbade drinking from vessels of silver. The category of drinking vessels is more restricted than that of clothing and adornment. Therefore, it is permitted for women as clothing and as adornment, whereas its use is forbidden to them in the form of drinking vessels. For the unlawfulness of drinking vessels does not entail the unlawfulness of clothing and adornment.

In the *Sunan*, on the authority of the Prophet ﷺ, is found: 'As for silver, use it as a plaything.' For prohibition needs some proof to confirm it, whether a text or by way of general consensus. If one of these is established, well and good; otherwise, there is in the heart some doubt concerning its prohibition, for the Prophet ﷺ grasped in one hand gold, in the other silk, and said: 'These two are forbidden to the men of my community, but permitted for their women.'[328]

Silver is one of God's secrets in the earth, and the talisman of needs, and used as a measure of value between the people of this world. One who owns it is well regarded among people, held in great esteem and respected in assemblies; no doors are shut against him, none finds his company dull nor his presence tiresome; fingers point to him, eyes are turned upon him; if he speaks, his words are heeded; any intercession of his is accepted, any witness he gives is attested; if he speaks, that is appropriate, and he is not blamed; if he has white hair, that is more comely upon him than the adornment of youth.

It is among those medicines which bring joy and are beneficial for anxiety, worry and grief, for weakness of the heart or palpitation. It is a component of the great electuaries (*maʿjūnāt*), and through its special property, it draws out such corrupting humours as may be generated in the heart, especially when it is added to purified honey and saffron.

Its temperament is towards cold and dryness, and a certain amount of heat and moisture is generated from it.

Now the Gardens which God, Exalted and Glorious, has prepared for His friends on the day when they meet Him, are four: two Gardens of gold and two Gardens of silver, with their drinking vessels, their adornment and all they contain.

It has been established on the authority of the Prophet ﷺ, in the *Ṣaḥīḥ*, that he said: 'If anyone drinks from vessels of gold or silver, the fire of hell will gurgle in his belly.'[329] It is reliably reported that he said: 'Do not drink from vessels of gold and silver, nor eat from plates thereof. Others will have these in this world and you in the next.'[330]

It has been said that the reason for their prohibition was the restriction of metal coin, for when these were taken for vessels the reason for their making was lost: upholding the interests of mankind. It has been said, also, that the reason was to avoid pride and haughtiness, and because the hearts of the poor and indigent would break when they saw them.

So much for these reasons. An explanation of restriction of coin also prevents its use as adornment, and making it into ingots and the like, which are neither vessels nor coin. Now pride and haughtiness are forbidden in all circumstances. Breaking the hearts of the needy is not necessarily a reason; for they can be crushed also seeing spacious houses, wonderful gardens, swift steeds, ostentatious garments, delicious foods, and other permitted objects. All these are disputed reasons for the prohibition of silver, as in the preceding example the effect (ie. their hearts being broken) is present, while the presumed cause (the silver) is absent.

The true reason—and God knows best—is that the use of silver brings to the heart a certain disposition and condition, very clearly contrary to the attitude appropriate for a servant's worship of his Lord. For this reason, the Prophet ﷺ explained that it is for the unbelievers in this world, since they had no share of servanthood whereby to obtain it in the afterlife. So its use is not fitting for God's servants in this world, but it is only used by one who has departed from his status as servant and is content with this world and gives it precedence over the afterlife. And God knows best.

Qāf

1. *Qur'ān*

The Most High said: *We send down of the Qur'ān that which is a healing and mercy to those who believe* (XVII:82). The word 'of' is specificative, not partitive. The Most High said: *O mankind! there hath come to you a direction* (mawʿiẓa) *from your Lord and a healing for what is in your hearts* (X:57).

The *Qur'ān* is the complete healing for all illnesses of heart and body and ills of this world and the next.[24] Not everyone is given the qualification nor the success to seek healing thereby. When the sick person is able to treat himself with it, and uses it for his illness with trust and faith and complete acceptance and certain belief, fulfilling the right conditions, the illness can never resist it.

For how could any illness resist the Word of the Lord of Earth and Heaven, whose Word if sent down upon the mountains would shatter them, or upon the earth would flatten it? For whatever illness of heart or body, the *Qur'ān* contains the way pointing to its remedy, its cause, and protection from it, for whomsoever God grants understanding of His Book.

At the start of the discussion on medicine we have already explained that the *Qur'ān* contains guidance to the sources of medicine and all its contents, these being: preservation of health, protection, expelling what is harmful, and the use of such knowledge to identify the detailed elements of these. As for medicines of the heart, it recounts these in detail, and gives the causes of the ills of hearts and their treatment. He said: *And is it not sufficient for them that We have sent down to thee the Book which is recited to them?* (XXIX:51). Anyone not healed by the *Qur'ān* may God not heal him; the one for whom it is not sufficient may God not suffice him.

2. *Qiththā'* (Cucumis sativa L. Cucurbitaceae. Cucumber)

In the *Sunan*, from *ḥadīth* of ʿAbd-Allāh b. Jaʿfar, it is related that the Messenger of God used to eat *qiththā'* with *ruṭab* (fresh dates).[331] This is related by al-Tirmidhī and others.

The *qiththā'* is cold and dry in the second degree, and extinguishes the heat of the inflamed stomach, slow to change in it, beneficial for pains of the bladder. Its scent is beneficial for swooning. The seeds are diuretic. Its leaves made into a poultice are beneficial for dog bite.

It is slow in its descent from the stomach, and its coldness is harmful to part of the stomach. So it should be taken together with something which will rectify

24 Reciting of the *Qur'ān* and its spiritual value, cf. Chapter 31.

it, and break its coldness and moisture, as the Prophet did when he ate it with *ruṭab*. If it is eaten with dates or raisins or honey, these rectify it.

3. *Qusṭ*, or *kust* (?Costus speciosus (J. König) Sm. Zingiberaceae. Costus, crepe ginger)

In the two books of the *Ṣaḥīḥ*, from *ḥadīth* of Anas on the authority of the Prophet ﷺ, is related: The best things you can use as medication are cupping and the sea *qusṭ*.[332]

And in the *Musnad*, from *ḥadīth* of Umm Qays, from the Prophet ﷺ: You should use this Indian *ʿūd*, for it contains healing for seven complaints, one of which is pleurisy.'[333]

Qusṭ[25] is of two types: the white, which is called sea *qusṭ*, and the Indian, which is the hotter of the two, the white being the softer. They are exceedingly beneficial. Both types are hot and dry in the third degree. They dry the phlegm, and reduce catarrh; when drunk, they are beneficial for weakness of the liver and stomach, for cold in them, and for periodic fever (*ḥummā al-dawr*) and quartan fever; they relieve pain of pleurisy, and are beneficial against poisons. Used as a plaster on the face kneaded with water and honey, they remove freckles.

Galen said: *Qusṭ* is beneficial for tetanus and pain of pleurisy, and kills round worm.

Its beneficial effect in pleurisy is hidden from ignorant physicians, so they deny it. If such an ignorant one were to obtain this quotation from Galen he would assign to it the status of a text; for any of the ancient physicians have written that the *qusṭ* is suitable for the phlegmatic type of pleurisy. Al-Khaṭṭābī spoke of this, on the authority of Muḥammad b. al-Jahm.

It has already been noted that the difference in rank between the medicine of physicians, in relation to the medicine of prophets, is far greater than that of the medicine of itinerants and old women compared to physicians' medicine: also, there is a greater difference between what is sent down by revelation and what is discovered by experiment and analogy, than there is between the stupid and the intelligent.

Were these ignorant ones to find a medicine in a text from a physician of the Jews, Christians or heathens, they would eagerly and willingly accept it, and would not refrain from experimenting with it.

Indeed, we do not deny that custom has an influence on whether or not benefit can be gained from a medicine. Any medicine or food is more beneficial and suitable for one accustomed to it than it is for one not so accustomed, and this latter sometimes will not benefit from it at all.

25 Cf. *ʿūd*. According to W. Miki, *Index of the Arab Herbalist's Materials, India* the white or sea-*qusṭ* is Hyacinthus sp. (Liliaceae), No. 512, and the Indian is Saussurea lappa Benth., Compositae, No. 884.

The words of the excellent physicians, while generally applicable are restricted in accordance with constitutions and seasons, places and customs. If such restriction prevents us from belittling their speech and their learning, then how can one belittle the words of the truthful, the trusted? But the souls of mankind are compounded with ignorance and darkness except the one whom God strengthens with the spirit of faith, and whose insight is illuminated by the Light of guidance.

4. *Qaṣab al-sukkar* (Saccharum officinarum L. Graminae. Sugar cane)

Among the words of the true *Sunna*, it is said of the Pool (*ḥawḍ*: ie. the pool of Paradise) that 'its water is sweeter than sugar'. I know of no other place in the *ḥadīth* where sugar is mentioned.

Sugar is modern: the earlier physicians do not speak of it, nor indeed did they know it or describe it among drinks; for they knew only honey, which they used medicinally.

Sugar cane is hot and moist; it is beneficial for cough, clears moisture, cleanses the bladder and the trachea. It is more emollient than plain sugar. It is helpful in emesis; it is diuretic and aphrodisiac.

Said ʿAffān b. Muslim al-Ṣaffār: Whoever sucks sugar cane after his food will feel in a pleasant mood all day.

When it is roasted it is beneficial for congestion of the chest and throat. It generates winds, but this can be avoided by peeling the cane and washing it in hot water.

Cane sugar is hot and moist, as is generally agreed, but it is also said to be cold. The best sort is the white, transparent, hard candy (*ṭabarzadh*). Old cane sugar is subtler than new. When it is cooked and the scum removed, it quenches thirst and soothes a cough. It harms the stomach in which yellow bile is generated by itself changing into bile. This harmful effect is repelled by juice of lemon or orange, or plumb pomegranate. Some people prefer cane sugar to honey because it is soft and less hot. But this is prejudice against honey; for honey has many times the benefits of sugar. God made honey as a healing remedy, as a condiment and a sweetmeat. What then are the benefits of sugar, in comparison with those of honey? Honey strengthens the stomach; softens the constitution; sharpens the sight by clearing away its obscurity; wards off choking when used as a gargle; and it cures paralysis and facial paralysis, and all cold diseases in all parts of the body which are caused by moistures, for it draws them forth from the depths of the body and from any part. The benefits of honey include preserving the body's health and warming it; its aphrodisiac quality; its dissoluent and clearing action; its ability to open the mouths of the veins, cleanse the intestines and expel worms and to prevent indigestion and other kinds of decomposition; its use as a beneficial condiment, and its suitability for those overcome by phlegm, for old people, and for those of cold temperaments.

In brief, there is naught more beneficial than honey for the body and in treatment; for kneading with medicines and preserving their powers, and for strengthening the stomach. There are countless more advantages. Where do we find any benefits contained in sugar to rival these, or even coming close to them?

Kāf

1. *Kitāb* (Written amulet)

(a) *For fever*

Said al-Marwazī: Abū ᶜAbd-Allāh heard that I was fevered, so he wrote for me, as protection from fever, on a scrap of paper: 'In the Name of God, the Merciful, the Compassionate. In the Name of God, and by God, and Muḥammad is the Messenger of God. *We said: O fire! be thou cool, and safe for Abraham! And they sought a strategem against him; but We made them the ones to lose most!* (XXI: 69–70). O God! Lord of Jibrā'īl and Mīkā'īl and Isrāfīl, heal the possessor of this writing by Your power and strength and might. O God of creation. Amen.'

Said al-Marwazī: This was recited over Abū ᶜAbd-Allāh, while I listened. Abū al-Mundhir ᶜAmr b. Majmaᶜ said to us, from Yūnus b. Ḥibān: I asked Abū Jaᶜfar Muḥammad b. ᶜAlī if I might wear the talisman (*taᶜwīdh*), and he said: 'If it is from God's Book or words from God's Prophet, then wear it, and ask healing with it as much as you can.' I asked: 'Did he write this (or: may I write this) for quartan fever?' He replied: 'Yes.'

Imām Aḥmad said, on authority of ᶜĀ'isha and others, that they were lenient concerning this practice. Said Ḥarb: Aḥmad b. Ḥanbal was not strict about it. Said Aḥmad: Ibn Masᶜūd disliked it very greatly. When asked about amulets (*tamā'im*) which were worn after the onset of affliction, Aḥmad said: 'I trust that there should be no harm therein.' Said al-Khallāl: ᶜAbd-Allāh b. Aḥmad narrated to us saying: I saw my father write a talisman for one who suffers fear, and for fever after the onset of the affliction.

(b) *For childbirth*

Talisman for difficult childbirth: Said al-Khallāl: ᶜAbd-Allāh b. Aḥmad narrated to me: I saw my father write a talisman for a woman, when she had difficulty in childbirth, on a white jar or something clean; he wrote the *ḥadīth* of Ibn ᶜAbbās. 'There is no god but God, the Clement the Gracious; praise be to God the Lord of the mighty Throne. *Praise be to God the Lord of the Worlds* (I: 1). *The Day they see it, it will be as if they tarried but a single day, or the morn thereof!*

(LXXIX:46). *The day they see (the punishment) promised them it will be as if they had not tarried more than an hour in a single day. (Thine but to proclaim the) Message; but shall any be destroyed except those who transgress?* (XLVI:35).

Said al-Khallāl: Abū Bakr al-Marwazī informed us that a man came to Abū ʿAbd-Allāh, and asked: O Abū ʿAbd-Allāh, would you write a talisman for a woman who had a difficult childbirth two days ago? He told him to bring a wide jar and some saffron. And I saw him write more than one. It is mentioned on the authority of ʿIkrima, from Ibn ʿAbbās, that ʿĪsā, peace be on our Prophet and on him, passed by a cow, whose young had become obstructed in her abdomen. The cow cried: 'O Word of God! Call upon God for me, that He may release me from my trouble.' He said: 'O Creator of life from life! O You Who save life from life, O You Who bring forth life from life, release her.' And she cast forth her young, and there she stood, sniffing at it. So when a woman is in difficult labour, write this for her.

The writing of all the above mentioned amulets may be useful. A number of earlier scholars have permitted that part of the Qur'ān be written down in ink, immersed in water, and the liquid drunk; they have considered that to be part of the healing property which God placed within it.

Another talisman for the same:

To be written inside a clean vessel: *When the sky is rent asunder, and harkens to the command of its Lord, and it must needs do so; and when the earth is flattened out, and casts forth what is within it and becomes empty* (LXXXIV:1–4). Then the pregnant woman drinks from it, and it is sprinkled on her abdomen.

(c) *For other ailments*

Talisman for nosebleed:

Shaykh al-Islām Ibn Taymiyya, may God sanctify his spirit, used to write upon the forehead: *It was said: O earth! Swallow up thy water; and O sky! Withhold thy rain, and the water abated, and the matter was ended...* (XI:44). And I heard him say: 'I have written it for several, who have been cured.' And he said: 'It is not permitted to be written in the blood of the patient, as the ignorant do. For blood is impure and thus it may not be used for writing the words of God the Most High.'

Another talisman for the same:

Moses, peace be on him, went out with a cloak and found a spring and stopped it with his cloak. *God wipes out or confirms what He pleases; with Him is the Mother of the Book* (XIII:39).

A talisman for scurf:

One writes on it: *And it was struck by a whirlwind, with fire in it, and was burnt up* (II:266). By the power and strength of God.

Another talisman for the same:

At a time the sun is pale, one writes *O ye that believe! Fear God, and believe in His Messenger, and He will bestow on you a double portion of His mercy; He will provide you with a Light whereby ye will walk, and He will forgive you. For God is most forgiving and most merciful!'* (LVII: 28).

Another talisman for tertian fever:

One writes on three thin sheets: 'In the Name of God it has fled, in the Name of God it has passed, in the Name of God it has diminished.' Each day one takes one sheet, puts it in the patient's mouth, and he swallows it with water.

A talisman for sciatica:

In the Name of God the Merciful the Compassionate: O God, Lord of all, Ruler of all, Creator of all! Thou didst create me, and Thou didst create sciatica in me. So let not its harm overwhelm me, nor give me power over it through incision. And heal me with a healing that leaves no sickness! There is no healer but Thee.

Talisman for a throbbing vein:

Al-Tirmidhī relates in his *Jāmiʿ* from *ḥadīth* of Ibn ʿAbbās that the Messenger of God ﷺ used to teach them that for fever and for all pains they should say: In the Name of God the Great, I take refuge with God the Mighty, from the evil of a vein agitated, and from the evil of the heat of fire.

Talisman for toothache:

One writes on the cheek which is near the pain: *In the name of God the Merciful the Compassionate! Say: It is He Who has created you, and made for you the faculties of hearing and seeing, feeling and understanding; but little thanks do you give* (LXVII: 23). And one could also write: *To Him belong all that dwell in the night and the day; for He is the One who hears and knows* (VI: 13).

Talisman for an abscess:

One writes upon it *They ask thee concerning the mountains. Say: My Lord will uproot them and scatter them as dust. He will leave them as plains smooth and level: nothing crooked or curved wilt thou see in them* (XX: 105–7).

2. *Kam'a* (?Tuber brumele. Tuberales. Truffles)

It is reliably reported that the Prophet ﷺ said: Truffles are a type of manna, and their juice is healing for the eye. [334] This is found in the two books of the *Ṣaḥīḥ*.

Said Ibn al-ʿArābī: *Kam'a* is plural, the singular being *kam'*. But this is contrary to the analogy in Arabic, for the difference is marked by there being a *tā marbūṭa* in the singular. So its absence indicates the plural. As to whether this is plural, or a plural noun, there are two well-known opinions. They say: There are only two exceptions: *kam'a/kam'*, and *khab'a/khab'*. Someone else said: But this is by analogy. *Kam'a* is for the singular and *kam'* for a quantity. Others again have said: *kam'a* is both for singular and plural.'

But those holding the former opinion argue that there is a plural form of *kam'*, namely *akmū'*.

Said the poet:

> I have picked for you truffles (*akmū'*) and onions,
> for I have forbidden you the smaller truffles.

This indicates that *kam'* is singular, and *kam'a* plural.

Kam'a grow wild in the earth without being cultivated. They are called *kam'a* because they are concealed; thence comes *kama'a al-shahāda* to 'conceal the testimony', when one veils or hides it. Truffles are hidden under the ground, having neither leaves nor stalk.

Their substance is of an earthy, vaporous essence, retained beneath the earth and about level with it. They are kept in it by the cold of winter, and the spring rains cause them to grow. Thus they come into being and are pushed upwards towards the surface of the earth as they take shape and grow. They are called smallpox of the earth because they resemble the shape and substance of smallpox (*judarī*). Their substance is a sanguineous moisture which is pushed back during the time of their flourishing and at the beginning of the predominance of heat and the growth of strength.

They are among the produce of the springtime and are eaten both raw and cooked. The bedouin call them 'thunder plants' because they are plentiful at the time of much thunder, and the earth breaks away from them. They are a food of the desert people and are plentiful in the land of the bedouin. The best are those which grow in sandy soil with little water. Their varieties include a deadly variety whose colour is reddish and which causes asphyxiation.

They are cold and moist in the third degree, bad for the stomach and slow to digest. If eaten frequently they cause colic, apoplexy and paralysis, stomach pains and dysuria. The moist is less harmful than the dry; if anyone wishes to eat them he should bury them in damp clay, boil them in water with salt and thyme and eat them with oil and hot spices. Their essence is earthy and thick; their nourishment is bad; but they contain a watery subtle essence which indicates that they are light. Their use as *koḥl* is beneficial in cases of darkness of the sight and for hot ophthalmia. The excellent physicians have recognised that their juice cleanses the eye; among those who mentioned this are al-Masīḥī, the author of the *Qānūn* [Ibn Sīnā], and others.

Concerning the words of the Prophet ﷺ: '*Kam'a* are a type of *mann*', there are two opinions:

1. The manna which was sent down to the Children of Israel did not mean this sweet substance only, but many things which God granted (*mann*) to them in the manner of plants found freely, without any work, tending nor ploughing. So the root *mann* is used in the sense of a passive particle, that is, what is

granted *(mamnūn bihi)*. For everything which God grants His servant freely, without any attention nor work on his part, is among the gifts (*mann*) of God Most High to him; for it does not resemble the servant's remuneration, and he is not troubled by the fatigue of work. This is pure gift even though all God's blessings are also a gift from Him to His servant. Yet the name of 'gift' (*mann*) is applied in particular to what entails no earning nor work on his part. For it is a gift with no effort on the part of the servant. For God, praised be He, gave the Children of Israel freely truffles for their food, so that they should take the place of bread. As their seasoning He gave them quails, taking the place of meat; and for their sweetmeats He gave them 'dew' (*ṭall*) which falls upon the trees, and so it took the place of sweetmeats for them. Thus did He give them a complete sustenance. So reflect on the words of the Prophet: 'Truffles are a kind of *mann* which God sent down upon the Children of Israel.' He considered truffles as part of the whole of His gift (*mann*), and as one of the individual elements. *Turanjubīn* which falls upon the trees is a type of *mann*; but recently it has become the custom to refer to it as *mann*.

2. He likened *kam'a* to *mann* which is sent down from heaven because it is gathered with neither fatigue nor trouble, nor sowing of seeds nor irrigation. One may ask: If this is the case of *kam'a*, then how do you explain the harm they contain? And whence did they acquire that? Know, then, that God, praised be He, perfected the creation of every thing, and made faultless all that He configured at the beginning of His creative activity, free of defects and ailments, complete in the beneficial property for which it was prepared and created. Defects come into it, after that, only by some contingency: contiguity, mixture, intermingling, or other causes which bring about its pollution. Were it left in its orginal nature, without the causes of corruption becoming attached to it, it would not be corrupt.

Whoever has knowledge of the conditions of the world and its original state knows that all pollution in its atmosphere, its flora and fauna, and the conditions of its people, have come about subsequent to its creation, due to recent factors that provoked such a change. Still man's continuous interference and his opposition to the prophets cause such widespread pollution that penetrates both public and private life and brings about suffering, illnesses, diseases, plagues, famines and droughts, spoiling the natural produce of the earth, its fruits and plants, thus destroying the goodness of the earth and reducing its benefits—these are interlinked phenomena that perpetually follow one upon another.

If your knowledge does not encompass such affairs, then be satisfied with the words of the Most High: *Pollution* (fasād) *has appeared on land and sea because of what the hands of men have earned (through their actions)* (XXX:41). Apply this verse to the state of things, and compare that with what the verse implies. So you see how at all times disasters and failures happen to fruit and crops and animals, and how from these disasters arise other consequent disasters, one following upon another. Whenever people cause oppression and evil, their Lord, blessed and exalted, brings upon them disasters and failures in their food crops and their fruit, their air and water, their bodies and their constitutions, their appearences and shapes; leaving for them such loss and disaster as a just consequence of their actions, their wrong-doing and evil.

The grains of corn and other cereals used to be larger than they are today, just as the blessing they contained was greater. Imām Aḥmad related, with his chain of transmission, that a bundle was found in the treasuries of one of the Umayyads, containing wheat the size of date stones, where there was written: this used to grow during the days of justice. He mentioned this story in his *musnad* following a *ḥadīth* he related.

Most of these general diseases and illnesses are what remains of a punishment meted out to former nations; some has remained, kept ready for anyone who still carries out any of their deeds. This is justice and right judgement. The Prophet ﷺ indicated that, in his words concerning plague: 'It is a remainder of a divine retribution sent down on the Children of Israel.'

Likewise God, praised be He, sent a wind of destruction over the people of ʿĀd, for seven nights and eight days; then, He left a portion of it, which He occasionally sends as a warning and admonition.

God, praised be He, has so ordained that the actions of the righteous and of the sinner have their own inexorable and inevitable results in this world. He ordained that the prevention of acts of charity and almsgiving should be a reason for withholding rain, and a cause of drought and of dearth. He ordained that oppression of the poor, stinting in measures and weights, and injury of the weak by the strong should be a cause for tyranny on the part of kings and rulers, who do not grant mercy when they are asked for mercy and are not generous when this is asked of them. Yet these—in reality—are the deeds of the subjects, which appear in the form of their rulers. For God praised be He, in His wisdom and justice, shows the people their deeds in forms which are appropriate to them: sometimes by drought and dearth, sometimes through an enemy, sometimes through rulers who oppress their subjects, sometimes through widespread diseases, and sometimes through worries, pains, and troubles which they constantly suffer and find no way to escape; sometimes by holding back the blessings of heaven and earth from them, sometimes allowing satans to have power over them, and to incite them with fury to commit that which will bring them punishment so that the decree duly befits them, and each one may move towards the purpose for which he was created.

The intelligent person lets his gaze travel over all parts of the world, and so he contemplates it, and recognizes the manifestations of God's justice and wisdom. Then, it becomes clear to him that the Messengers and their followers in particular are on the path of deliverance, while the rest of the people are travelling on the path of destruction, moving towards the abode of perdition.

God is able to accomplish what He decrees; there is none to reverse His decree, none to reject His orders. And through God comes success.

The Prophet's words concerning truffles: 'Their juice is healing for the eye', is a matter in which there are three opinions: (1) Their juice is a component of medicines which are used for eye treatment, i.e. it is not used alone. Thus said Abū ʿUbayd; (2) it is used unmixed after being roasted and its juice filtered. For fire refines and cooks it, melts away its harmful superfluities and moistures, leaving the useful part; (3) 'juice' (*mā'*) refers to the rain water which comes into contact with it. So the construct state (*iḍāfa*) is one of contiguity, not partitive. This is Ibn al-Jawzī's opinion; it is the more remote and the weakest.

It has been said that when their juice is used for cooling, then it is a simple. If, on the other hand, it is used for other purposes, it becomes a compound.

Al-Ghāfiqī said: Truffle-juice is the most suitable medicament for the eye, when it is kneaded with antimony and used as a *koḥl*. It strengthens the eyelids and increases the strength and force of the perceptive spirit and wards off from it the descent of catarrhs (*nawāzil*).

3. *Kabāth* (fruit of Salvadora persica L. Salvadoraceae)

In the two books of the *Ṣaḥīḥ*, from *ḥadīth* of Jābir b. ʿAbd-Allāh, it says: We were with the Messenger of God ﷺ, picking *kabāth* and he said: 'Make for the black ones, for they are the best.'[335]

Kabāth is the fruit of the *arāk* tree. It is found in the land of Ḥijāz; its constitution is hot and dry. Its benefits are the same as for the *arāk*: it strengthens the stomach, improves the digestion, clears the phlegm, and is beneficial for pains of the back, and for many illnesses.

Ibn Juljul said: A drink of its cooked juice is diuretic and cleanses the bladder. And Ibn Riḍwān said: It strengthens the stomach and is costive.

4. *Katam* (Indigofera tinctoria L. Legominosae. Indigo)

Al-Bukhārī related in his *Ṣaḥīḥ*, from ʿUthmān b. ʿAbd-Allāh b. Mawhab: We went in to Umm Salma, and she brought out for us some of the hair of the Messenger of God ﷺ, and lo, it was dyed with henna and indigo.[336] And in the four *Sunan*, from the Prophet ﷺ, it is related that he said: 'The best you can use for changing the colour of white hair are henna and *katam*.'[337]

In the two books of the *Ṣaḥīḥ*, from Anas, it is quoted that Abū Bakr used hair dye of both henna and *katam*.[338] In the *Sunan* of Abū Dāwūd, from Ibn ʿAbbās, it says: A man dyed with henna passed by the Prophet ﷺ, and he said: 'How pleasing is this one!' Then another passed by, dyed with henna and *katam*, and he said: 'This one is more pleasing than the other.' Then another passed, one dyed with yellow, and he said: 'This is the most pleasing of them all.'[339]

Said al-Ghāfiqī: *Katam* is a plant which grows on the plains; its leaves are like olive leaves, and it grows to a good height. It has a fruit about the size of a peppercorn, with a kernel inside it. When it is cracked it turns black. If the juice of its leaves is extracted, and one *awqiya* of it drunk, it brings on severe vomiting. It is beneficial for dog bite. When its root is cooked in water, it produces ink which can be used for writing.

Said al-Kindī: The seeds of *katam*, when used as a *koḥl*, dissolve the fluid descending in the eye and heal it.

Some people have thought that *katam* is the *wasma*, which is the leaf of *nīl* (indigo). But this is wrong. For *wasma* is not *katam*. Said the author of *al-Ṣaḥḥāḥ*: *katam* is a plant mixed with *wasma*, and is used for dyeing. It has been said that *wasma* is a plant with long leaves, of a colour tending to blue, larger than the leaves of poplar, resembling leaves of the bean but larger; it is brought from the Ḥijāz and Yemen.

It may be said that it is established in the *Ṣaḥīḥ*, from Anas, that the Prophet ﷺ did not use any dyestuff.

The reply to this has been given by the Imām Aḥmad b. Ḥanbal, saying: Others than Anas have testified that the Prophet ﷺ did dye his hair. Now the one who testifies is not in the position of one who has not testified. Aḥmad, and a group of *ḥadīth* experts, have confirmed that the Prophet ﷺ did use dyestuff, while Mālik denied this.

It may be said that in Muslim's *Ṣaḥīḥ*, the prohibition of using black dyestuff has been confirmed, concerning Abū Quḥāfa, when it was brought to him; his head and beard were white as the hoar-frost. So he said: Change this white hair, but avoid turning it black. *Katam* makes hair black.

The answer is twofold: (1) The prohibition refers to black dye on its own; but when something else, like *katam*, is added to henna, there is no harm. For *katam* and henna give the hair a colour between red and black, contrary to the *wasma*, for that makes it coal-black. This is the more correct answer; (2) the kind of dyeing with black which is forbidden is the dyeing meant as deception, like dyeing the hair of an older slave woman or free woman, deceiving the husband or master thereby; and an old man's dyeing his hair to deceive the woman thereby. This is in the category of cheating and deception. As for the kind where no fraud nor deceit is involved, it is reliably reported of Ḥasan and Ḥusayn that they used black dyestuff. Ibn Jarīr reports this, in the book of *Tahdhīb al-Āthār.*

He reported this of ʿUthmān b. ʿAffān, of ʿAbd-Allāh b. Jaʿfar, Saʿd b. Abī Waqqāṣ, ʿUqba b. ʿĀmir, al-Mughīra b. Shuʿba, Jarīr b. ʿAbd-Allāh, ʿAmr b. al-ʿĀs. He spoke of this concerning the authority of a number of the followers, including ʿAmr b. ʿUthmān, ʿAlī b. ʿAbd-Allāh b. ʿAbbās, Abū Salama b. ʿAbd al-Raḥmān, ʿAbd al-Raḥmān b. al-Aswad, Mūsā b. Ṭalḥa, al-Zuhrī, Ayyūb, Ismāʿīl b. Maʿdikarib. Ibn al-Jawzī related this of Muḥārib b. Dithār, Yazīd, Ibn

Jurayj, Abū Yūsuf and Abū Isḥāq, Ibn Abī Laylā, Ziyād b. ʿAlāqa, Ghaylān b. Jāmiʿ, Nāfiʿ b. Jubayr, ʿAmr b. ʿAli b. al-Muqaddamī, and al-Qāsim b. Sallām.

5. *Karm* (Vitis vinifera L. Vitaceae. Vine)

Vine of the grape; also known as *ḥabala* (vinestock). It is not approved to call it *karm* because of Muslim's narrative in his *Ṣaḥīḥ*, from the Prophet ﷺ, saying: 'Let none of you call grapes *karm*; *karm* signifies the Muslim man.'[340] And in another narration it says: The word *karm* is only used for the heart of the believer.[341] And again: Do not say *karm*, but say *ʿinab* (grapes) and *ḥabala*.[342]

In this there are two meanings: (1) The bedouin used to name the grape-vine *karm* because of its great benefits and goodness (*karam*). The Prophet ﷺ did not like it to be called by a name which could incite men's minds to desire it and also its produce, which is an intoxicant and the originator of evil deeds. So he did not wish to call its source by a name which is so fine and so inclusive of good; (2) it is in the same category as his saying: 'The strong is not one to overthrow others, nor is the wretched a wanderer asking charity.' This means that although one names the grape-vine *karm* because of its many benefits, this name more appropriately describes the heart of the believer, or the Muslim. For in all his affairs the believer is a source of goodness and beneficence. Such a description is used as an indication to reveal all that is contained in the heart of the believer of goodness and generosity, faith and light, guidance and piety, and all other similar qualities which make him more worthy of this name than the *ḥabala*.

Further the power of the *ḥabala* is cold and dry, and its leaves, tendrils (*ʿalāʾiq*) and vines (*ʿurūsh*) are cooling at the limit of the first degree. When pounded and used as a poultice it quietens headache and can be used for hot inflammations and burning of the stomach.

Drinking juice of vine branches settles emesis and constrains the abdomen. The effect is the same if the moist insides of the branches are chewed. The juice of its leaves is beneficial for ulcers of the intestines, haemopthysis and haematemesis, and pain of the stomach. The 'tears' of the veins are like gum, borne in the branches; when drunk they expel stone; used as ointment, they clear tetters and ulcerated scab and other ailments. Before using this medicament, one must wash the limb with water and natron. Mixed with oil and used as a massage it removes hair.

The ashes of its branches, used as a poultice with vinegar, oil of roses and rue, are beneficial for inflammation occurring in the spleen. Oil of the flowers of vine has a costive power, similar to that of rose oil. Its beneficial properties are many, being close to those of the palm.

6. *Karafs* (Apium graveolens L. Umbelliferae. Wild celery.)

It is related in a *ḥadīth*, not genuine, that the Messenger of God ﷺ said: 'Whoever eats *karafs* and then sleeps upon it, sleeps with a good breath and is safe from pain of molars and toothache.' This is falsely attributed to the Messenger of God ﷺ. But the garden variety sweetens the breath greatly, and if the stem is worn around the neck, it is beneficial for toothache.

It is hot and dry, though some say it is moist. It opens obstructions of the liver and spleen. Its leaves, when moist, are beneficial for cold stomach and liver, are diuretic and emmenagogue, and break stone. Its seeds have a stronger effect in this and are aphrodisiac and beneficial for bad breath. Al-Rāzī said: One should avoid eating it when there is a danger of the scorpion's sting.

7. *Kurrāth* (Allium porrum L., A. rosaceae. Liliaceae. Leeks)

There is an inauthentic *ḥadīth* concerning leeks, falsely attributed to God's Messenger ﷺ: 'Whoever eats it, then sleeps upon it, sleeps secure from the wind of haemorrhoids; but the angel avoids him because of his putrid breath until the morning.'

Leeks are of two species: Nabatean and Syrian. The Nabatean is the one eaten at table, and the Syrian the one with heads. It is hot and dry and can cause headache. When it is cooked and eaten, or its juice drunk, it is beneficial for cold haemorrhoids. If its seeds are pounded, kneaded with pitch (*qaṭrān*), and used as a fumigation for molar teeth containing decay (lit. worms), it disperses and expels them and quietens the pain. When the anus is fumigated with seeds of leeks, haemorrhoids are dried up. All of this refers to the Nabatean leek.

However, it can cause decay to teeth and gums, cause headache, and bring on bad dreams; it darkens the sight and makes the breath putrid. It has a certain quality as diuretic and emmenagogue, and as an aphrodisiac. It is slow to digest.

Lām

1. *Laḥm* (Meat)

The Most High said: *We give them fruit, and meat such as they desire* (LII:22). And He said: *Meat of birds, such as they desire* (LVI:21). In the *Sunan* of Ibn Māja, from *ḥadīth* of Abū al-Dardā', from the Messenger of God ﷺ, it says: The chief food of the people of this world and the people of Paradise is meat.[343] And from *ḥadīth* of Burayda (*marfūʿ*): The best seasoning in this world and the next is meat.[344]

And in the *Ṣaḥīḥ*, from the Prophet ﷺ: 'The superiority of ʿĀ'isha over other women is like the superiority of *tharīd* over all other food.'[345] Now *tharīd* consists of bread and meat. The poet said:

When you season bread with meat,
that—God be my witness—is *tharīd*

Al-Zuhrī said: Eating meat nourishes seventy faculties. And Muḥammad b. Wāsiʿ said: Meat improves the sight. It is related from ʿAlī b. Abī Ṭālib: Eat meat, for it clears the complexion, empties the belly, and improves the character. Said Nāfiʿ: Ibn ʿUmar, during Ramaḍān, never missed having meat, nor when he was travelling. And it is said, on the authority of ʿAlī, that if anyone refrains from eating it for forty days, his character deteriorates.

As for *ḥadīth* of ʿĀ'isha, related by Abū Dāwūd (*marfūʿ*): 'Do not cut meat with a knife, for that is the practice of non-Arabs, but bite it, for this is more healthy and digestible,' this was rejected by the Imām Aḥmad, because it was reliably reported of the Prophet ﷺ that he cut it with a knife: this is found in two *ḥadīth* already reported.

Meat is of many kinds, differing by reason of its source and constitution. So we shall give a short account of each kind and its constitution, its benefits and its harmful properties.

Sheep's meat is hot in the second, moist in the first degree. Good meat is from a yearling, for it generates good blood when it is well digested. It is suitable for those of cold and moderate temperament, and for those who take vigorous exercise, in cold places and seasons. It is beneficial for those of black bile, and it strengthens the mind and the memory; meat of an old sheep or a thin one is bad, and so is meat of the ewe.

The best meat comes from the black male, for this is the lightest, most delicious and most beneficial. The castrated male is more beneficial and of superior quality. The meat of red fat animals is lighter and gives better nourishment; while that from a young one is less nourishing and floats on the stomach.

The most excellent meat sits nearest to the bone. The right side is lighter and better than the left, and the fore parts superior to the rear. The part of the sheep preferred by God's Messenger ﷺ was the fore part. All higher parts, except the head, are lighter and better than the lower. Al-Farazdaq gave some money to a man to buy meat for him and said: Take the front part, but beware of the head and the abdomen, for these contain illness.

Meat from the neck is good and delicious, light and easy to digest. Meat from the forelegs is the lightest, most delicious and subtlest meat, the least likely to cause harm, the swiftest to digest. In the two books of the *Ṣaḥīḥ* it is said that the Messenger of God ﷺ used to enjoy it.

Meat from the back is very nourishing and generates laudable blood. In the *Sunan* of Ibn Māja (*marfūʿ*) it says: 'The best meat is meat from the back.'

Goat's meat has little heat and is dry. The humour generated from it is not excellent, nor is it good to digest, nor does it give laudable nourishment. Meat of the he-goat is bad, without exception: exceedingly dry, hard to digest, and generating atrabilious humour.

Said al-Jāḥiẓ: An outstanding physician said to me: O Abū ʿUthmān, beware of goat's meat for it causes anxiety, stirs up the black bile, and causes forgetfulness and spoils the blood. Moreover, by God, it causes mental disturbance in children.

A certain physician said: the goat's meat is only bad when it is from an old animal, and then it is especially bad for the aged. It brings no harm to those accustomed to it. Galen placed meat of yearlings among the moderate foods, able to modify the laudable chyme. The female is more beneficial than the male. Al-Nisāʾī has related in his *Sunan,* from the Prophet ﷺ: 'Treat the goat well and protect it from harm, for it is one of the animals of Paradise.' There is speculation as to the reliability of this *ḥadīth*.

However, the physicians' judgement that it is harmful is a particular judgement, not a comprehensive nor general one. For it concerns the weak stomach and weak temperaments, which are not accustomed to it but are used to subtle foods. These are city dwellers who are accustomed to refined food, and they are in the minority.

Meat of kid is near to the mean, especially while it is still suckling but is not newly born. It is swifter to digest because of the strength of the milk it contains. It softens the constitution and is agreeable for most people in most conditions. It is more subtle than camel meat; blood generated from it is moderate.

Cow's meat is cold, dry, hard to digest, slow to flow down, and generates atrabilious blood; it is suitable only for those doing strenuous work. Eating it in excess brings about atrabilious illnesses such as leukoderma, scab, tetters, leprosy, elephantiasis, cancer, melancholic delusions, quartan fever, and many kinds of swellings. This refers to one who is not accustomed to it, or who has not removed its harm with pepper, garlic, cinnamon, ginger and suchlike. The male is less cold, the female less dry.

Meat of calf, especially a fat one, is one of the best and most moderate foods, the most delicious and laudable. It is hot and moist. When it is digested, it gives exceedingly good nourishment.

Concerning meat of mare, it is confirmed in the *Ṣaḥīḥ*, from Asmāʾ, who said: We slaughtered a mare and ate it, in the time of the Messenger of God ﷺ.[346] And it is reliably reported of him that he permitted the meat of horses but prohibited the meat of donkeys.[347] These two *ḥadīth* are reported in both the books of the *Ṣaḥīḥ*. But there is no confirmation from him of the *ḥadīth* of al-Miqdām b. Maʿdikarib 'that he prohibited it', as was said by Abū Dāwūd and other specialists in *ḥadīth*. Its association with the mule and the donkey in the Qur'ān does not indicate that the Judgement concerning its meat is the same as that for their meat, in any way whatever, just as it does not indicate that the Judgement concerning its share in the booty is the same as the Judgement for the mare. For God, praised be He, sometimes joins together things similar or those which differ, or opposites. His remark *That ye ride them* (XVI:8) contains nothing to prevent their being eaten, just as it does not prevent using them in any other way than riding, but it simply prescribes the most valuable of their uses, which is riding. The two *ḥadīth* regarding their lawfulness are sound, with naught to oppose them. Further, their meat is hot and dry, thick, atrabilious, harmful and not suitable for delicate bodies.

As to camel meat, there is a difference between the Rāfiḍites and the people of the *Sunna*, similar to one of the differences between Jews and Muslims; for the Jews and the Rāfiḍites think it objectionable and do not eat it. But its lawfulness is accepted in Islam, when this is necessary. For many a time did the Messenger of God ﷺ and his Companions eat this, both when at home and while travelling.

Meat of the young, weaned camel is among the best and most delicious of meats and gives the best nourishment. For those used to it, it is similar to meat of sheep; it has no harmful effect on them, nor does it generate any illness. Certain physicians have found fault with it, but only in relation to those people who lead a comfortable life in settled areas, who are not accustomed to it. For it contains heat and dryness, generates black bile, and is hard to digest.

It contains an objectional characteristic, on account of which the Prophet ﷺ ordered *wuḍū'* , in two separate, unopposed sound *ḥadīth*. The order to perform *wuḍū'* here cannot correctly be interpreted as merely washing the hands, for the following reasons: (1) It is not what is generally understood as the meaning of *wuḍū'* in the speech of the Prophet ﷺ; (2) he made a clear distinction between eating the meat of sheep and goats and eating the meat of camel; in the former case it is optional, while in the latter it is obligatory. If *wuḍū'* were to be interpreted as washing the hands only, then why does not the same interpretation apply to his words: 'If anyone touches his private parts, he must perform *wuḍū'*.'[348]

Moreover, a man could eat camel's meat without having to touch it directly with his hand (by using a fork, or having it put into his mouth). Hence it would be pointless, and would amount to an interpretation of the words of the Lawgiver which is neither customary nor accepted.

It cannot validly be opposed by the *ḥadīth* that says that the last of the two commands of the Messenger of God ﷺ was to omit *wuḍū'* for what has been touched by fire. This is for several reasons: (1) this is a general command, while the order for *wuḍū'* after eating camel's meat is particular; (2) the order for *wuḍū'* after eating camel's meat relates only to the fact that it is meat of camel, regardless of whether it be raw, cooked or sun-dried. Thus fire as cooking agent has no effect on the necessity for *wuḍū'*. On the other hand, not performing *wuḍū'* after eating what is cooked by fire is indicative of the fact that cooking by fire is not a reason for performing *wuḍū'*. Both *ḥadīth* deal with totally unrelated aspects of the reasons for *wuḍū'*, its being camel's meat; while the other concerns the reasons for exemption from *wuḍū'*, ie. its being touched by fire. So there is no contradiction whatever between them; (3) this contains no general pronouncement on the authority of the Lawgiver, but it is simply information given about the performance of a certain action, one of which is prior to the other; similarly, the same *ḥadīth* contained a clarification: that they bought the Prophet ﷺ some meat, and he ate of it and then the time came for prayer; he performed *wuḍū'* and prayed. Later they brought him meat and he ate; then he prayed but did not perform *wuḍū'*. And the latter occasion was the omission of *wuḍū'* with respect to what had been touched by fire. Thus the *ḥadīth* runs. The narrator has shortened it to use it as an example. There is no indication in this *ḥadīth* to validate the abrogation of the command to perform *wuḍū'* after eating camel's meat. Even if it were a general and subsequent pronouncement it is still imperative to give precedence to the specific over the general. This is exceedingly obvious.

As to meat of lizard (*ḍabb*),[26] the *ḥadīth* concerning its lawfulness has already been noted. Its meat is hot and dry and is aphrodisiac.

Gazelle is the most suitable of game and has the most laudable meat. It is hot and dry, said to be very moderate; beneficial for healthy, moderate bodies. The good is the young (*khishf*). Meat of female gazelle (*ẓabiy*): hot and dry in the first degree, dessicative to the body, appropriate for moist bodies. Ibn Sīnā said: the best of the wild game meat is the female gazelle, despite its tendency to be atrabilious.

Concerning meat of hare or rabbit (*arnab*), it is reliably reported in the two books of the *Ṣaḥīḥ*, from Anas b. Mālik, saying: We started up a hare, so they ran after it and caught it. Then Abū Ṭalḥa sent its haunch to the Messenger of God ﷺ, and he accepted it.[349]

Rabbit's meat is moderate, tending towards heat and dryness. The best part is the haunch, and the most laudable of its meat is eaten roasted. It constrains the abdomen, is diuretic, and disperses stone. Eating the rabbit's head is beneficial for tremor.

For meat of wild asses, it is reliably reported in the two books of the *Ṣaḥīḥ*, from *ḥadīth* of Abū Qutāda, that they were with the Messenger of God ﷺ when he was once making the *ʿumra*; and he hunted a wild ass, and the Prophet ﷺ ordered them to eat it while they were in the state of *iḥrām* (for the *ʿumra*) but Abu Qutāda was not.[350]

In the *Sunan* of Ibn Māja, from Jābir, it says that at the time of Khaybar, we ate horses and wild asses.[351]

Its meat is hot and dry, very nourishing, generating thick atrabilious blood. However its fat is beneficial, with oil of costus, for pain of molar teeth, and for the thick wind which slackens the kidney. Its fat as an embrocation is good for freckles. In short, meats of all wild beasts generate thick atrabilious blood. The most laudable is gazelle, followed by rabbit.

Meat of unborn animals is not commendable because of the blood being restricted within them; but it is not unlawful, because of the saying of the

26 See Chapter 34.

Prophet ﷺ: The legal slaughter of the foetus is the legal slaughter of its mother.[352] The jurists of Iraq prohibited eating it, except when it was obtained live and then killed. They have interpreted the *ḥadīth* as meaning that its legal slaughter is the same as that of its mother, saying: It is an argument indicative of its being unlawful.

This interpretation is not valid, as in the first part of the *ḥadīth*: They asked the Messenger of God ﷺ, saying: 'O Messenger of God, when we slaughter a sheep and find within its belly a foetus, should we eat it?' and he replied: 'Eat it if you wish, for its legal slaughter is the legal slaughter of its mother.'

Moreover, analogy enforces its lawfulness; for as long as it is unborn, it is an integral part of its mother, the legal slaughter of which extends to all its parts. This is what was indicated by the Lawgiver, in his words: 'Its legal slaughter is that of its mother,' just as its slaughter is the slaughter of all its parts. So even if the *sunna* did not give a clear statement about eating the foetus, the use of correct analogy would confirm its lawfulness. And from God comes success.

Concerning dried meat (*qadīd*) it says in the *Sunan*, from *ḥadīth* of Bilāl: I slaughtered a sheep for the Messenger of God ﷺ, while we were on a journey, and he said: 'Prepare its meat suitably.' And I continued to give him of that meat until we came to Madīna.[353]

Qadīd is more beneficial than hung meat (*maksūd*); it strengthens the body but causes itching. Its harm is removed by cold, moist spices. It is moderate for hot temperaments. Hung meat is hot and dry, dessicative, the best being from fat, moist meat; it is bad for colic. Its harmful effect is removed by cooking it with milk and oil. It is appropriate for a hot, moist temperament.

Concerning the meat of birds The Most High said: *And flesh of birds, such as they desire . . .* (LVI:21). In the *Musnad* of al-Bazzār and elsewhere (*marfūʿ*) it says: Indeed you will regard birds in Paradise, and will desire them, and they will fall down, ready roast before you.

Some birds are lawful, others unlawful. The unlawful ones are those with claws, like hawk and falcon and Indian falcon, and those which eat carrion, like eagle and Egyptian vulture, stork magpie, spotted crow, and the large black crow. And there are those which must not be killed, such as the hoopoe and wild crow, and those which must be killed, like the kite and the carrion crow.

Lawful birds are numerous and include chicken. In the two books of the *Ṣaḥīḥ*, from *ḥadīth* of Abū Mūsa, it is related that the Prophet ﷺ ate the meat of chicken.[354] It is hot and moist in the first degree, light upon the stomach, swift to digest, good of humour; it fortifies the brain and the semen, clears the voice, improves the complexion, strengthens the intellect and generates good blood. It inclines towards moisture; it is said that eating it in excess brings on gout; but that is unconfirmed.

Cockerels are warmer in temperament, and less moist. The old sort is a beneficial remedy for colic, asthma, and dense winds, when cooked with juice of carthamus, cinnamon and dill; flesh of the capon gives excellent nourishment and is swiftly digested. Pullet flesh is swift to digest and has a laxative effect. Its blood is subtle and good blood.

Francolins are hot and dry in the second degree, light, subtle, swiftly digested, generating moderate blood. Frequent consumption sharpens the sight.

Partridges (*ḥajal* and *qabaj*) generate good blood and are swiftly digested.

Goose is hot and dry and gives bad nourishment when eaten frequently. It does not have much superfluity.

Duck is hot and moist, with much superfluity. It is hard to digest, and not suitable for the stomach.

As regards bustard it says in the *Sunan*, from *ḥadīth* of Burayya b. ʿUmar b. Safīna, from his father, from his grandfather: Together with the Messenger of God ﷺ I ate the flesh of bustard.[355] It is hot, dry, hard to digest, and beneficial for those who take exercise and do hard labour.

Cranes are dry and light. There is dispute as to the heat or coldness of the meat. It generates atribilious blood and is suitable for those who do hard physical labour. After being slaughtered the birds should be left for a day or two before being eaten.

As to sparrows and larks al-Nisāʾī related in his *Sunan*, from *ḥadīth* of ʿAbd-Allāh b. ʿUmar, that the Prophet ﷺ said: 'If anyone kills a sparrow or a larger bird, without observing its due right, then the Exalted One will call him to task.' He was asked: 'O Messenger of God, what is its due right?' He replied: 'That you slaughter it and eat it, and do not cut off its head and throw the bird away [i.e. do not hunt it just for sport].'[356] And his *Sunan*, from ʿUmar b. al-Sharīd, from his father, it also says: I heard the Messenger of God ﷺ say: 'Whenever anyone kills a sparrow in vain, it cries out to God, saying: O Lord, such a one killed me in vain, not for any good purpose.'[357] The meat is hot and dry, constrains the constitution and is aphrodisiac. Gravy made from it is laxative and is beneficial for the joints. When the brains of these birds are eaten, with ginger and onion, they arouse the appetite for sexual intercourse. The humour it generates is not commendable.

Pigeons are hot and moist but the wild variety is less moist. The young are moister, especially those reared in pigeon cotes. The part-grown young have lighter flesh, and give more laudable nourishment. Flesh of the males is a healing for flaccidity and torpor, for apoplexy and tremor; so does smelling the scent of their breathing. Eating their young is prescribed for women. They are good for the kidney and increase the blood.

A false unfounded *ḥadīth* has been related concerning pigeons that a man complained of loneliness to the Messenger of God ﷺ, and he replied: 'Take a pair of pigeons.' A better *ḥadīth* is that he saw a man pursuing a female pigeon and said: 'A satan following a female satan.'

ʿUthmān b. ʿAffān, in his preaching, would order the killing of dogs and the slaughter of pigeons.

Sandgrouse is dry, generates black bile, and is costive. It is one of the worst foods, though it is beneficial for dropsy.

Quails are hot, dry, beneficial for the joints, and are harmful to the hot liver, which can be averted by vinegar and coriander.

One should avoid such meat of birds as are nesting in jars or in putrid places. Meat of all birds is more swiftly digested than meat of cattle. The swiftest to digest is the least nourishing, namely the necks and wings. Birds' brains are more laudable than the brains of cattle.

On the subject of locusts (*jarād*) it says in the two books of the *Ṣaḥīḥ*, from ʿAbd-Allāh b. Abī Awfā: We went out on seven raids with the Messenger of God ﷺ, and we ate locusts.[358] And in the *Musnad*, on his authority: Made lawful to us were two dead creatures and two kinds of blood: large sea fish and locusts, liver and spleen.[359] This is related both with a full chain of transmission and stopping at Ibn ʿUmar.

Locusts are hot and dry, of slight nourishment. Constant eating of them causes emaciation. When used for fumigation, they are beneficial for dripping of urine and for dysuria, and especially for women; they are used as a fumigant for haemorrhoids. The fat ones (those without wings) are roasted and eaten for cases of scorpion bite. They are harmful for epileptics and for bad humour.

Concerning the lawfulness of those which are found dead for no known reason, there are two opinions: the majority of jurists agree on their lawfulness, while Mālik considered them unlawful. There is no dispute as to their lawfulness when they died for some reason such as being crushed or burnt and so forth.

One should take care not to eat meat in excess, for this causes illnesses of a sanguineous nature or of repletion and severe fevers. ʿUmar b. al-Khaṭṭāb said: 'Beware of meat, for there is in it a greed like that of wine. And God finds hateful the people of any house who constantly eat meat.' Mālik records this, on the authority of the Prophet, in the *Muwaṭṭa'*. Hippocrates said: Do not make your stomach a grave for animals.

2. *Laban* (Milk)

Said God the Most High: *And there is a lesson for you in cattle: from what their bellies contain, among excrement and blood, We produce for you milk, pure and agreeable* (XVI:66); and He said concerning Paradise: *Therein are rivers of water, never of bad odour and rivers of milk whose taste does not alter . . .* (XLVII:15).

In the *Sunan* (*marfūʿ*) it says: Anyone to whom God gives food should say: O God! bless our food and sustain us with goodness from it! And one to whom God gives milk to drink should say: O God! bless our milk, and through it give us increase. For I do not know any food or drink which has such recompense, except milk.'[360]

Although milk in outward appearance is simple, it is compound in its very origin, by a natural composition, from three essential elements: caseous, fatty and watery. Now the caseous component is cold and moist, nourishing to the body; the fatty is moderate in heat and moisture, suitable for the healthy human body, and extremely beneficial; and the watery is hot and moist, releases the constitution and moistens the body. Milk, in an absolute sense, is colder and moister than the mean. It has been said that its power, when just obtained, is of heat and moisture; it is also said that it is moderate in both heat and cold.

Milk is at its best when freshly milked. After that, its goodness continues to decrease as time passes; at the time of milking it is less cold and moister; the acrid sort is the reverse. Milk is at its best for forty days after parturition. The best kind is that which is intensely white, with a good odour, delicious to taste, with a slight sweetness, a moderate fattiness, its substance moderate, neither thin nor thick; and that which is milked from young healthy animals, of moderate flesh, which have had excellent pasturage and water. It is laudable and generates good blood, moistens the dry body and gives good nourishment; it is beneficial for melancholy delusions, anxiety, and atrabilious diseases. When drunk with honey, it cleanses internal ulcers arising from putrid humours. Drunk with sugar it much improves the complexion.

Milk (*ḥalīb*) rectifies the harm of sexual intercourse, is suitable for chest and lungs and is excellent for consumptives; it is bad for the head, stomach, liver and spleen. Drinking it in quantity is harmful to the teeth and gums. Therefore the mouth should be rinsed afterwards with water. In the two books of the *Ṣaḥīḥ* we find that the Prophet ﷺ drank milk, then called for water and rinsed his mouth, saying: 'It contains some fat.'[361]

Milk is bad for sufferers from fever and headache, hurtful to the brain and the weak head. Constant use brings about darkness of the sight and the mucosa, and pain of the joints, obstruction of the liver, and distension in the stomach and intestines. Its rectification is with honey and ginger *robb* (concentrate), and similar. All this refers to those people not accustomed to it.

Sheep's milk is the heaviest and moistest of milks, containing such fattiness and odour as is not found in milk of goat and cow. It generates phlegmatic superfluities, and causes whiteness on the skin when it is taken constantly. Therefore, this milk should be drunk with water, so that the body may obtain a smaller proportion of it, and it is quicker to quench thirst, and better to cool the body.

Goat's milk is subtle, moderate, releases the abdomen and moistens the dry body. It is beneficial for ulcers of the throat, for dry cough and haemopthysis.

Milk in general is the most beneficial drink for the human body, by virtue of the nutritive and sanguineous elements contained in it, and its being habitual to the state of childhood, and its suitability for the original nature (*fiṭra*) of the human being. In the two books of the *Ṣaḥīḥ* we find that the Messenger of

God ﷺ, during his Night Journey, was proferred a cup of wine and a cup of milk. He looked at them both, then took the milk. Then Jibrīl said: 'Praise be to God Who has guided you to *fiṭra*, the original nature of man, for had you taken the wine, your community would have gone astray.'[362]

Acid milk is slow to digest, raw of humour. A hot stomach digests it and benefits from it.

Cow's milk nourishes the body, makes it fat and releases the abdomen in moderation. It is among the most moderate and excellent of milks, between sheep's and goat's milk, as to its thinness, thickness and fattiness. In the *Sunan*, from *ḥadīth* of ʿAbd-Allāh b. Masʿūd (*marfūʿ*), it says: See that you have cow's milk, for they pastured from all the trees.

Camel's milk has been mentioned at the beginning of the section, together with its benefits which need not be repeated.

3. *Lubān* (*kundur*) (Boswellia, B. carterii. Burseraceae. Frankincense)

From the Prophet ﷺ we find the following: 'Fumigate your houses with frankincense and thyme.' But this is not reliable. However it is related of ʿAlī that he said to a man who complained to him of forgetfulness: 'You should take *lubān*, for it encourages the heart and cures forgetfulness.' It is said on the authority of Ibn ʿAbbās, that it is good to drink it with sugar, on an empty stomach; it is good for the urine, and helpful for forgetfulness. And it is said, on the authority of Anas, that a man complained to him of forgetfulness and he replied: 'you must take *kundur*, and soak it overnight, and in the morning take a draught on it on an empty stomach: it is good for forgetfulness.'

For this there is an obvious, natural reason. If forgetfulness is caused by the harm of a cold moist temperament which predominates over the brain, so that it does not retain what is imprinted upon it, then *lubān* can be of benefit for it. But when forgetfulness is caused by the predominance of something contingent, it can swiftly be brought to an end by moistening agents. The difference between them is that the kind caused by dryness is followed by sleeplessness and remembering of matters long past but not those present, while for the kind caused by moisture the reverse is true.

Now forgetfulness can be brought on by certain things in particular: like cupping at the nape of the neck; excessive eating of coriander and sour apples; and much anxiety and grief; looking at stagnant water; and urinating in it; looking at a crucified form and much reading of gravestones; walking between two camels linked together; removing lice during menstruation; and eating heads of rats; most of which is known from experience.

The meaning is that *lubān* is warming in the second degree, dessicative in the first, and contains slight costiveness. It is very beneficial, and has little harm. Among its benefits is that it is useful for haemorrhages, for stomach winds, and clears ulcers of the eye, causes flesh to grow on most ulcers, strengthens and warms the weak stomach, dries up phlegm, dries moistures of the chest, clears darkness of the sight, and prevents foul ulcers from spreading. When chewed, alone or with Persian thyme, it draws the phlegm, and is beneficial for speech impediment, increases and brightens the intellect. Used as a fumigant, it is beneficial for pestilence and sweetens the smell of the air.

Mīm

1. *Mā'* (Water)

Water is the substance of life, the chief of drinks, one of the four elements of the world, indeed its chief element. For the heavens were created from its vapour, and the earth from its foam (*zabad*). From it God made every living creature.

As to whether it nourishes on its own account or merely conveys the nourishment, there are two differing opinions which have already been mentioned, along with the most likely opinion and its supporting argument. It is cold and moist and moderates heat; it preserves the body's moistures and restores whatever has been dissolved from it; and it dilutes the food and causes it to penetrate to the veins.

The goodness of water can be seen in ten ways: (1) from its colour, which should be clear; (2) from its smell, that it should have no smell at all; (3) from its taste, that it should be soft and sweet, like the water of the Nile and Euphrates; (4) from its weight, that it be light and thin in substance; (5) from its course, that it should have a pure course and path; (6) from its source, that it should be from a distant source; (7) from its being open to sun and wind, that it be not hidden beneath the earth, when the sun and wind would not be able to blanch it; (8) from its movement, that it should run and move swiftly; (9) from its abundance, that it be of quantity to repel any superfluities mixed with it; (10) from its flowing, that it should take the direction from north to south, or from west to east.

When these attributes are considered, you will find that they exist as a totality only in the four rivers: Nile, Euphrates, Sayḥūn, Jayḥūn. In the two books of the *Ṣaḥīḥ*, from *ḥadīth* of Abū Hurayra, it says: The Messenger of God ﷺ said: 'Sayḥān, Jayḥān, Nile and Euphrates are all of them rivers of Paradise.'[363]

The lightness of water can be tested by three of its qualities: (1) its swiftness to accept heat and cold. Hippocrates said: Water which swiftly becomes warm and becomes cold is the lightest of waters; (2) its weight; (3) two pieces of cotton of equal weight, should be made wet with two different waters, then completely dried and weighed; whichever of them is lighter, this indicates that its water is lighter.

Even if in origin it is cold and moist, the strength of water can be transmitted through contingent causes which bring about its reaction. For water opened out to the north and not exposed to other directions will be cold, containing a dryness acquired from the north wind. And the same will apply for the other directions. Water which comes forth from metal mines is of the constitution of that metal and will have an effect upon the body similar to that of the metal.

Sweet water is beneficial for both the sick and the healthy, and when cold is more beneficial and delicious. It should not be drunk to break one's fast nor just after sexual intercourse, nor on awakening from sleep, nor just after the bath nor eating fruit as has been stated. As for drinking it close upon food there is no harm when this is from necessity, but rather it is prescribed. One should not take a great deal but should sip it slowly. For it causes no harm whatever, but strengthens the stomach, arouses the appetite and quenches thirst.

Warm water distends and has the opposite effect to what we have just described. That which has rested overnight is preferable to freshly drawn, as has already been stated. Cold water is more beneficial internally than externally; for hot water the reverse holds. Cold is beneficial for putrefaction of the blood, and ascent of vapours to the head. It dispels putrefactions, is appropriate to all temperaments and ages, times, and hot places. But it is harmful for any condition which needs coction and dissolution, such as catarrh and inflammations. Water exceedingly cold hurts the teeth. An excess brings about eruption (*infijār*) of the blood, catarrhs (*nazalāt*) and pains of the chest.

Water both excessively hot and cold is harmful to the nerves and most of the organs; for one of them is dissoluent and the other thickening; hot water quietens the sting of hot humours, dissolves and cocts, expels superfluities, moistens and warms; drinking it spoils the digestion, and it rises with the food to the upper part of the stomach and slackens it. It does not quickly quench thirst, and it causes the body to wither and leads to grave illnesses, and is harmful in most illnesses; yet it is suitable for old people and those who suffer from epilepsy, cold headache and ophthalmia. It is more beneficial when used externally.

Concerning water warmed by the sun there is neither *ḥadīth* nor report; the ancient physicians neither disliked it nor were they critical about it. Very warm water melts the fat of the kidney. Rain water has already been discussed under the letter *ghayn* (*ghayth*).

As to water from snow and ice it is confirmed in the two books of the *Ṣaḥīḥ* from the Prophet ﷺ, that he used to supplicate at the opening prayers or elsewhere: 'O God! Wash me from my sins in water of snow and ice.'[364]

Snow has in itself a fierce smoky quality, and so its water is like it. We have already referred to the wisdom and motive of seeking to be cleansed from sins in its water, because the heart needs to be made cool and firm and strong. From this can be profitably inferred the basic principles of medicine for bodies and hearts, and the treatment of their ailments by opposites.

Water from hail is subtler and more delicious than water from snow. As for frozen water, that is ice, its properties depend on its source. Likewise snow acquires the quality, whether for good or ill, of the mountains and earth upon which it falls.

One should avoid drinking ice-cooled water after the bath or sexual intercourse, exercise, or hot food; and it should be avoided by sufferers from cough, pain in the chest and weak liver, and those of cold temperaments.

Water from wells has little refinement; water from underground conduits is heavy. For the one is confined and cannot be free from putrefaction, and the other is kept away from the air. It is necessary that they should not be drunk at once, but left overnight to absorb some air. The worst sort is that which runs through lead pipes, or from a well out of use, especially if its earth is bad, for such water is pestilential and raw.

Water of Zamzam is the noblest of all waters, the most pleasing to souls, the most highly prized and the most valued by people. It is the well of Jibrīl and the watering place of Ismāʿīl.

It is confirmed in the two books of the *Ṣaḥīḥ* from the Prophet ﷺ: when Abū Dharr had stood up between the Kaʿba and its covering for forty sessions, between night and day, and had no other food, the Prophet ﷺ said: 'Indeed it is the food of nourishment.'[365] Another, not Muslim, added, with his chain of transmission: 'And healing of sickness.'

In the *Sunan* of Ibn Māja, from *ḥadīth* of Jābir b. ʿAbd-Allāh, from the Prophet ﷺ, it is related that he said: 'Zamzam water is effective for that for which it is drunk.'[366] Some *ḥadīth* scholars have called this a weak *ḥadīth*, because ʿAbd-Allāh b. al-Mu'ammal is included in the chain of transmission from Muḥammad b. Muslim al-Makkī.

We have related from ʿAbd-Allāh b. al-Mubārak that when he went on pilgrimage, he came to Zamzam and said: 'O God! Ibn Abī'l-Mawālī related to us, from Muḥammad b. al-Munkadir, from Jābir, from your Prophet ﷺ, that he said: "Water of Zamzam is effective for that for which it is drunk." So I drink anticipating the thirst of the Day of Resurrection.' Now Ibn Abī'l-Muwālī is reliable, so the *ḥadīth* thus is sound. Some have confirmed it, while others have called it fabricated. In both opinions there is some uncertainty.

Now I myself and others have experienced marvels in the drinking of Zamzam water and I have sought healing by it for many illnesses and received healing by God's permission. I have seen one who took nothing else for days on end, about half a month or more and experienced no hunger; he performed *ṭawāf* (circumambulation of the Kaʿba) with the people. He told me that he sometimes remained thus for forty days, and had good strength, so as to have intercourse with his wives, and fast, and perform *ṭawāf* several times.

Water of the Nile comes from one of the rivers of Paradise, originating beyond the Mountains of the Moon, in the furthest reaches of Abyssinia, from rain waters which are collected there and watercourses which replenish one another. For God the Most High sends it towards the harsh dry land which has no plants and thereby He makes crops spring forth which feed both animals and human beings.

Now the earth to which He sends it is of hard alluvial deposits, so if average amounts of rain for that part of the earth were to fall, it would not receive moisture and would not be prepared for plant life; and if it rained above the average amount, then it would damage dwellings and injure their inhabitants and interrupt people's livelihood and spoil their interests. So He made rain to fall on distant lands, then He sent those rains to this earth in a mighty river; and He made it to overflow at appointed times, in amounts able to irrigate the land sufficiently. When it gave the land its irrigation and it went over every part, He permitted it to decrease gradually and dry up, so that its benefit might be completed by the possibility of cultivation. And this water has the ten aspects already mentioned; it is among the subtlest and lightest of waters, the choicest and the sweetest.

Concerning sea water it is confirmed that the Prophet ﷺ said concerning the sea: 'Its water and its dead creatures are lawful.'[367]

God, praised be He, has made it salty, bitter, too harsh to drink, in the best interests of all who dwell on the earth, both humans and animals. It is always peaceful, with many living creatures. These are many which die within it and are not buried. If it were sweet water, then its lack of movement and the creatures dying in it would make it go bad and putrid. Then the air surrounding the world would acquire that character from it, and would go bad and putrid and so the world would be polluted. The Lord in His wisdom, praised and exalted be He, saw fit to make it like the salty brine: so, if all the corpses, rottenness and dead things of the world were to be thrown into it, they would not alter it in any way; nor will it be altered, despite its enduring from the time it was created until God the Most High will fold up the world at the end of time. This is the final cause (*ghā'ī*), which requires its saltiness; and its effective cause (*fāʿilī*) is the fact that its ground is briny and salty.

Further, washing with sea water is beneficial for numerous external ills of the skin, while drinking it causes damage both internally and externally. It releases the abdomen, emaciates, causes itching and scab, distension and thirst.

If one is compelled to drink it, there are ways of treating it to remove its harmful qualities. For instance, one can pour some into a cauldron, placing over the cauldron some reeds, and over them a new fluffy woollen cloth. One lights a fire beneath the cauldron, so that its vapour rises up to the woollen cloth. When there is plenty, this is wrung out, and one continues thus until the required amount has collected, for the vapour obtained from the wool is the sweet water while the undrinkable element remains in the cauldron. Or again, one can dig a wide hole at the edge of the sea, so that the water will percolate into it, then, at the side of it nearby, another hole to which the water of the first hole will percolate, then a third hole and so on until the water is sweet. When necessity compels one to drink water which is muddy, the treatment is to throw apricot stones into it, or a piece of teak wood, or lighted embers, which are extinguished in it, or Armenian clay, or gruel of wheat; then the muddiness sinks to the bottom.

2. *Misk*

It is confirmed in Muslim's *Ṣaḥīḥ*, from Abū Saᶜīd al-Khudrī, from the Prophet ﷺ, that he said: 'The best of scents is musk.'[368]

In the two books of the *Ṣaḥīḥ*, from ᶜĀ'isha, it says: I used to perfume the Messenger of God ﷺ before he went into a state of *iḥrām*, and on the day of Sacrifice, and before he performed *ṭawāf* around the Kaᶜba, with scent containing musk.'[369]

Musk is the king among perfumes, the best and noblest and used in metaphorical speech: for other things are compared to it, yet it is not compared to others. It is the stuff of the hills of Paradise.

It is hot and dry in the second degree; it gladdens and strengthens the soul, and fortifies all the internal organs, whether it is drunk or sniffed, and the external organs, when placed upon them. It is beneficial for old people, those made cold or moist, especially in winter; it is good for swooning, palpitation and weakness of the faculty by the way it arouses the innate heat.

It clears the white of the eye and dries up its moisture, makes wind subside from it, and from all the organs, and is an antidote for poisons, and is beneficial for serpent bites. Its benefits are very numerous. It is the strongest of the substances which bring gladness.

3. *Marzanjūsh* (Origanum majorana L., Majorana hortensis Moench. Labiatae. Marjoram)

There is a *ḥadīth* concerning this, but we do not know if it is genuine: Take *marzanjūsh*, for it is good for *khushām* (which is catarrh).

It is hot in the third, dry in the second degree. Sniffing it is beneficial for cold headache and headache arising from phlegm, black bile, catarrh and thick winds; it opens obstructions which occur in the head and the nostrils. It dissolves most cold inflammations and is beneficial for most inflammations and cold, moist pains.

Used as a pessary, it is emmenagogue and helps a woman to conceive. When its dry leaves are pounded and used as a compress, this disperses traces of blood occurring beneath the eye. When made into a poultice with vinegar, it is beneficial for scorpion sting.

Its oil is beneficial for pain of the back and the knees, and dispels fatigue. If a man sniffs it continuously, then no water descends in his eyes. When its juice is used as a sternutatory with bitter almond oil, it opens obstructions of the nostrils, and is beneficial for wind occurring there and in the head.

4. *Milḥ* (Salt)

Ibn Māja relates in his *Sunan*, from *ḥadīth* of Anas (*marfūᶜ*): Your chief seasoning is salt.[370] The 'chief' of anything is that which adjusts and governs it. The majority of seasonings are rectified by salt.

In the *Musnad* of al-Bazzār (*marfūᶜ*) it says: It is as if you should be in the midst of people like salt in food; for food is only rectified by salt.

Al-Baghawī mentions in his *tafsīr*, from ᶜAbd-Allāh b. ᶜUmar (*marfūᶜ*): God sent down four blessings from heaven to earth: iron, fire, water and salt.[371] The shortened version of the *ḥadīth* also resembles this.

Salt preserves man's food, guards his body and improves everything it is mixed with, even gold and silver; for it contains a power which increases the yellowness of the gold and the whiteness of the silver. It contains powers to cleanse and dissolve, and expel the thick moistures and dry them up, to strengthen bodies and prevent their putrefaction and corruption; it is beneficial for ulcerated scab.

When used as a *koḥl*, it removes superfluous flesh from the eye, and eradicates yellowness. *Andarānī* salt has a stronger effect of that kind and prevents foul ulcers from spreading and is a laxative. When used as an embrocation on the abdomen of one suffering from dropsy, it is beneficial. It cleanses the teeth, expels decay from them, firms and strengthens the gums. Its benefits are numerous.

Nūn

1. *Nakhl* (Phoenix dactylifera L. Palmae. Date palm)

This is mentioned in the Qur'ān in several places. In the two books of the *Ṣaḥīḥ*, from Ibn ᶜUmar, it says: While we were seated with the Messenger of God ﷺ he was brought the spathe (*jummār*) of a date palm. The Prophet ﷺ said: 'Among the trees there is one which is likened to the Muslim man, for its leaves do not fall. Now tell me, which is it?' So people thought of various trees of the desert places, but it occurred to me that it was the date palm. I wanted to say: 'It is the date palm!' Then I looked around and lo! I was the youngest of those present, so I kept silence. Then the Messenger of God ﷺ said: 'It is the date palm.' So I later mentioned that to ᶜUmar, and he said: 'If you had said this, it would have pleased me more.'[372]

This *ḥadīth* contains an example of the learned man posing questions to his companions in order to exercise them and test their knowledge. It also demonstrates the making of a proverb and similitude, as well as the modesty of the Companions before their elders and their more distinguished members, and their refraining from speech in their presence, and the joy of a man when his son is successful in arriving at the correct answer. Also that it is in no way disapproved that a son should reply if he knows the answer in the presence of his father, even if the father does not know it; this contains no element of bad manners. The comparison of the Muslim with the palm encompasses the abundance of its benefits, the continuance of its shade, the delight of its fruit, and its long-lasting duration.

The fruit of the date palm is eaten moist or dry, as fresh (unripe) dates (*balaḥ*) and when fully ripe (*yāniᶜ*). It is food and medicine, sustenance and sweetmeat, drink and fruit. Its trunk is used for building, for implements and containers, and from its leaves (*khūs*) are made matting, large baskets, containers, fans and other objects. And from its fibres come ropes, mattresses, and other things. Finally, its stones are a food for camels, and they are included in medicines and eye medicaments (*koḥl*). To that we should add the beauty of its fruit and foliage, its excellent form, its splendid appearance, the marvellous arrangement of its fruit in layers, its shape and splendour and the joy that souls derive from seeing it. For its sight is a reminder of the One Who formed and created it, of His excellent workmanship, His perfect power, and His complete wisdom. No object is more fittingly likened to it than the believer, since he contains goodness in all his affairs and benefit is generated at his hand both outwardly and inwardly.

This is the tree whose trunk sighed after the Messenger of God ﷺ when he left it, longing to be near him and hear his words. This is the tree beneath which Mary gave birth to Jesus.

We find in a *ḥadīth* about whose chain of transmission there is some speculation: Honour your aunt the palm tree, for she was created of the same clay as was Adam. [373]

As to whether or not it is to be preferred to the vine (*ḥabala*), people are of two opinions; for God in His Book has put them together, in several places, indeed how close are they to each other! Nevertheless each one, in the place where it is predominant and in its appropriate habitat, is the more excellent and more salutary.

2. *Narjis* (Narcissus poeticus L., N. pseudo-narcissus L. Amaryllidaceae. Narcissus)

Concerning this plant there is an unconfirmed *ḥadīth*: See that you sniff the narcissus. For the heart contains the seed of madness, leprosy and vitiligo, which can only be prevented by smelling narcissus.

It is hot and dry in the second degree. Its root puts flesh on ulcers which go deep into the nerves. It has a cleansing, attracting, drawing power. When cooked, and its juice drunk, or eaten boiled, it provokes emesis and draws moistures from the depth of the stomach. When cooked with vetch (*karsanna*) and honey, it cleanses the dirt of ulcers, and draws abscesses which are hard of coction.

Its flower is of a moderate heat and subtle; it is beneficial for cold catarrh. It contains a strong dissoluent power, opens up obstructions of the brain and nostrils, is beneficial for moist and atrabilious headache, but causes pain to heads which are heated. When the bulb of burnt narcissus is split, firm, and planted, it multiplies. If a man smells it continuously in winter, this protects him from pleurisy in the summer. It is beneficial for pains of the head caused by phlegm and black bile. It has a scent which strengthens the heart and the brain, being beneficial for many of their illnesses. The author of the *Taysīr* said: 'Smelling it dispels epilepsy in children.'

3. *Nūra* (Quick-lime)

Ibn Māja related, from *ḥadīth* of Umm Salma, that the Prophet ﷺ when he used to anoint himself, began with his private parts, anointed them with *nūra*, and then the rest of his body. On this subject there are a number of *ḥadīth*, this being a good example.

It has been said that Solomon, son of David, was the first person to enter the bath and have *nūra* made for him.

It consists of two parts lime plaster (*kils*), one part zinc (*zarnīkh*), mixed with water. It is left in the sun or in the bath, according to the coction and how blue it is. Then it is used as an embrocation, and one sits for an hour until it takes effect, without letting water touch it. Then one washes, and anoints that place with henna to remove its fiery quality.

4. *Nabq* (fruit of Zizyphus spina-Christi (L.) Desf. Rhamnaceae. Zizyphus)

Abū Nuᶜaym mentioned in his book 'Medicine of the Prophet' (*marfūᶜ*) that when Adam fell to earth, the first fruit that he ate there was the *nabq*. The Prophet ﷺ mentioned the *nabq* in a *ḥadīth*, agreed to be authentic: that on his Night Journey he saw the zizyphus tree of the Boundary, and lo, its fruits were like the clay jugs of Hajar.[374]

Nabq is the fruit of the zizyphus tree (*sidr*); it constrains the constitution, is beneficial for diarrhoea, tans the stomach, settles the yellow bile, nourishes the body, awakens the appetite, generates phlegm, and is beneficial for bilious diarrhoea (*darab*).

It is slow to digest; its gruel strengthens the intestines; it is suitable for bilious temperaments. Its harm is rectified by comb honey.

There are two opinions as to whether it is moist or cold, the correct one being that the moist sort is cold and moist, while the dry kind is cold and dry.

Hā'

1. *Hindibā'* (Cichorium intybus L. Compositae. Chicory)

There are three *ḥadīth* concerning this, but these are not genuinely from the Prophet ﷺ, though they have a full chain of transmission: (1) 'Eat chicory, but do not shake it violently, for on every single day drops fall onto it from Paradise.' (2) 'If anyone eats chicory, then sleeps afterwards, neither poison nor magic can have any power over him.' (3) 'On every leaf of chicory there is a drop from Paradise.'

Morover, it changes its temperament, differing with the seasons as they change. So in winter it is cold and moist, in summer hot and dry, in spring and autumn moderate; in most of its states it tends towards cold and dryness. It is costive, cooling, excellent for the stomach. When cooked and eaten with vinegar, it constrains the abdomen. This applies particularly to the wild (*barrī*) variety, which is better for the stomach and more costive, and is beneficial for weakness of the stomach.

Used as a poultice, it settles inflammation arising in the stomach, is beneficial for gout and for hot inflammations of the eye. A poultice made from its leaves and roots is beneficial for scorpion bite.

It strengthens the stomach, opens obstructions occurring in the liver, is beneficial for pains of the liver, both hot and cold, opens obstructions of the spleen, the veins and the intestines, and cleanses the passages of the kidneys.

The more bitter sort is more beneficial for the liver. Its pressed out juice is beneficial for obstructive jaundice, especially when mixed with juice of moist fennel (*rāziyānaj*). When its leaves are pounded and placed on hot inflammations they cool and dissolve them; they cleanse the contents of the chest, and extinguish the heat of the blood and the yellow bile.

It is best eaten neither washed nor shaken, for when this is done its power departs from it, despite the fact that it has a power as antidote (*tiryāq*) beneficial for all poisons.

When its juice is used as a *koḥl*, it is good for night blindness. Its leaves are used in *tiryāq*, and it is beneficial for scorpion stings and counteracts most poisons. Its juice mixed with oil gives release from all deadly drugs. When its root is pressed and the juice drunk, it is beneficial for viper and scorpion bites and hornet stings. The milk of its root clears the white of the eye.

Wāw

1. *Wars* (Memecyclon tinctorium Willd. Melastomataceae. Dye Plant)

Al-Tirmidhī mentioned in his *Jāmiᶜ*, from *ḥadīth* of Zayd b. Arqam, from the Prophet ﷺ, that he used to prescribe oil with *wars* for pleurisy.[375] Said Qutāda: It is given at the side of the mouth (*yuladdu bihi*) and it is administered from the side of the body of which he complains. Ibn Māja related in his *Sunan*, also from *ḥadīth* of Zayd b. Arqam, that the Messenger of God ﷺ prescribed for pleurisy *wars*, costus and oil, to be given at the side of the mouth.[376]

It is reliably reported from Umm Salma: One who gave birth would rest for forty days after childbirth, and one of us would anoint her on her face with *wars* for freckles.[377]

Abū Ḥanifa the philologist said: *wars* is a cultivated plant, and does not occur wild. I do not know of it outside the bedouin regions, nor any land apart from Yemen.

Its strength is heat and dryness at the beginning of the second degree. The best sort is the red, soft to the touch, with little rough residue. When used as an embrocation, it is beneficial for freckles, itching, and pustules occurring on the surface of the body. It has a costive staining faculty and when drunk it is beneficial for leprous whiteness (*waḍaḥ*). The dosage is one *dirham*'s weight.

In its temperament and benefits it is close to the benefits of sea costus. It is beneficial when smeared on leukoderma, itching, pustules and mange (*saᶜfa*). A robe dyed with *wars* has an aphrodisiac effect.

2. *Wasma* (?Indigofera tinctoria L. Leguminosae. Indigo)

This is the leaves of *nīl*. It blackens the hair. We have but recently discussed the controversy regarding the permissibility of using a black dye and those who did this, cf. under *katam* above.

Yā'

1. *Yaqṭīn* (Cucurbita sp. Cucurbitaceae. Gourd)

This is the *dubbā'* and the *qarᶜ*, although the name *yaqṭīn* is more general. For in classical Arabic it indicates any shrub that does not have an upright stalk, like the watermelon (*biṭṭīkh*) and cucumbers (*qiththā', khiyār*).

Said God Most High: *We made there to grow up over him a shrub of gourd* (yaqṭīn). (XXXVII: 146)

It may be said that what does not grow upright on a stalk is called herbage (*najm*), not shrub (*shajar*). *Shajar* indicates that which has a stem. Philologists have raised the question of how He could have said: 'A shrub of *yaqṭīn*.'

The answer is that shrubs (*shajar*) in the general sense means that which stands upon a stem, but when restricted in any way, it becomes qualified accordingly. The difference between the general and the restricted usage of nomenclature is a most important and useful division in the comprehension and classification of language. The *yaqṭīn* mentioned in the Qur'ān is the plant of the *dubbā'*, and its fruit is called *dubbā'* and *qarᶜ*, and shrub of *yaqṭīn*.

It is confirmed in the two books of the *Ṣaḥīḥ*, from *ḥadīth* of Anas b. Mālik, that a tailor invited the Messenger of God ﷺ to a meal he had prepared. 'And I (Anas) went with the Messenger of God ﷺ. He was brought barley bread and a gravy containing *dubbā'* and dried meat (*qadīd*).' Said Anas: 'And I saw the Messenger of God ﷺ picking pieces of the *dubbā'* from round the dish; and I have always liked *dubbā'* from that day onwards.'[378]

Abū Ṭālūt said: I went to see Anas b. Mālik when he was eating gourd, and he said: 'What a shrub! How much I like you! For the Messenger of God ﷺ liked you.' It is related in the *Ghaylāniyyāt*, from *ḥadīth* of Hishām b. ʿUrwa, from his father, from ʿĀ'isha, who said: The Messenger of God ﷺ said to me: 'O ʿĀ'isha, when you cook a cauldron of food, put in plenty of *dubbā'*, for it strengthens the heart of the sad.'

Yaqṭīn is cold and moist, gives slight nourishment, and is swift to descend. If it is not corrupt before digestion, a laudable humour is generated from it. And one of its characteristics is that this humour is of the same kind as whatever accompanies it. For if it is eaten with mustard, a pungent humour is generated; with salt, a salty humour; and with something costive, a costive humour. If cooked with quince it gives the body excellent nourishment.

It is subtle, watery and gives a moist phlegmy nourishment and is good for those of heated temperaments, but is not appropriate for those of cold temperaments, and those in whom phlegm is predominant. Its juice quenches thirst, removes headache when drunk or used for washing the head. It softens the abdomen in whatever way it is used. Its like cannot be found for treating those of hot temperaments, nor is anything swifter to bring relief.

Among its benefits is that when it is smeared with dough and roasted in the stove or oven, and its juice extracted, and it is then drunk with one of the subtle drinks, it calms the heat of inflammatory fever, quenches thirst and gives good nourishment.

When drunk with *turanjabīn* and quince as a *rubb* (concentrate), it expels an unmixed yellow bile.

When the gourd (*qar*ʿ) is cooked, and its juice drunk with a little honey and natron, it brings down phlegm and bile together. When pounded and a poultice made from it is put on the crown of the head it is beneficial for hot inflammations in the brain.

When juice is extracted from its peelings, and the juice mixed with rose oil and drops are instilled into the ear, it is beneficial for hot inflammations. And its peelings are useful for hot inflammations of the eye and for hot gout.

It is very useful for those of hot temperaments and the fevered. When it encounters in the stomach an evil humour, it adapts its nature and becomes corrupt, and generates an evil humour in the body. Its harm can be removed by vinegar and salt fish.

In short it is one of the subtlest and most quickly-reacting of foods.

It is mentioned, from Anas, that the Messenger of God ﷺ used to eat it frequently.

Conclusion: General Principles

Now I have seen fit to end my words on this subject with an abbreviated section of great value, containing warnings and exhortations, general and useful, so that the benefit of this book may be complete.

I have seen some remarks by Ibn Māsawayh, in the book *al-Maḥādhīr* ('Warnings'), which I have quoted in his own words. He says: If a man eats onions for forty days, and his face becomes freckled, then he has none to blame but himself. If anyone undergoes venesection and eats salty food, and then is afflicted by leukoderma or scab, he has only himself to blame. If anyone combines eating eggs and fish, and is afflicted by paralysis or facial paralysis, he has none to blame but himself. If anyone enters the bath while he is replete and is afflicted by paralysis, let him blame none but himself. If anyone combines eating milk and fish into his stomach, and is afflicted by leprosy or vitiligo or gout, let him blame only himself. If anyone combines in his stomach both milk and date wine (*nabīdh*), and is afflicted by vitiligo or gout, the fault is his alone. Whoever has emission of semen in his sleep and does not perform *ghusl* before sexual intercourse with his wife, and she gives birth to one mad or of confused mind, the blame is on him alone. Anyone who eats cold boiled eggs to repletion, and is afflicted by asthma, let him blame none but himself. Whoever has sexual intercourse, without waiting for ejaculation, and is afflicted by stone, let him blame none but himself. If one looks into a mirror at night, and is afflicted by facial paralysis or by some illness, then he has none but himself to blame.

Said Ibn Bukhtīshūʿ: Be careful not to combine eggs and fish, for these two cause colic, the winds of haemorrhoids, and the pain of the molars. Continual eating of eggs generates freckles on the face.

Eating salted food and salt fish, and undergoing venesection after the bath, generate leukoderma and scab. Excessive eating of sheeps' or goats' kidneys damages the bladder. Washing in cold water, after eating fresh fish, generates paralysis. To have sexual intercourse with a menstruating woman generates leprosy. Sexual intercourse, without complete voiding of the seminal fluid afterwards, generates stone. Delaying evacuation of food residues causes windy illness.

Hippocrates said: To have but little of what is harmful is better than to have much of what is useful. And he said: Safeguard your health by taking physical exercise, and avoiding excessive consumption of food and drink.

A philosopher once said: Whoever wishes to be in good health should take good food, and eat when in a clean state, drink when thirsty, take only a little water, rest at ease after the midday meal, go for a walk after the evening meal, and not sleep until he has evacuated the superfluities; and let him beware of entering the bath in a state of repletion; one occasion in summer is better than ten in winter. Eating dried meat at night aids destruction of health. Sexual intercourse with an old woman shortens the life span and makes ill the bodies of healthy people. This is related on the authority of ʿAlī, but it is not confirmed; however, it is partially from the words of al-Ḥārith b. Kalada, the physician of the Arabs, and others.

Al-Ḥārith said: Whoever wishes to live long—for naught is permanent—let him come early to the noon meal, and hasten to his evening meal, have light clothing and have little to do with women.

And he said: There are four things which destroy the body: sexual intercourse following too large a meal; entering the bath when replete; eating of dried meat; and sexual intercourse with an old woman.

When al-Ḥārith was near to death, the people came to him and said: 'Give us a command which we can follow after you have left us.' He replied: 'Of women, marry only one who is young; and eat of fruit only in the seasons they are ripe; and let no one of you receive treatment so long as his body is able to bear the illness. See that you cleanse your stomach every month; for it will melt phlegm, destroy bile, and cause flesh to grow. After the midday meal, let one sleep for an hour afterwards; after supper, let him walk forty paces.'

A certain king said to his physician: 'You might pass away, so give me a prescription which I may follow.' He replied: 'Marry none but a young woman; eat of meat only that which is young; take medicine only for an ailment; eat fruit only when it is ripe. Chew your food well. When you have eaten by day, then you may sleep; but when you eat at night, do not sleep until you have walked, even only fifty paces. Never eat until you are hungry; do not have sexual intercourse unless you desire it; do not retain urine. Make use of the benefits of the bath, lest you may be harmed by the lack of it. Do not eat food when there is already food in your stomach. Take care not to eat any food that your teeth are not able to masticate with the result that your stomach would be unable to digest it. See that every week by emesis you cleanse your body. Take good care of the blood in your body, and do not let it forth except when necessary. And be sure to bathe, for this will expel such obstructions as medicines cannot reach.'

Al-Shāfiʿī said: There are four things that strengthen the body: eating meat; smelling scent; frequent *ghusl* without sexual intercourse; and wearing of linen. And four which weaken the body: frequent sexual intercourse; much anxiety; drinking much water on an empty stomach; and too much eating of sour things. There are four which strengthen the sight: sitting down facing the direction of the Kaʿba; using *koḥl* when going to sleep; looking at greenery; and keeping clean the place where you sit. And four which weaken the sight: looking upon filth; upon one crucified; upon the private parts of a woman; and sitting with one's back to the *qibla*. Four things promote sexual intercourse: eating sparrows; the great *uṭrīfil* (electuary); pistachios; and carob. Four which strengthen the intellect: leaving aside any superfluous talk; using the *siwāk*; sitting in company with the righteous; and sitting with the learned.

Plato said: There are five which reduce the body, and sometimes destroy it: inferiority because of poverty; parting with loved ones; repressing anger; rejection of advice; and the laughter of the ignorant at the intelligent.

The physician of al-Ma'mūn said: You must hold to certain principles; if one observes these, he should never suffer any illness save the illness of death. Do not eat food when there is already food in your stomach; see that you eat no food which your molars cannot thoroughly masticate for your stomach will be unable to digest it. See that you do not over-practise sexual intercourse, for this takes from the light of life; beware of sexual intercourse with an old woman, for this can lead to sudden death. See that you do not undergo venesection unless there is a need for it. And use emesis in the summer.

Among the sayings of Hippocrates is the following: Every excess is harmful to the human constitution.

Galen was asked: 'Wherefore is it that you do not fall sick?' He replied: 'Because I never combine two foods which are bad; I never let one food follow close upon another, and I do not retain in the stomach any food which could harm me.'

Four things make the body ill: excessive talking; too much sleep; over-eating; and over-indulging in sexual intercourse. For excessive talking reduces and weakens the marrow of the brain, and hastens white hair: too much sleep makes the face pale, blinds the heart, and agitates the eye, causes aversion to work, and generates moistures in the body. Over-eating harms the mouth of the stomach, weakens the body, and generates thick winds and severe illnesses. Over-indulging in sexual intercourse undermines the body, weakens the faculties, dries up the moistures of the body, slackens the nerves, causes obstruction, and its harm spreads to the whole body, and in particular the brain, because of the amount of the bodily essence it disssolves. Its weakening effect is greater than that of all the other evacuating agents, and it evacuates a large amount of the spirit's essence.

The most beneficial of intercourse is an encounter of true desire, with a young beautiful woman in a lawful relationship at the age of youth, and combined with the heat and moisture of temperament, and after a period of abstinence. Also, when the heart is free from mental distraction, and without excess, and when one does not combine it with such things as should be avoided at this time: excessive repletion, emptiness and evacuation, or violent exercise, or excessive heat or cold. When one takes care of all these ten factors, it becomes exceedingly beneficial. If one of them is missing, he is subject to harm accordingly; if all, or most are missing, then this brings speedy destruction.

Excessive precaution in a state of health is similar to complications in a state of illness. But moderate precaution is beneficial.

Galen said to his friends: Avoid three things and make sure you have four, and you will have no need of a physician. Avoid dust, smoke and putrefaction. And see you have fatness, scent, sweetness and the bath. Do not eat more than enough to satisfy you and do not clean your teeth with the sticks of basil nor ocimum; do not eat walnuts at night. Let the one with catarrh not sleep upon his back, nor the one with anxiety eat sour things. Let the one who undergoes venesection not walk hurriedly for that runs the risk of death. Let the one who suffers from an illness of the eyes avoid emesis; do not eat too much meat in the summer. Let the one with cold fever not sleep in the sun. Do not consume aubergine with old seeds. If a man drinks a cup of hot water each day in winter, he is secure from illnesses. If he rubs his body in the bath with pomegranate peel, he is secure from scab and itching.

If he eats five corms of iris with a little Greek mastic and raw aloe wood and musk, for his whole life his stomach will not be weak nor corrupt. If he eats seeds of watermelon with sugar, he cleanses the stone from his stomach and will not suffer from burning of the urine.

Four things ruin the body: anxiety, grief, hunger, sleeplessness. And four things bring joy to the body: looking at greenery, at running water, at the beloved, and at fruits.

Four darken the sight: walking barefoot; keeping company with one hated, or disliked, or an enemy; excessive weeping; and too much looking at fine script.

Four strengthen the body: wearing soft clothes; taking a moderate bath; eating sweet and fatty food; and smelling sweet scents.

Four darken the face and conceal its honour, its beauty and its radiance: lying; insolence; arguing without knowledge; and indulging in immorality. Four illuminate the face and increase its dignity: chivalry (*murū'a*); loyalty; generosity; and piety; and four bring on hatred and loathing: pride; envy; lying; and slander.

Four bring one's sustenance: standing for prayer at night; asking forgiveness before dawn; habitual almsgiving; and remembrance of God at the beginning and end of the night. And four prevent the sustenance: sleep in the morning; insufficient worship; laziness; and treachery.

Four harm the understanding and intelligence: excessive eating of sour foods and of fruits; sleeping upon the nape of the neck; anxiety; and worry. And four increase the intellect: protecting the heart (from distractions); reducing intake of food and drink; careful organisation of the diet with sweet and fatty things; and expulsion of superfluities which make the body heavy.

Among those which harm the intelligence are: excessive eating of onions, beans, olives and aubergines; too much sexual intercourse; solitude; brooding; inebriation; excessive laughing; and worry.

One of the philosophers said: 'My train of thought was interrupted in three sessions and I saw no good reason for that except that I ate too many aubergines on one of those days, and olives on another, and beans on the third.'

We have now come to the end of a useful collection of the excerpts of scientific medicine; perhaps one who reads them will not find many of them elsewhere than in this book. So we have shown you how closely linked it is to the *sharīʿa*, and that the relationship of the scientists to the medicine of the Prophet ﷺ is less than the relationship of old wives' medicine to theirs.

The matter is even more than we mentioned, and far greater than we have described. But what we have said gives some indication of what is behind it. If anyone is not given by God perception to distinguish this, then let him know the status of the power which is assisted by revelation from God, and the knowledge which God has granted to the prophets, and the understanding and visions which God has bestowed on them, when compared with that which others have.

Now one might ask: What is the connection between the guidance of the Messenger ﷺ, and the contents of this book which deals with the powers of medicines, the rules of treatment, and the preservation of health?

However, anyone who says this has an inadequate understanding of what the Messenger ﷺ brought. For what we have mentioned in this book and many, many times as much is but a glimpse of his teaching and guidance. Deep understanding of God and what the Prophet ﷺ has brought is a gift which God grants to such of His servants as He wishes.

We have shown you the three foundations of medicine in the Qur'ān. So how could you deny that the Law of the Messenger, sent with the welfare of this world and the next, should be concerned with bodily welfare, as well as the welfare of hearts; and that it guides towards the preservation of bodily health, repelling afflictions, by comprehensive ways? The deduction of its details has been entrusted to the healthy intellect and the sound nature through analogy and many signs. The same applies to many questions in the branches of jurisprudence as well. So do not be one of those who are hostile to what they do not know.

Were the servant to be granted thorough familiarity with the Book of God and the *sunna* of His Messenger, and full understanding concerning the texts and their requirements, he would need no further writings and would be able to derive and deduce all the sound sciences therefrom.

All the sciences find their centre and foundation in knowledge of God, of His command and His creation. That was entrusted to the Messengers, may God's blessings and peace be on them. For they of all humankind have the best knowledge of God, His command and His creation and His wisdom in His creation and His decree.

The medicine of the followers of the Prophet ﷺ is more sound and more beneficial than that of any others. Thus the medicine of the followers of the Seal and Master and Leader of the prophets, Muḥammad b. ʿAbd-Allāh, God's blessings and peace be on him, is the most perfect medicine, the soundest and the most beneficial.

This will only be recognised by one who knows both the medicine of other people and that of the followers of the Prophet ﷺ, and then compares them; whereupon the difference will become clear to him. For they are the soundest of people, in intellect and nature, and the most learned, and in all things the nearest of them to the truth. For they are God's choicest blessing among the peoples, just as their Prophet ﷺ is His choicest blessing among the prophets. He has given them such knowledge, discernment and wisdom as none other can rival.

The Imām Aḥmad related in his *Musnad*, from *ḥadīth* of Bahz b. Ḥakīm, from his father, from his grandfather: The Messenger of God ﷺ said: 'You will be summoned at death as seventy communities; you are the best of them, and the noblest in God's sight.'[379]

So the effect of their nobility in God's sight appears in their learning, their intelligence, their insight and nature. They are the ones to whom have been offered the sciences of the nations before them, and their works and their degrees. So they thereby increased in knowledge, discernment and intelligence up to that of His knowledge and discernment which God, praised and exalted be He, poured out upon them.

Therefore they have the sanguineous constitution, while the Jews have the bilious and the Christians the phlegmatic.

Thus it is that the Christians' chief characteristics are gullibility and lack of understanding and of perspicacity; and the Jews are chiefly characterised by grief and anxiety, worry and servility. But the Muslims' chief characteristics are intelligence and courage, understanding and intrepidity, joy and gladness.

These are secrets and truths the extent of which will be known only to one with good understanding, subtle intellect, abundant knowledge, and who recognises the truth of people.

And with God is success.

The book is ended, praise be to God.

Index of Qur'ānic Quotations
References to *Ḥadīth*
English-Arabic Technical Glossary
English-Arabic *Materia Medica* Glossary
Bibliography of Works Cited
General Index

Index of Qur'ānic Quotations

(*Sūra* in Roman numerals; verse in Arabic numerals)

PART ONE

PART TWO

References to *Ḥadīth*

1 Muslim, *Salām*, 69.
2 Bukhārī, *Ṭibb*, 1.
3 Ibn Ḥanbal, *Musnad*, I. 377, 413, 443.
4 Ibn Ḥanbal, *Musnad*, I. 377, 413, 443.
5 Tirmidhī, *Ṭibb*, 21.
6 Tirmidhī, *Zuhd*, 47; Ibn Māja, *Aṭʿima*, 50.
7 Muslim, *Zuhd*, 60.
8 Bukhārī, *Ṭibb*, 28.
9 Tirmidhī, *Ṭahāra*, 6.
10 Tirmidhī, *Ṣalāt*, 139.
11 Bukhārī, *Ṭibb*, 28.
12 Ibn Māja, *Ṭibb*, 19.
13 Ibn Ḥanbal, *Musnad*, I. 377, 413, 443.
14 See also Muslim, *Birr*, 53.
15 See *Jāmiʿ Ṣaghīr*, III. 421.
16 Muslim, *Salām*, 125; Abū Dāwūd, *Ashriba*, 5.
17 The narrator of the *ḥadīth* is Thawbān, not Rāfiʿ ibn Khudīj, Tirmidhī, *Ṭibb*, 33; Ibn Ḥanbal, *Musnad*, IV. 281.
18 Bukhārī, *Ṭibb*, 4, 24.
19 Ibn Māja, *Ṭibb*, 7. The *isnād* includes al-Zubayr ibn Saʿīd who is *matrūk*.
20 Ibn Māja, *Ṭibb*, 7.
21 Bukhārī, *Ṭibb*, 4, 24.
22 Bukhārī, *Anbiyā'*, 54.
23 Bukhārī, *Jihād*, 306, *Ṭibb*, 30.
24 Ibn Ḥanbal, *Musnad*, VI. 145, 255.
25 Ibn Ḥanbal, *Musnad*, IV. 295.
26 Bukhārī, *Anbiyā'*, 54.
27 Abū Dāwūd, *Ṭibb*, 24. 26 & 27 not found.
28 Bukhārī, *Anbiyā'*, 54; *Tibb*, 30.
29 Bukhārī, *Ḥudūd*, 15.
30 Nisā'ī, *Ṭahāra*, 190; *Taḥrīm*, 9.
31 Bukhārī, *Jihād*, 85.
32 Bukhārī, *Ṭibb*, 3.
33 Bukhārī, *Ṭibb*, 15 & 17.
34 Bukhārī, *Ṭibb*, 28.
35 Ibn Māja, *Ṭibb*, 20. The *isnād* includes Jabāra and Kathīr ibn Salīm and they are both weak.
36 Tirmidhī, *Ṭibb*, 12. The *isnād* includes ʿAbbād ibn Manṣūr, who is weak.
37 Bukhārī, *Ṭibb*, 9, 14, 16.
38 Tirmidhī, *Ṭibb*, 13.
39 Tirmidhī, *Ṭibb*, 9 and 12.
40 Abū Dāwūd, *Ṭibb*, 4. In Abū Dāwūd there is an extra 'three times'.
41 Ibn Ḥanbal, *Musnad*, III. 119, 192. This *ḥadīth* is neither in Bukhārī, nor Muslim by Anas. A similar narration comes from Ibn ʿAbbās.
42 Abū Dāwūd, *Manāsik*, 35. Ibn Ḥanbal, *Musnad*, I. 260, 372.

43 Ibn Māja, *Ṭibb*, 21. The *isnād* is weak because of Aṣbagh ibn Nabāta.
44 Abū Dāwūd, *Ṭibb*, 5.
45 Tirmidhī, *Ṭibb*, 12.
46 Ibn Ḥanbal, *Musnad*, I. 354.
47 Ibn Māja, *Ṭibb*, 22.
48 Abū Dāwūd, *Ṭibb*, 5. In the *isnād* Saᶜīd bin ᶜAbd al-Raḥmān al-Jumaḥī is weak.
49 The *isnad* is weak.
50 Ibn Māja, *Ṭibb*, 22. The *isnad* is weak.
51 Abū Dāwūd, *Ṭibb*, 5. The *isnād* is weak.
52 Bukhārī, *Ṭibb*, 11.
53 Bukhārī, *Ṣawm*, 32.
54 Muslim, *Salām*, 73.
55 Abū Dāwūd, *Ṭibb*, 7.
56 Ibn Ḥanbal, *Musnad*, I. 377, 413, 443.
57 Ibn Ḥanbal, *Musnad*, I. 377, 413, 443.
58 Muslim, *Salām*, 73.
59 Bukhārī, *Ṭibb*, 26
60 Tirmidhī, *Ṭibb*, 11.
61 Bukhārī, *Ṭibb*, 15 & 17.
62 Bukhārī, *Ṭibb*, 3.
63 Tirmidhī, *Ṭibb*, 10.
64 Bukhārī, *Ṭibb*, 17.
65 Bukhārī, *Marḍā*, 6.
66 Ibn Ḥanbal. *Musnad*, IV. 170 & 172.
67 Ibn Māja, *Ṭibb*, 14.
68 Tirmidhī, *Ṭibb*, 30.
69 Ibn Māja, *Ṭibb*, 9, 5.
70 Tirmidhī, *Ṭibb*, 9, 12.
71 Bukhārī, *Jihād*, 91.
72 Tirmidhī, *Libās*, 1
73 Bukhārī, *Libās*, 25.
74 Tirmidhī, *Ṭibb*, 28.
75 Ibn Ḥanbal, *Musnad*, VI. 118 & 438.
76 Bukhārī, *Maghāzī*, 83.
77 Ibn Māja, *Ṭibb*, 29, 32; *Libās*, 34.
78 See also Bukhārī, *Jumuᶜa*, 29.
79 Bukhārī, *Marḍā*, 16; *Aḥkām*, 51.
80 Abū Dāwūd, *Tarajjul*, 4, 18, 19; *Ṭalāq*, 46.
81 Tirmidhī, *Ṭibb*, 13. Both *ḥadīth* are weak in *isnād*.
82 Tirmidhī, *Ṭibb*, 4.
83 Bukhārī, *Ṣawm*, 20, 48, 50.
84 Bukhārī, *Ṭibb*, 13.
85 Ibn Ḥanbal, *Musnad*, III. 315.
86 Abū Dāwūd, *Ṭibb*, 8.
87 Abū Dāwūd, *Ṭibb*, 13.
88 Bukhārī, *Aṭᶜima*, 39, 45, 47.
89 See also Tirmidhī, *Mawāqīt*, 182.
90 Bukharī, *Aṭᶜima*, 39, 45, 47.
91 Ibn Māja, *Ṭibb*, 3.
92 Ibn Māja, *Ṭibb*, 3.
93 Tirmidhī, *Ṭibb*, 1.
94 Abu Nuᶜaym, *Ṭibb*, with *isnād ḥasan*.
95 Ibn Māja, *Ṭibb*, 2; *Janā'iz*, 1.
96 Abū Dāwūd, *Ṭibb*, 17, 19.
97 Bukhārī, *Ṭibb*, 58.
98 Ibn Māja, *Ṭibb*, 31.
99 See also Ibn Ḥanbal, *Musnad*, V. 370.
100 Bukhārī, *Libās*, 81.
101 Ibn Māja, *Janā'iz*, 1.
102 Muslim, *Salām*, 90.
103 Ibn Māja, *Ṭibb*, 5.
104 Ibn Ḥanbal, *Musnad*, IV. 79, 152.
105 Abū Dāwūd, *Diyāt*, 6.
106 Dārimī, *Muqaddima*, 11.
107 Bukhārī, *Ṭibb*, 50, 47, 49, 74.
108 Ibn Ḥanbal, *Musnad*, VI. 57, 63, 96; V. 211; IV. 367.
109 Tirmidhī, *Ṭahāra*, 64.

110 Mālik, *Muwaṭṭa'*, *ʿAyn*, 12.
111 Ibn Ḥanbal, *Musnad*, I. 42.
112 Abū Dāwūd, *Diyāt*, 23.
113 Bukhārī, *Ṭibb*, 47, 49, 50.
114 Muslim, *Salām*, 126.
115 Bukhārī, *Ṭibb*, 19.
116 Ibn Māja, *Ṭibb*, 44.
117 Bukhārī, *Ṭibb*, 53.
118 Suyūṭī, *Jāmiʿ Ṣaghīr*, V. 41. In the *isnād* Yaḥyā al-Ḥamānī is weak.
119 Tirmidhī, *Aṭʿima*, 19. Tirmidhī said the *ḥadīth* is *gharīb*, only known through *ḥadīth* al-Mufḍil ibn Fuḍala.
120 Bukhārī, *Ṭibb*, 19, 43.
121 Abū Dāwūd, *Ṭibb*, 11.
122 Bukhārī, *Ashriba*, 15.
123 Ibn Ḥanbal, *Musnad*, II. 305.
124 Muslim, *Ashriba*, 12.
125 Abū Dāwūd, *Ṭibb*, 11.
126 Ibn Ḥanbal, *Musnad*, IV. 311.
127 Ibn Ḥanbal, *Musnad*, III. 453.
128 Abū Nuʿaym in his *Ṭibb*, see also *Jāmiʿ Ṣaghīr*, VI. 100.
129 Muslim, *Ḥajj*, 80, 85.
130 Nisā'ī, *Zinā*, 57.
131 Ibn Ḥanbal, *Musnad*, III. 198.
132 Muslim, *Salām*, 42.
133 Tirmidhī, *Ṭibb*, 15.
134 Muslim, *Salām*, 41.
135 Abū Dāwūd, *Ṭibb*, 15.
136 Muslim, *Salām*, 49.
137 Ibn Ḥanbal, *Musnad*, VI. 438.
138 Mālik, *Muwaṭṭa'*, *ʿAyn*, 2.
139 Mālik, *Muwaṭṭa'*, *ʿAyn*, 1.
140 Bukhārī, *Ṭibb*, 35.
141 Al-Bazzār in *al-Musnad* also mentioned the meaning of this *ḥadīth* with *isnād ḥasan*.
142 Tirmidhī, *Ṭibb*, 16.
143 Bukhārī, *Bad' al-Khalq*, 14, 15.
144 Abū Dāwūd, *Ṭibb*, 17, 18.
145 Muslim, *Salām*, 39.
146 Abū Dāwūd, *Ṭibb*, 19.
147 Muslim, *Salām*, 39.
148 Abū Dāwūd, *Ṭibb*, 17, 18.
149 Abū Dāwūd, *Ṭibb*, 17, 18.
150 Muslim, *Salām*, 56, 57.
151 Bukhārī, *Ṭibb*, 33.
152 Ibn Māja, *Ṭibb*, 28, 41.
153 Ibn Māja, *Iqāma*, 146.
154 Muslim, *Dhikr*, 55.
155 Bukhārī, *Ṭibb*, 39.
156 Bukhārī, *Maghāzī*, 12.
157 Muslim, *Dhikr*, 54.
158 Abū Dāwūd, *Jihād*, 75.
159 Muslim, *Salām*, 57, 58.
160 Abū Dāwūd, *Ṭibb*, 18.
161 Ibn Māja, *Ṭibb*, 35.
162 Bukhārī, *Ṭibb*, 33, 34.
163 Bukhārī, *Ṭibb*, 38.
164 Muslim, *Salām*, 67.
165 Bukhārī, *Marḍā*, 20.
166 Ibn Ḥanbal, *Musnad*, IV. 27.
167 Tirmidhī, *Zuhd*.
168 Ibn Ḥanbal, *Musnad*, V. 427, 429.
169 Bukhārī, *Janā'iz*, 32, 42.
170 Bukhārī, *Daʿawāt*, 27.
171 Tirmidhī, *Daʿawāt*, 19.
172 Abū Dāwūd, *Adab*, 18, 103.
173 Abū Dāwūd, *Adab*, 101.
174 Abū Dāwūd, *Witr*, 26.
175 Ibn Ḥanbal, *Musnad*, I. 391, 452.
176 Ibn Ḥanbal, *Musnad*, I. 170.
177 Abū Dāwūd, *Witr*, 32.
178 Ibn Māja, *Adab*, 57.
179 Ibn Ḥanbal, *Musnad*, I. 206, 268.
180 Bukhārī, *Daʿawāt*, 50, 51.
181 Ibn Ḥanbal, *Musnad*, XI. 461.
182 Tirmidhī, *Daʿawāt*, 63, 99.
183 Ibn Māja, *Ṭibb*, 10.
184 Tirmidhī, *Daʿawāt*, 90.

185 Tirmidī, *Da^cawāt*, 90.
186 Ibn al-Sunnī, *Amal al-Yawm wa'l-Layla*.
187 Bukhārī, *Riqāq*, 1.
188 Tirmidhī, *Zuhd*, 34.
189 Tirmidhī, *Tafsīr, sūra* no. 102, 5.
190 Ibn Ḥanbal, *Musnad*, I. 5, 7.
191 Ibn Ḥanbal, *Musnad*, I. 3, 4.
192 Tirmidhī, *Daʿawāt*, 101, 84.
193 Bukhārī, *Aṭʿima*, 21.
194 Bukhārī, *Aṭʿima*, 10, 24.
195 Bukhārī, *Anbiyā'*, 3.
196 Ibn Ḥanbal, *Musnad*, VI. 360, 361.
197 Ibn Māja, *Aṭʿima*, 24.
198 Ibn Māja, *Aṭʿima*, 33.
199 Tirmidhī, *Nikāḥ*, 5.
200 Bukhārī, *Aṭʿima*, 13.
201 Ibn ʿAdī, *al-Kāmil fi Ḍuʿafa' al-Rijāl*.
202 Abū Dāwūd, *Aṭʿima*, 18.
203 Tirmidhī, *Aṭʿima*, 46.
204 Bukhārī, *Ashriba*, 14, 20.
205 Ibn Ḥanbal, *Musnad*, VI. 100, 108.
206 Ibn Ḥanbal, *Musnad*, VI. 38.
207 Ibn Māja, *Ashriba*, 25.
208 Muslim, *Ashriba*, 123.
209 Ibn Ḥanbal, *Musnad*, III. 26.
210 Tirmidhī, *Ashriba*, 13.
211 Muslim, *Ashriba*, 99.
212 Bukhārī, *Ashriba*, 24.
213 Abū Dāwūd, *Ashriba*, 16.
214 Muslim, *Faḍā'il*, 63.
215 Tirmidhī, *Daʿawāt*, 54.
216 Muslim, *Ashriba*, 79.
217 Ibn Ḥanbal, *Musnad*, II. 287.
218 Abū Dāwūd, *Adab*, 13.
219 Ibn Māja, *Adab*, 26.
220 Bukhārī, *Wuḍū'*, 75.
221 Bukhārī, *Tahajjud*, 12.
222 Bukhārī, *Tahajjud*, 23.
223 Ibn Ḥanbal, *Musnad*, III. 128.
224 Nisā'ī, *Nikāḥ*, 11.
225 Bukhārī, *Nikāḥ*, 4.
226 See also Bukhārī, *Nikāḥ*, 1.
227 Bukhārī, *Ṣawm*, 10.
228 Bukhārī, *Buyūʿ*, 34.
229 Ibn Māja, *Nikāḥ*, 8.
230 Ibn Māja, *Nikāḥ*, 1.
231 Muslim, *Raḍāʿa*, 59,.
232 Ibn Ḥanbal, *Musnad*, V. 432, 438.
233 Bukhārī, *Nikāḥ*, 15.
234 Abū Dāwūd, *Nikāḥ*, 3.
235 Tirmidhī, *Nikāḥ*, 1.
236 Abū Dāwūd, *Ṣawm*, 34.
237 Muslim, *Ḥayḍ*, 28.
238 Abū Dāwūd, *Ṭahāra*, 85.
239 Tirmidhī, *Ṭahāra*, 107.
240 Bukhārī, *Nikāḥ*, 9.
241 Bukhārī, *Waṣāyā*, 4.
242 Bukhārī, *Tafsīr, sūra* no. 2, 39.
243 Muslim, *Nikāḥ*, 119.
244 Abū Dāwūd, *Nikāḥ*, 45.
245 Tirmidhī, *Ṭahāra*, 102.
246 Tirmidhī, *Raḍāʿa*, 12.
247 Ibn Ḥanbal, *Musnad*, II. 182.
248 Ibn Ḥanbal, *Musnad*, I. 268.
249 Ibn Ḥanbal, *Musnad*, I. 297.
250 Tirmidhī, *Raḍaʿa*, 12.
251 Suyūṭī, *Jāmiʿ Ṣaghīr*.
252 *Ḥadīth ṣaḥīḥ* mentioned by Shāfiʿī.
253 See also Tirmidhī, *Manāqib*, 14, 16.
254 Bukhārī, *Anbiyā'*, 2.
255 See also Ibn Ḥanbal, *Musnad*, VI. 145, 160.
256 Bukhārī, *Ṣawm*, 10.
257 Ibn Māja, *Nikāḥ*, 1.
258 Bukhārī, *Libās*, 80.
259 Muslim, *Alfāẓ*, 20.
260 Nisā'ī, *Zinā*, 73.
261 See also Bukhārī, *Jumuʿa*, 12.

262 Abū Dāwud, *Ṣawm*, 31.
263 Ibn Ḥanbal, *Musnad*, I. 354.
264 Ibn Māja, *Ṭibb*, 25.
265 See also Ṭabarānī; the *isnād* of the *ḥadīth is ḥasan*.
266 Ibn Māja, *Ṭibb*, 25.
267 Bukhārī, *Aṭʿima*, 30.
268 Bukhārī, *Marḍā*, 1.
269 Bukhārī, *ʿIlm*, 39.
270 Ibn Māja, *Aṭʿima*, 40.
271 Muslim, *Ashriba*, 140.
272 Abū Dāwūd, *Aṭʿima*, 40.
273 Bukhārī, *Aṭʿima*, 43.
274 Bukhārī, *Aṭʿima*, 49.
275 Muslim, *Ashriba*, 153.
276 Bukhārī, *Adhān*, 89.
277 Ibn Ḥanbal, *Musnad*, I. 15, 28.
278 Bukhārī, *Iʿtiṣām*, 24.
279 Bukhārī, *Aṭʿima*, 25, 30.
280 Bukhārī, *Adab*, 79, 89.
281 Abū Dāwūd, *Aṭʿima*, 38.
282 Bukhārī, *Ṭibb*, 7.
283 Ibn al-Dībaʿ said 'Razīn in the *isnad* is weak'.
284 Bukhārī, *Riqāq*, 44.
285 Abū Dāwūd, *Aṭʿima*, 22. Abū Dāwūd said the *ḥadīth* is weak.
286 Abū Dāwūd, *Aṭʿima*, 37.
287 Ibn Ḥanbal, *Musnad*, V. 252, 255.
288 Muslim, *Ashriba*, 167, 168.
289 Tirmidhī, *Aṭʿima*, 34.
290 Bukhārī, *Libās*, 81.
291 Ibn Ḥanbal, *Musnad*, V. 23.
292 Tirmidhī, *Jihād*, 18.
293 Bukhārī, *Riqāq*, 10, 49.
294 Bukhārī, *Aṭʿima*, 39.
295 Ibn Ḥanbal, *Musnad*, III. 164.
296 Muslim, *Alfāẓ*, 20.
297 Ibn Māja, *Zuhd*, 39.
298 Muḥammad ibn al-Walīd ibn Ibbān al-Qalānis, in the *isnād* of the *ḥadīth* and he is a liar who makes up *ḥadīth*.
299 Tirmidhī, *Aṭʿima*, 43.
300 Ibn Māja, *Aṭʿima*, 34.
301 Abū Dāwūd, *Aṭʿima*, 44.
302 Ibn Māja, *Aṭʿima*, 61.
303 Bukhārī, *Jumuʿa*, 8.
304 Bukhārī, *Wuḍū'*, 73.
305 Bukhārī, *Ṣawm*, 27.
306 Muslim, *Ṭahāra*, 43, 44.
307 Ibn Ḥanbal, *Musnad*, III. 445.
308 Ibn Ḥanbal, *Musnad*, II. 97.
309 Bukhārī, *Dhabā'iḥ*, 12.
310 Tirmidhī, *Ṭibb*, 1.
311 Tirmidhī, *Ṭibb*, 30.
312 Tirmidhī, *Ṭibb*, 3.
313 Tirmidhī, *Aṭʿima*, 27.
314 Ibn Ḥanbal, *Musnad*, III. 211.
315 Muslim, *Jihād*, 72.
316 Ibn Ḥanbal, *Musnad*, I. 206, 268.
317 Abū Dāwūd, *Ṭalāq*, 46.
318 Bukhārī, *Aṭʿima*, 10, 24.
319 Muslim, *Ṣayd*, 40.
320 Ibn Ḥanbal, *Musnad*, III. 453, 499.
321 Nisā'ī, *Nisā'*, 1.
322 Muslim, *Faḍā'il*, 139, 140.
323 Bukhārī, *Aṭʿima*, 43.
324 Ibn Māja, *Ṭibb*, 8.
325 Muslim, *Alfāẓ*, 21.
326 Abū Dāwūd, *Adab*, 105.
327 See also Bukhārī, *Libās*, 45–8.
328 Abū Dāwūd, *Libās*, 10.
329 Bukhārī, *Aṭʿima*, 28.
330 Bukhārī, *Aṭʿima*, 29.
331 Tirmidhī, *Aṭʿima*, 37.
332 Bukhārī, *Ṭibb*, 13.
333 Ibn Ḥanbal, *Musnad*, VI. 356.
334 Bukhārī, *Ṭibb*, 20.
335 Bukhārī, *Aṭʿima*, 50.
336 Bukhārī, *Libās*, 66.
337 Tirmidhī, *Libās*, 20.
338 Muslim, *Faḍā'il*, 100.
339 Ibn Māja, *Libās*, 34.

340 Muslim, *Alfāẓ*, 6.
341 Muslim, *A ˌāẓ*, 10.
342 Muslim, *Alfāẓ*, 12.
343 Ibn Māja, *Aṭʿima, Bāb al-Laḥm* and in the *isnād* one weak and two unknown narrators.
344 See Bayhaqī, Ibn al-ʿAbbas ibn Baḥār in the *isnād* and he makes up *ḥadīth*; see Shawkānī's *al-Fawā'id*, p. 168.
345 Bukhārī, *Aṭʿima*, 25.
346 Bukhārī, *Dhabā'iḥ*, 24.
347 Bukhārī, *Dhabā'iḥ*, 27, 28.
348 Nisā'ī, *Ghusl*, 30.
349 Muslim, *Ṣayd*, 53.
350 Muslim, *Ḥajj*, 62.
351 Ibn Māja, *Dhabā'iḥ*, 12.
352 Tirmidhī, *Ṣayd*, 10.
353 Muslim, *Aḍāḥī*, 35, 36.
354 Bukhārī, *Dhabā'iḥ*, 26.
355 Abū Dāwūd, *Aṭʿima*, 28.
356 Nisā'ī, *Ṣayd*, 34.
357 Nisā'ī, *Ḍaḥāyā*, 42. All men of the *isnād* are trustworthy except Ṣāliḥ ibn Dīnār; only Ibn Ḥanbal places him among the trustworthy, but the *ḥadīth* is *ḥasan*.
358 Bukhārī, *Dhabā'iḥ*, 13.
359 Ibn Ḥanbal, *Musnad*, II. 97.
360 Abū Dāwūd, *Ashriba*, 21.
361 Bukhārī, *Wuḍū'*, 52.
362 Bukhārī, *Ashriba*, 1 and 12.
363 Muslim, *al-Janna wa Ṣifat Naʿīmuhā, Bāb mā fī al-Dunyā min Anhār al-Janna*.
364 Bukhārī, *Daʿawāt*, 39.
365 Muslim, *Faḍā'il al-Ṣaḥāba*, 132.
366 Ibn Māja, *Manāsik*, 78.
367 Abū Dāwūd, *Ṭahāra*, 41; Tirmidhī, *Ṭahāra*, 52.
368 Muslim, *Alfāẓ*, 19.
369 Muslim, *Ḥajj*, 46.
370 Ibn Māja, *Aṭʿima*, 32.
371 Haythamī, *Majmaʿ*, x.18.
372 Bukhārī, *Aṭʿima*, 46.
373 See al-Ḥamawī's *Aḥkām* II. 111.
374 Bukhārī, *Manāqib al-Anṣār*, 42.
375 Tirmidhī, *Ṭibb*, 28.
376 Ibn Māja, *Ṭibb*, 17.
377 Ibn Ḥanbal, *Musnad*, VI. 300.
378 Bukhārī, *Aṭʿima*, 4 and 25.
379 Ibn Ḥanbal, *Musnad*, V. 5.

English-Arabic Technical Glossary

Abdomen *baṭn*
Abdomen, sickness of *ijtawā*
Abrasions *saḥaj*
Abscess *khurāj*
Accidental *ʿaraḍiyy*
Adventitious *ʿaraḍiyy*
Alopecia *dā' al-thaʿlab*
Aorta *abhar*
Apoplexy *sakta*
Arteries *sharāyīn*
Asthma *rabw*

Back, upper part *kāhil*
Belly *baṭn*
Bite *ladgha*
Bladder *mathāna*
Blindness, night *ghashā*
Blister(s) *sulāq, naffāṭāt*
Blistering *tanaffuṭ*
Blood *dam*
Bloodletting *faṣd*
Body *badn*
Boil *dubayla*
Boil, furuncle *dummal*
Brain *dimāgh*
Breath *nafas*
Buttocks *maqʿada*

Cancer *saraṭān*
Catarrh *zukām, nazla*
Cautery *kayy*
Chest *ṣadr*
Choking *khunāq, ghuṣṣa*
Chyme *kaymūs*
Colic *qūlanj*
Compress *naṭūl*
Confusion *takhlīṭ*
Conjuction *ittiṣāl*
Constipation *ḥuṣr, yubs al-ṭabʿ*
Constitution *ṭabʿ, mizāj*
Consumption *sill, sull*
Convulsions *tashannuj*
Costiveness *qabḍ*
Cough *suʿāl*
Coughing *sharaq*
Crisis *buḥrān*
Cupping *ḥijāma*
Cyst *silʿa*

Delusion, melancholic *waswās*
Dermis *ṣifāqāt*
Diaphragm *ḥijāb*
Diarrhoea *dharab, ishāl*
Diet *ḥimya*
Digestion *istimrā'*
Disease *maraḍ*
Disjunction *tafarruq al-ittiṣāl*
Diuretic *mudirr al-bawl*
Dropsy *istisqā'*
Dysentery *zaḥīr*
Dysuria *ʿasr al-bawl*

Element(s) *ʿunṣur, ʿanāṣir*
Elephantiasis *dā' al-fīl*
Emesis *qayy'*
Emmenagogue *mudirr al-ṭamth*

Epilepsy *ṣarᶜ*
Erysipelas *ḥumra*
Excoriation *saᶜfa, safᶜa*
Eye *ᶜayn*

Faculty *quwwa*
Fainting *ighmā', ghashiy*
Fauces *ᶜudhra*
Fester (vb) *naghila*
Fever *ḥummā*; hectic: *ḥummā diqq*; quartan: *ḥumma al-rabᶜ*; quotidian: *ḥumma yawm*
Fissures *shuqāq*
Fistula *nāsūr*
Forehead *jabha*
Forgetfulness *nisyān*
Freckles *kalaf, namash*
Frenitis *sirsām*

Gangrene *ākila*
Gland (swelling) *ghudda*
Gout *niqris*
Gullet *marī'*
Gums *litha*

Haemorrhoids *bawāsīr*
Hair (in eye) *shaᶜra*
Headache *bayḍa; khūdha; ṣudāᶜ*
Heart *fu'ād; qalb*
Heat, innate *ḥarāra gharīziyya*
Hemiplegia *fālij*
Humour(s) *khilṭ, akhlāṭ*

Incision *baṭṭ*
Incontinence *salas al-bawl*
Indigestion *tukhām; maghṣ*
Infatuation *ᶜishq*
Inflammations *iltihāb; waram; awrām*
Insomnia *araq*
Intestines *aḥshā'; marāq, marrā; amᶜā'*
Itch *ḥikka*; itching, *namla*

Jaundice *yaraqān*
Joint *mafṣil*

Kidney(s) *kilā, kilyatān*
Kidneys, two veins of *ḥālabayn*

Lancing *bazl*
Leprosy *judhām*
Leucoma *bayāḍ; b. al-ᶜayn*
Leukoderma *bahaq*
Lice *qaml*
Lichen *ḥazāz*
Liver *kabid*
Lung *ri'a*

Madness *junūn*
Magic *siḥr*
Measles *ḥaṣba*
Melancholia *mālīkhūliyā*
Melancholic delusions *waswās*
Membrane *ṭabl*
Memory *ḥifẓ*
Menses *ṭamth*
Migraine *shaqīqa*
Moles *khīlān*
Mouth *fam*

Nails *aẓāfīr*
Nature *ṭabīᶜa*
Nausea *ghathayān*
Neck, nape of *qafā'*
Nerve(s) *aᶜṣāb*
Night blindness *ghashā'*
Nose *khayāshīm; mankharān* (nostrils)
Nosebleed *ruᶜāf*

Obstruction *sadad*
Ophiasis *dā' al-ḥayya*
Ophthalmia *ramad*

Pallor *ṣafar*
Palpitations *khafaqān*
Paralysis, total *khadarān*

Paralysis, facial *laqwa*
Paralysis, one-sided (hemiplegia) *fālij*
Plague *ṭāʿūn*
Pleurisy *birsām; dhāt al-janb; shawṣa*
Poison *samm*
Pores *masāmm*
Power *quwwa*
Pulse *nabḍ*
Purging *ishāl*
Pus *qayḥ; midda*
Pustules *buthūr*

Respiration, difficult *buhr*
Rib area *janb*
Rib cage *bahw*
Rumblings *qarāqīr*

Scab, moist *nuqba*
Scabies *jarab*
Scarring *khushkharīsha*
Sciatica *ʿirq al-nasā*
Scorpion *ʿaqrab*
Semen *minan*
Serpent *ḥayya*
Sexual potency *bāh*
Sexual intercourse *jimāʿ*
Sight *baṣar*
Similar disease *mutashābih*
Skin *bashara*
Skin eruption *sharā*
Sleeplessness *sahar*
Smallpox *jadarī*
Sneezing *ʿuṭās*
Spasm *tashannuj*
Spirit *rūḥ*
Spleen *ṭuḥāl*
Spots *barash*
Sting *ladgha*
Stomach *miʿda*
Stone *ḥaṣā*
Stroke *khabṭa*
Superfluity *faḍl*
Sweat *ʿaraq*

Temperament *mizāj*
Tetanus *kazāz*
Tetter *qubā'*
Thrush *qulāʿ*
Tinnitus *al-dā' al-dawwiyy*
Trachea *qaṣbat al-ri'a*
Trachoma *jarab al-ʿayn*
Tremor(s) *riʿsha; rajafān*
Trembling *tashannuj*

Ulcer *qarḥ*
Urine *bawl*
Urine, retention of *taqṭīr al-miyāh*
Uterus *raḥim*

Vapour *bukhār*
Vein *ʿirq*
Vein, medial arm *akḥal*
Venesection *faṣd*
Vertigo *sadar*
Vitiligo *baraṣ*

Waking *yaqẓa*
Warts *thalīl*
Whitening, hair *shayb*
Whitlow *dāḥis*
Wounds *jarḥ*

English-Arabic *Materia Medica* Glossary

Acacia *ṭalḥ*
Achillea *qayṣūm*, cf. *shīḥ*
Acorus *dharīra*
Almond *lawz*
Aloe *ṣabir*
Aloe wood *ʿūd*
Alum *shabb*
Ambergris *ʿanbar*
Antimony *ithmid*
Apple *tuffāḥ*
Artemisia *shīḥ*, cf. *qayṣūm*
Astragalus *anzarūt*
Aubergine *bādhinjān*

Banana *mauz* cf. *ṭalḥ*
Barley *shaʿīr*
Basil *bādharūj, rayḥān*
Beet *silq*
Bean (Lupinus angustifolia) *bāqillā*; (Phaseolus vulgaris) *lūbyā*
Ben nut *bān*
Bread (white bread) *khubz*; (special type) *ḥawāriyy*
Broth of barley *talbīna*
Broth of meat and bread *tharīd*
Broth made from parched barley or wheat *sawīq*
Broth made with dates, curd, and bread *ḥays*
Butter *zubd*; clarified butter (ghee) *samn*

Camomile *uqḥuwān, bābūnaj*
Camphor *kāfūr*
Cedar of Lebanon *arz*
Celery *karafs*
Chicory *hindibā', baql*
Citron *utrujj, laymūn*
Costus *qusṭ*
Cotton *quṭn*
Cress *thuffā', ḥurf, rashād*
Cucumber *khiyār, qiththā'*
Cumin *kammūn*; (black cumin, Nigella) *ḥabba sawdā'*

Dates (unripe) *busr*; (fresh) *balaḥ, ruṭab*; (dried) *tamr*; (pressed dried) *ʿajwa*; (clusters) *dawālī*
Dill *shībith*
'Dragon's blood' (Dracaena draco, Calamus draco, Liliac.) *dam al-akhawayn*

Electuaries *jawārishāt*; *maʿjūn*, pl. *maʿājīn*; *laʿūq*
Euphorbia *shubrum*

Fennel *rāziyānaj*
Fenugreek *ḥulba*
Figs *tīn*
Flax *kittān*
Flour (coursely ground) *khashkār*
Fumitory *shāhtaraj*

Garlic *thūm*
Ghee (clarified butter) *samn*
Ginger *zanjabīl*
Gourd (Citrullus colocynthis) *ḥanẓal*; (Cucurbita maxima, Lagenaria vulgaris) *qarʿ*; (Cucurbita sp.) *yaqṭīn*
Grapes *ʿinab*; (raisins) *zabīb*; (juice of unripe grapes) *ḥiṣrim*; (cooked and concentrated) *mayūfakhtaj*

Halva (sweetmeat) *ḥalwā'*
Henna *ḥinnā'*; (blossoms) *fāghiya*
Hiera *iyārij*

Ice/snow *thalj*
Incense *kundur, lubān*
Indigo *nīl, katam, wasma*
Iris *sawsan*
Iron *ḥadīd*

Kohl *kuḥl*; (black kohl) *ithmid*

Lavender *khuzāma*
Leeks *kurrāth*
Lemon-grass *idhkhir*
Lentils *ʿadas*

Manna *taranjabīn*
Marjoram *marzanjūsh*
Mastic (Pistacia terebinthus, Anacard.) *buṭm, ḥabba khaḍrā'*; (gum mastic) *maṣṭikā*
Melon *biṭṭīkh*
Mint *ḥabaq*
Mulberrry *tūt*
Mushroom *fuṭr*
Musk *misk*
Mustard *khardal*
Myrtle *ās*

Narcissus *narjis*
Nigella *ḥabba sawdā'*

Oil (vegetable) *duhn, adhān*; (olive) *zayt*
Olives *zaytūn*
Onion *baṣal*
Oxymel (vinegar and honey) *sakanjabīn*

Palm (tree) *nakhl*; (core) *jummār*; (spadix) *kufurrī*; (spathe) *ṭalʿ*, (fibres, matting) *ḥaṣīr*
Pepper *filfil*
Pickles *kawāmij*
Pine *ṣanawbar*
Pistachio *fustuq*
Pomegranate *rummān*; (flowers) *jundhub*
Poplar *khilāf*
Poppy *khashkhāsh, shūnīz*

Quince *safarjal*

Raisins *zabīb*
Rice *aruzz*
Rose *ward*
Rue *sadhāb*

Safflower *qurṭum*
Saffron *zaʿfarān*
Salvadora *arāk*; (fruit) *kabāth*
Semolina *samīd*, see wheat
Senna *sanna*
Sesame oil *shīraj*
Sherbet *sharāb*
Silk *ḥarīr*; (raw silk) *ibrīsim*
Smilax *mughlā*
Snow/ice *thalj*
Spinach *isfānākh*
Squash *qiththā'*
Sugar *sukkar*; (cane) *qaṣab*; (sugar candy) *fānīdh*
Sulphur *kibrīt*

Sweet flag *dharīra*

Tar (pitch from Coniferae) *qiṭrān*
Terebinth *buṭm; ḥabba khaḍrā'*
Tragacanth *kathīrā'*
Toothpick twigs *khilāl*
Toothbrush (from twigs of Salvadora persica) *siwāk*
Truffles *kam'a*
Tutty (oxide of zinc) *tūtiyā'*

Valerian *fuwwa*
Vine *karm*
Vinegar *khall*; (vinegar sauce) *murrī, mirrī*
Violet *banafsaj*
Vipers *afāʿī*

Walnut *jauz*
Water lily (Nymphaea lotus, N. alba) *nīlūfar, līnūfar*
Wheat *ḥinṭa*
Wine *khamr*

Zizyphus (tree) *sidr*; (fruit) *nabq*

Bibliography of works cited

QUR'ĀN

An English interpretation of the Holy Qur'an with full Arabic text by Abdallah Yusuf Ali, Lahore.

ḤADĪTH

The translation of the meanings of Sahih al-Bukhari, by M.M. Khan, 7 vols, 2nd ed., Madīna, 1973.

REFERENCE AND HISTORY

EI: *The Encyclopaedia of Islam*, 2nd ed., Leiden-London, 1960– .

GAL: C. Brockelmann. *Geschichte der arabischen Litteratur*, Leiden, 1937.

Hajjī Khalīfa. *Kashf al-Ẓunūn ʿan asmā' al-kutub wa-l-funūn*, 2 vols., Istanbul, 1941–43.

Ibn Khaldūn. *The Muqaddimah: an introduction to history*, translated from the Arabic by Franz Rosenthal, 3 vols., London/New York, 1958.

Ibn Abī Uṣaybiʿa, *ʿUyūn al-anbā' fi ṭabaqāt al-aṭibbā'*, Cairo, 1882.

MEDICINE & PHARMACY: ARABIC

Abū Ḥanīfa: (1) *The Book of Plants of Abū Ḥanīfa ad-Dinawarī.* Part of the Alphabetical Section (*alif* to *zā'*), ed. B. Lewin, Uppsala, 1953; (2) *The Book of plants.* Part of the monograph section by Abū Ḥanīfa ad-Dinawarī, ed. B. Lewin (*Bibliotheca Islamica* 26), Wiesbaden, 1974.

al-Ghāfiqī: *The Abridged Version of 'The Book of Simple Drugs' of Aḥmad ibn Muḥammad al-Ghāfiqī*, ed. M. Meyerhof and G.P. Sobhy, Cairo, 1932–40.

Ibn Bayṭār, ʿAbd-Allāh b. Aḥmad. *al-Jāmiʿ li-mufradāt al-adwiya wa-l-aghdhiya*, Cairo, 1291/1874.

Ibn Juljul, Sulaymān b. Ḥasan. *Ṭabaqāt al-aṭibbā' wa-l-ḥukamā'*, ed. F. Sayyid, Cairo, 1955

Ibn Riḍwān: *Medieval Islamic Medicine: Ibn Ridwan's Treatise 'On the Prevention of Bodily Ills in Egypt'*, translated with introduction by M.W. Dols, Arabic text edited by A.S. Gamal, London, 1984.

Ibn Samajūn: P. Kahle, 'Ibn Samagun und sein Drogenbuch' in *Documenta Islamica Inedita*, Berlin, 1952.

Ibn Zuhr: *La Tedkirà d'Abû 'l-ʿAlâ'*, publiée et traduite par G. Colin, (*Publications de la Faculté des lettres d'Alger, Bulletin de correspondance africaine* 45) Paris, 1911.

Isaac Isrā'īlī. *Isaac Judaeus: on fevers* (the third discourse: on consumption), ed. J.D. Latham and H.D. Isaacs, *Arabic Technical and Scientific Texts* vol. 8, Cambridge, 1981.

al-Kindī: M. Levey. *The Medical Formulary or Aqrabadhin of al-Kindī*, Wisconsin, 1966.

al-Rāzī: *Kitābu'l-Ḥāwī fi'ṭ-Ṭibb, Continens of Rhazes*: an encyclopaedia of medicine, edited from the unique [sic] Escurial and other manuscripts, 23 parts, Dā'irat al-Maʿārif al-ʿUthmāniyya, Hyderabad, 1955–71.

al-Ṭabarī, ʿAlī b. Rabbān, *Firdaws al-ḥikma*, ed. M. Z. Siddiqi, Berlin, 1928.

Medicine & Pharmacy: European

Dols, *Medicine*, see Ibn Riḍwān.

Jones, W. H. S., ed. and trans. *Hippocrates*, The Loeb Classical Library, 4 vols, Cambridge-London, 1923–31.

Levey, M., *Early Arabic Pharmacology, an introduction based on ancient and medieval sources*, Leiden, 1973.

Levey, M., 'Medical Ethics of Medieval Islam with Special Reference to al-Ruhawi's "Practical Ethics of the Physicians"', *Transactions of the American Philosophical Society*, n.s., 57/3 (1967).

Opitz, K., *Die Medizin im Koran*, Stuttgart, 1906.

Temkin, O., *Galenism: rise and decline of a medical philosophy*, New York, 1974.

Ullmann, M., *Die Medizin im Islam, Handbuch der Orientalistik* Ergänzungsband VI, I Abschnitt, Leiden/Cologne, 1970.

Ullmann, M., *Islamic Medicine*, Islamic Surveys 11, Edinburgh, 1978.

Prophetic Medicine

Elgood, C., 'Tibb ul-Nabbi or Medicine of the Prophet. Being a translation of two works of the same name.'. *Osiris* 14 (1962).

Elgood, C., 'The Medicine of the Prophet', *Medical History* 6 (1962), pp. 146–53.

Burgel, J. C., 'Secular and Religious Features of Medieval Arabic Medicine', in *Asian Medical Systems: A Comparative Survey*, ed. C. Leslie, Berkeley, 1976, pp. 44–62.

Burgel, J. C., 'Prophetic Medicine' (unpublished paper, The Kaplan Lectures, University of Pennsylvania, September 1977).

Perron, A., *La médecine du prophète*, Paris/Algiers, 1860.

Dictionaries

Ghalab, E. *Dictionnaire des Sciences de la nature*, 3 vols., Beirut, 1965–66.

Hitti, Y. K., *Hitti's Medical Dictionary* English-Arabic with an Arabic-English Vocabulary, 2nd revised edition, Beirut, 1972.

Issa, A., *Dictionnaire des noms des plantes en latin, francais, anglais et arabe*, Cairo, 1930.

Miki, W., *Index of the Arab Herbalist's Materials, Studia Culturae Islamicae* No. 2, Institute for the study of Languages and Cultures of Asia and Africa, Tokyo, 1976.

Sharaf, M., *An English-Arabic Dictionary of Medicine, Biology, and Allied Sciences*, Cairo, 1926.

Index — subjects, places, *materia medica*

Numbers in italics indicate the main reference for the entry

Index of Qur'ānic Quotations
References to *Ḥadīth*
English-Arabic Technical Glossary
English-Arabic *Materia Medica* Glossary
Bibliography of Works Cited
General Index